frédéric delavier

STRENGTH TRAINING ANATOMY

THIRD EDITION

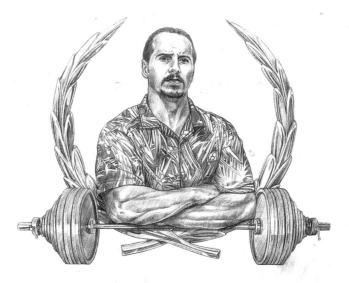

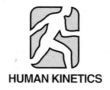

HUMAN KINETICS

For my father

Library of Congress Cataloging-in-Publication Data

Delavier, Frédéric.
  [Guide des mouvements de musculation. English]
  Strength training anatomy / Frédéric Delavier. -- 3rd ed.
      p. cm.
  ISBN-13: 978-0-7360-9226-5 (soft cover)
  ISBN-10: 0-7360-9226-9 (soft cover)
  1. Muscles--Anatomy. 2. Weight training. 3. Muscle strength. I. Title.
  QM151.D454 2010
  611'.73--dc22

                              2009045227

ISBN-10: 0-7360-9226-9 (print)
ISBN-13: 978-0-7360-9226-5 (print)

Copyright © 2010, 2006, 2001 by Éditions Vigot, 23 rue de l'École de Médecine, 75006 Paris, France

This publication is written and published to provide accurate and authoritative information relevant to the subject matter presented. It is published and sold with the understanding that the author and publisher are not engaged in rendering legal, medical, or other professional services by reason of their authorship or publication of this work. If medical or other expert assistance is required, the services of a competent professional person should be sought.

This book is a revised edition of *Guide des Mouvements de Musculation*, 5th edition, published in 2010 by Éditions Vigot.

Illustrator: Frédéric Delavier

Human Kinetics books are available at special discounts for bulk purchase. Special editions can also be created to specification. For details, contact the Special Sales Manager at Human Kinetics.

Printed in Singapore   10 9 8 7 6 5 4 3 2 1

Human Kinetics
Web site: www.HumanKinetics.com

United States: Human Kinetics
P.O. Box 5076
Champaign, IL 61825-5076
800-747-4457
e-mail: humank@hkusa.com

Canada: Human Kinetics
475 Devonshire Road Unit 100
Windsor, ON N8Y 2L5
800-465-7301 (in Canada only)
e-mail: info@hkcanada.com

Europe: Human Kinetics
107 Bradford Road
Stanningley
Leeds LS28 6AT, United Kingdom
+44 (0) 113 255 5665
e-mail: hk@hkeurope.com

Australia: Human Kinetics
57A Price Avenue
Lower Mitcham, South Australia 5062
08 8372 0999
e-mail: info@hkaustralia.com

New Zealand: Human Kinetics
P.O. Box 80
Torrens Park, South Australia 5062
0800 222 062
e-mail: info@hknewzealand.com

E5126

CONTENTS

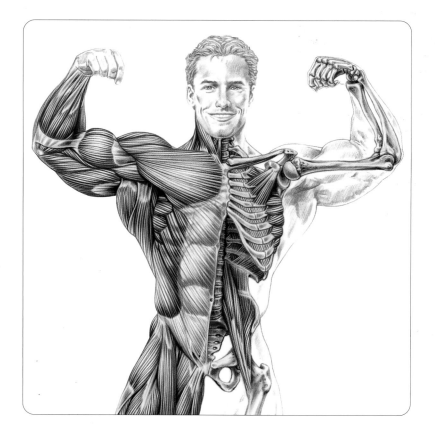

1
ARMS

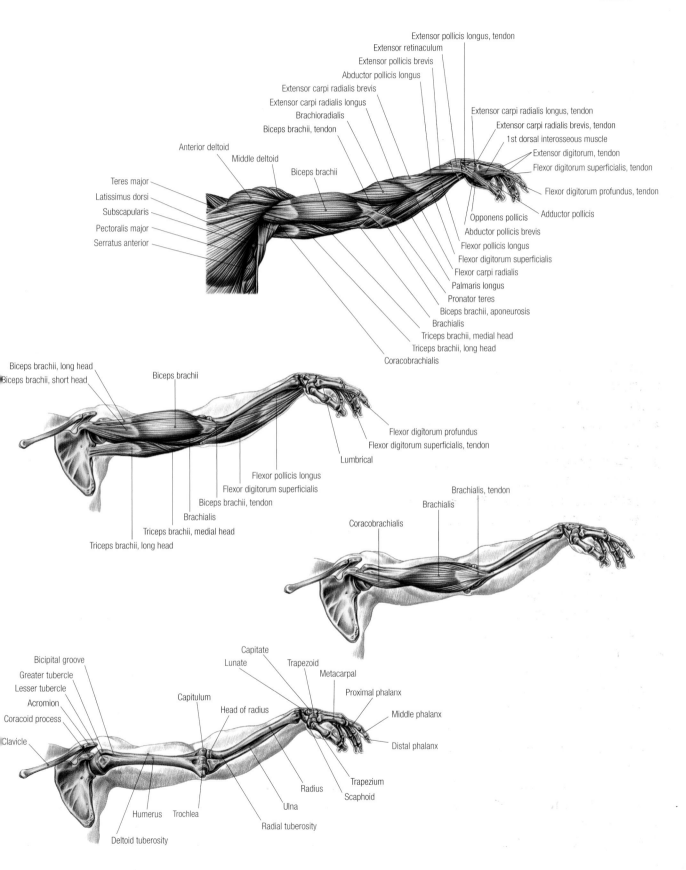

Extensor pollicis longus, tendon
Extensor retinaculum
Extensor pollicis brevis
Abductor pollicis longus
Extensor carpi radialis brevis
Extensor carpi radialis longus
Brachioradialis
Biceps brachii, tendon
Anterior deltoid
Middle deltoid
Biceps brachii
Teres major
Latissimus dorsi
Subscapularis
Pectoralis major
Serratus anterior

Extensor carpi radialis longus, tendon
Extensor carpi radialis brevis, tendon
1st dorsal interosseous muscle
Extensor digitorum, tendon
Flexor digitorum superficialis, tendon
Flexor digitorum profundus, tendon
Adductor pollicis
Opponens pollicis
Abductor pollicis brevis
Flexor pollicis longus
Flexor digitorum superficialis
Flexor carpi radialis
Palmaris longus
Pronator teres
Biceps brachii, aponeurosis
Brachialis
Triceps brachii, medial head
Triceps brachii, long head
Coracobrachialis

Biceps brachii, long head
Biceps brachii, short head
Biceps brachii

Flexor digitorum profundus
Flexor digitorum superficialis, tendon
Lumbrical
Flexor pollicis longus
Flexor digitorum superficialis
Biceps brachii, tendon
Brachialis
Triceps brachii, medial head
Triceps brachii, long head

Brachialis, tendon
Brachialis
Coracobrachialis

Capitate
Lunate
Trapezoid
Metacarpal
Proximal phalanx
Middle phalanx
Distal phalanx
Bicipital groove
Greater tubercle
Lesser tubercle
Acromion
Coracoid process
Clavicle
Capitulum
Head of radius
Trapezium
Scaphoid
Radius
Ulna
Radial tuberosity
Humerus
Trochlea
Deltoid tuberosity

1 DUMBBELL CURLS

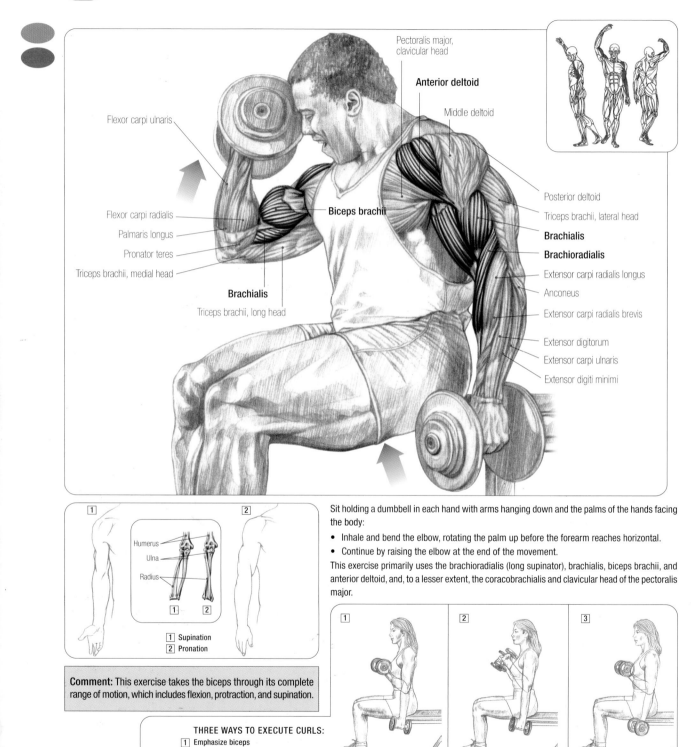

Pectoralis major, clavicular head

Anterior deltoid

Middle deltoid

Flexor carpi ulnaris

Posterior deltoid

Triceps brachii, lateral head

Flexor carpi radialis

Brachialis

Palmaris longus

Brachioradialis

Pronator teres

Extensor carpi radialis longus

Triceps brachii, medial head

Anconeus

Biceps brachii

Extensor carpi radialis brevis

Brachialis

Extensor digitorum

Triceps brachii, long head

Extensor carpi ulnaris

Extensor digiti minimi

1 | 2

Humerus
Ulna
Radius

1 | 2

1 Supination
2 Pronation

Sit holding a dumbbell in each hand with arms hanging down and the palms of the hands facing the body:

- Inhale and bend the elbow, rotating the palm up before the forearm reaches horizontal.
- Continue by raising the elbow at the end of the movement.

This exercise primarily uses the brachioradialis (long supinator), brachialis, biceps brachii, and anterior deltoid, and, to a lesser extent, the coracobrachialis and clavicular head of the pectoralis major.

Comment: This exercise takes the biceps through its complete range of motion, which includes flexion, protraction, and supination.

THREE WAYS TO EXECUTE CURLS:
1 Emphasize biceps
2 Work brachioradialis intensely
3 Work mainly biceps and brachialis

CONCENTRATION CURLS 2

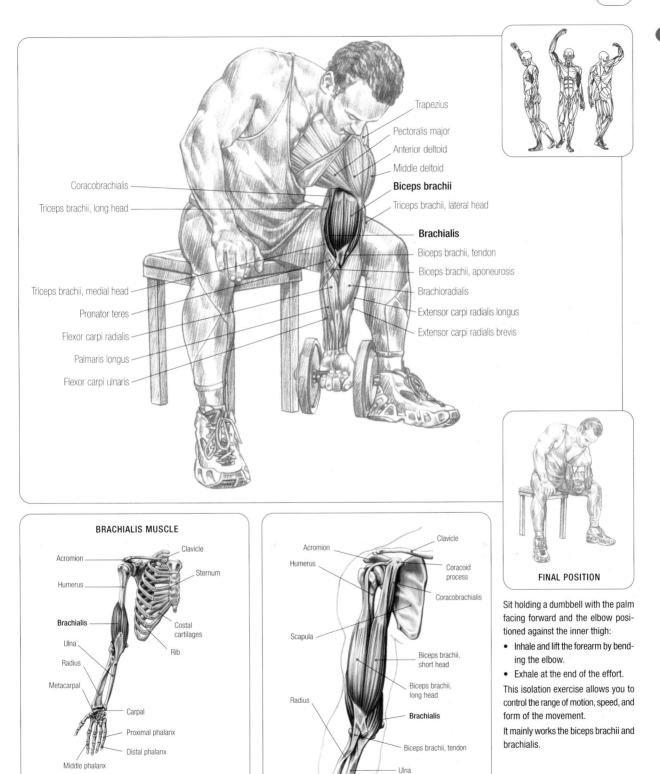

Trapezius

Pectoralis major

Anterior deltoid

Middle deltoid

Biceps brachii

Triceps brachii, lateral head

Brachialis

Biceps brachii, tendon

Biceps brachii, aponeurosis

Brachioradialis

Extensor carpi radialis longus

Extensor carpi radialis brevis

Coracobrachialis

Triceps brachii, long head

Triceps brachii, medial head

Pronator teres

Flexor carpi radialis

Palmaris longus

Flexor carpi ulnaris

FINAL POSITION

BRACHIALIS MUSCLE

Clavicle

Acromion

Sternum

Humerus

Brachialis

Ulna

Costal cartilages

Radius

Rib

Metacarpal

Carpal

Proximal phalanx

Distal phalanx

Middle phalanx

Clavicle

Acromion

Humerus

Coracoid process

Coracobrachialis

Scapula

Biceps brachii, short head

Biceps brachii, long head

Brachialis

Radius

Biceps brachii, tendon

Ulna

Sit holding a dumbbell with the palm facing forward and the elbow positioned against the inner thigh:

- Inhale and lift the forearm by bending the elbow.
- Exhale at the end of the effort.

This isolation exercise allows you to control the range of motion, speed, and form of the movement.

It mainly works the biceps brachii and brachialis.

3 INCLINE DUMBBELL CURLS

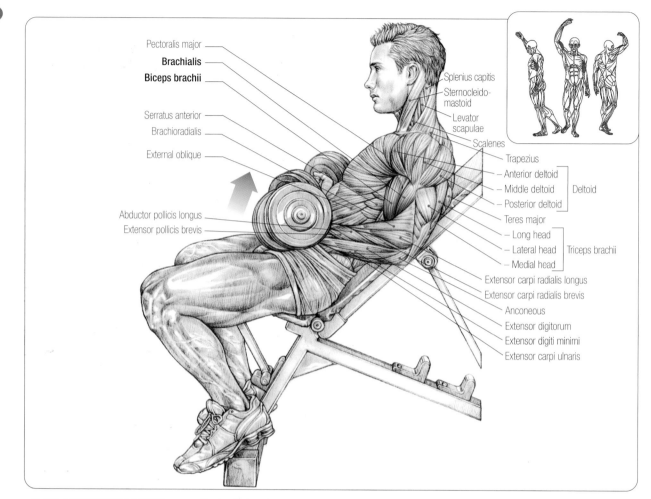

Pectoralis major
Brachialis
Biceps brachii

Serratus anterior
Brachioradialis

External oblique

Abductor pollicis longus
Extensor pollicis brevis

Splenius capitis
Sternocleido-mastoid
Levator scapulae
Scalenes
Trapezius
Anterior deltoid
Middle deltoid — Deltoid
Posterior deltoid
Teres major
Long head
Lateral head — Triceps brachii
Medial head
Extensor carpi radialis longus
Extensor carpi radialis brevis
Anconeous
Extensor digitorum
Extensor digiti minimi
Extensor carpi ulnaris

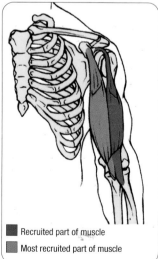

◼ Recruited part of muscle
◼ Most recruited part of muscle

Sit on an incline bench with your back leaning against the support. In each hand, hold a dumbbell with a relaxed overhand grip (thumbs face to the inside):

- Inhale and bend your elbows while externally rotating your wrists before your forearms reach horizontal so that at the end of the movement your hands are in an underhand grip (thumbs face to the outside).
- Exhale at the end of the movement.

This exercise targets the long head of the biceps (the lateral part of the muscle), which is stretched at the beginning of flexion of the elbow. This movement also works the brachioradialis and the brachialis.

Variations: Use alternating forearm curls. Increase the intensity of the effort by initiating the movement in an underhand grip.

⚠ **Attention:** Adjust the angle of the bench according to individual variations in shoulder flexibility. If the arm is too far back, the long head of the biceps will create excessive friction in the bicipital groove of the humerus and will strain the tendon.

INITIAL POSITION

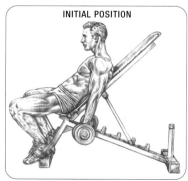

HAMMER CURLS 4

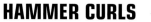

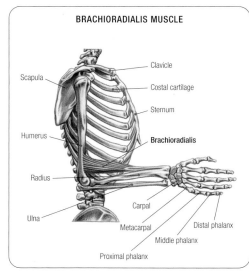

THE MOVEMENT

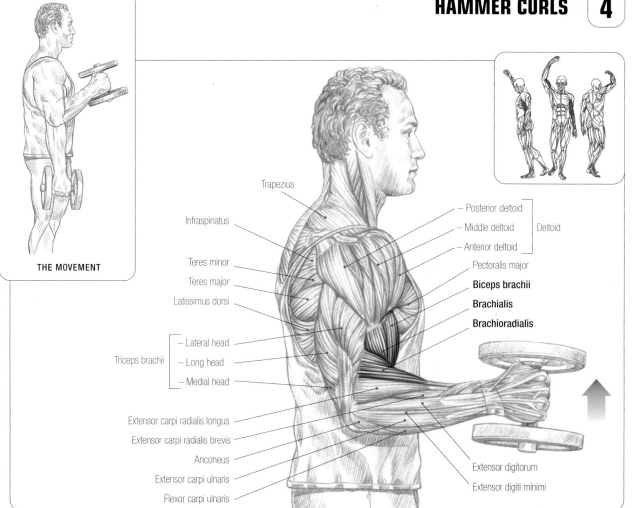

Trapezius

Infraspinatus

Teres minor

Teres major

Latissimus dorsi

Triceps brachii
- Lateral head
- Long head
- Medial head

Extensor carpi radialis longus

Extensor carpi radialis brevis

Anconeus

Extensor carpi ulnaris

Flexor carpi ulnaris

Posterior deltoid

Middle deltoid — Deltoid

Anterior deltoid

Pectoralis major

Biceps brachii

Brachialis

Brachioradialis

Extensor digitorum

Extensor digiti minimi

Stand or sit gripping a dumbbell in each hand with the palms facing each other:

- Inhale and raise the forearms together or alternately.
- Exhale at the end of the movement.

This is the best exercise for developing the brachioradialis. It also develops the biceps brachii, brachialis, and, to a lesser degree, the extensor carpi radialis brevis and longus.

BRACHIORADIALIS MUSCLE

Clavicle

Scapula

Costal cartilage

Sternum

Humerus

Brachioradialis

Radius

Carpal

Ulna

Metacarpal

Distal phalanx

Middle phalanx

Proximal phalanx

DISTRIBUTION OF THE MUSCLE FIBERS ACCORDING TO THEIR SPECIFIC ACTIONS

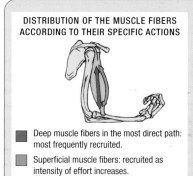

■ Deep muscle fibers in the most direct path: most frequently recruited.

■ Superficial muscle fibers: recruited as intensity of effort increases.

THE LAW OF LEAST EFFORT

To minimize effort when performing an action, the muscle will first recruit the fibers in the most direct path (that is, the most linear path located deep in the muscle).

A common belief is that the greater the force, the more the deep part of the muscle is worked. But in reality, the more the intensity of effort increases, the more the superficial muscles will be recruited to perform the movement.

Furthermore, the deep and linear muscles are generally slower to contract but more resistant to repetitive movements than the lateral, more curved, and longer muscles.

5 LOW-PULLEY CURLS

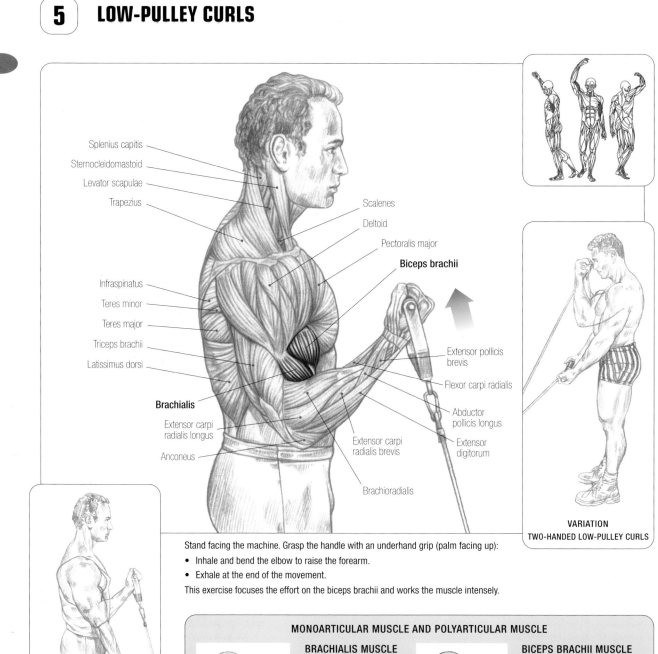

- Splenius capitis
- Sternocleidomastoid
- Levator scapulae
- Trapezius
- Scalenes
- Deltoid
- Pectoralis major
- **Biceps brachii**
- Infraspinatus
- Teres minor
- Teres major
- Triceps brachii
- Latissimus dorsi
- **Brachialis**
- Extensor carpi radialis longus
- Anconeus
- Extensor pollicis brevis
- Flexor carpi radialis
- Abductor pollicis longus
- Extensor digitorum
- Extensor carpi radialis brevis
- Brachioradialis

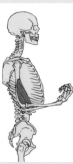

VARIATION
TWO-HANDED LOW-PULLEY CURLS

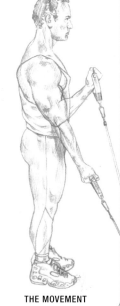

THE MOVEMENT

Stand facing the machine. Grasp the handle with an underhand grip (palm facing up):

- Inhale and bend the elbow to raise the forearm.
- Exhale at the end of the movement.

This exercise focuses the effort on the biceps brachii and works the muscle intensely.

MONOARTICULAR MUSCLE AND POLYARTICULAR MUSCLE

BRACHIALIS MUSCLE

The brachialis muscle crosses at only one articulation, the elbow. It is said to be monoarticular. Its simple action mobilizes this joint; it flexes only the forearm.

BICEPS BRACHII MUSCLE

The biceps brachii muscle crosses over at more than one articulation, that of the elbow and shoulder. It is said to be polyarticular. That is, it mobilizes more than one joint, and its action is complex. The biceps brachii can bend the elbow, raise the elbow, bring the arm to the thorax, and place the forearm into supination (underhand grip).

HIGH-PULLEY CURLS 6

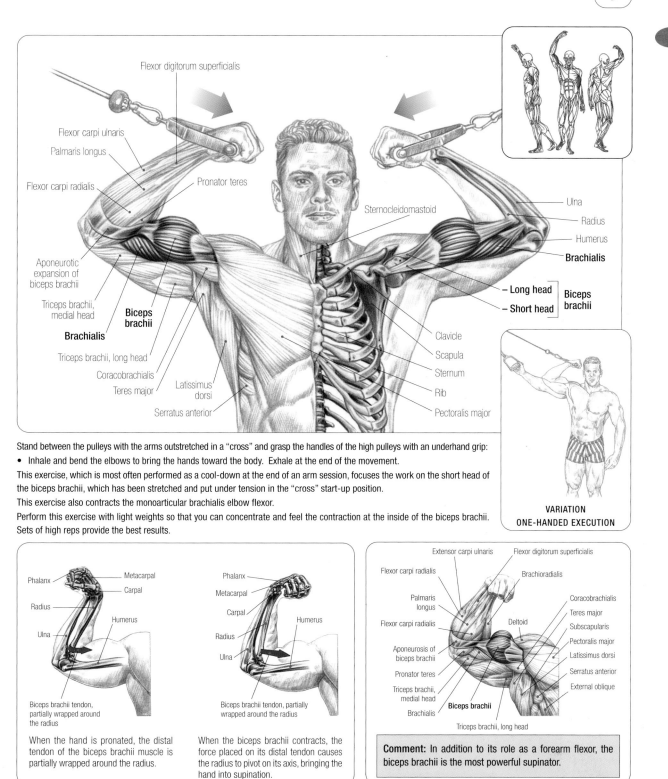

Stand between the pulleys with the arms outstretched in a "cross" and grasp the handles of the high pulleys with an underhand grip:
- Inhale and bend the elbows to bring the hands toward the body. Exhale at the end of the movement.

This exercise, which is most often performed as a cool-down at the end of an arm session, focuses the work on the short head of the biceps brachii, which has been stretched and put under tension in the "cross" start-up position.

This exercise also contracts the monoarticular brachialis elbow flexor.

Perform this exercise with light weights so that you can concentrate and feel the contraction at the inside of the biceps brachii. Sets of high reps provide the best results.

**VARIATION
ONE-HANDED EXECUTION**

When the hand is pronated, the distal tendon of the biceps brachii muscle is partially wrapped around the radius.

When the biceps brachii contracts, the force placed on its distal tendon causes the radius to pivot on its axis, bringing the hand into supination.

Comment: In addition to its role as a forearm flexor, the biceps brachii is the most powerful supinator.

7 BARBELL CURLS

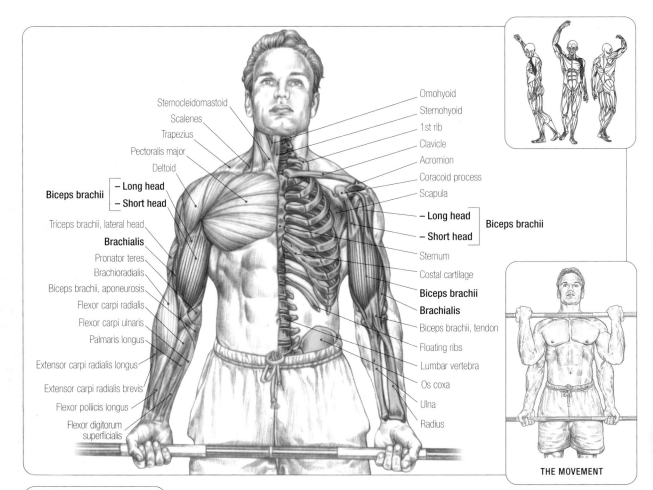

Sternocleidomastoid
Scalenes
Trapezius
Pectoralis major
Deltoid
Biceps brachii
— Long head
— Short head
Triceps brachii, lateral head
Brachialis
Pronator teres
Brachioradialis
Biceps brachii, aponeurosis
Flexor carpi radialis
Flexor carpi ulnaris
Palmaris longus
Extensor carpi radialis longus
Extensor carpi radialis brevis
Flexor pollicis longus
Flexor digitorum superficialis

Omohyoid
Sternohyoid
1st rib
Clavicle
Acromion
Coracoid process
Scapula
— Long head
— Short head
Biceps brachii
Sternum
Costal cartilage
Biceps brachii
Brachialis
Biceps brachii, tendon
Floating ribs
Lumbar vertebra
Os coxa
Ulna
Radius

THE MOVEMENT

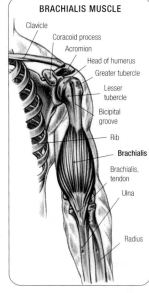

BRACHIALIS MUSCLE

Clavicle
Coracoid process
Acromion
Head of humerus
Greater tubercle
Lesser tubercle
Bicipital groove
Rib
Brachialis
Brachialis, tendon
Ulna
Radius

Stand with the back straight. Grasp the barbell with an underhand grip and hands slightly wider than shoulder-width apart:

- Inhale and raise the barbell by bending the elbows, taking care to stabilize the torso and spine by isometrically contracting the gluteal muscles, abdominal muscles, and spinal muscles.
- Exhale at the end of the movement.

This exercise mainly contracts the biceps brachii, brachialis, and, to a lesser degree, the brachioradialis, pronator teres, and the wrist flexor group.

Variations: Vary the width of the grip to work different parts of the muscle more intensely:

- Placing the hands farther apart isolates the short head of the biceps brachii.
- Placing the hands closer together isolates the long head of the biceps brachii.

Raising both elbows after they are flexed increases the contraction of the biceps brachii and contracts the anterior deltoid.

To make the exercise more difficult, perform the movement with the back against a wall so that the shoulder blades don't move.

You can lift more weight and gain strength by leaning the torso back while lifting the bar; however, to prevent injury, this requires good technique and well-developed abdominal and lumbar muscles.

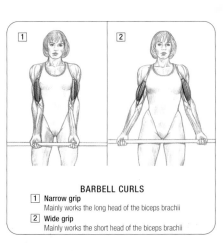

BARBELL CURLS

1 **Narrow grip**
Mainly works the long head of the biceps brachii

2 **Wide grip**
Mainly works the short head of the biceps brachii

ELBOW STRUCTURE AND ITS EFFECT ON TRAINING

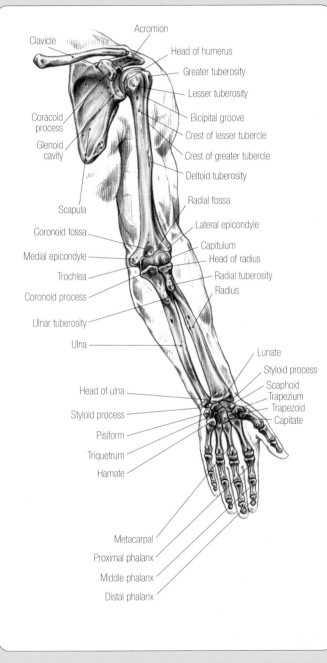

Acromion
Clavicle
Head of humerus
Greater tuberosity
Lesser tuberosity
Coracoid process
Bicipital groove
Crest of lesser tubercle
Glenoid cavity
Crest of greater tubercle
Deltoid tuberosity
Radial fossa
Scapula
Lateral epicondyle
Coronoid fossa
Capitulum
Medial epicondyle
Head of radius
Trochlea
Radial tuberosity
Coronoid process
Radius
Ulnar tuberosity
Ulna
Lunate
Styloid process
Head of ulna
Scaphoid
Trapezium
Styloid process
Trapezoid
Capitate
Pisiform
Triquetrum
Hamate
Metacarpal
Proximal phalanx
Middle phalanx
Distal phalanx

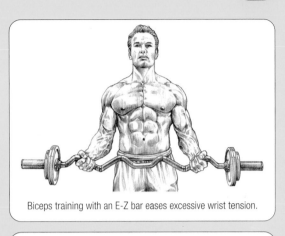

Biceps training with an E-Z bar eases excessive wrist tension.

1 2

1 Upper extremity with a small angle

2 Upper extremity with a significant valgus angle (more common in women)

When training the biceps brachii using a barbell, take into account variations in each person's physical structure.

In the anatomical position (arms hanging alongside the body, palms facing forward, and thumbs pointing laterally), the angle at the elbow between the upper arm and the forearm varies from person to person. Someone whose forearm hangs distinctly away from the body in a valgus position must break excessively at the wrist when performing a curl with a straight bar, which is painful. Therefore, these people should work with an E-Z bar to spare their wrists.

Comment: Valgus of the elbow is usually more pronounced in women.

8 MACHINE CURLS

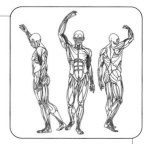

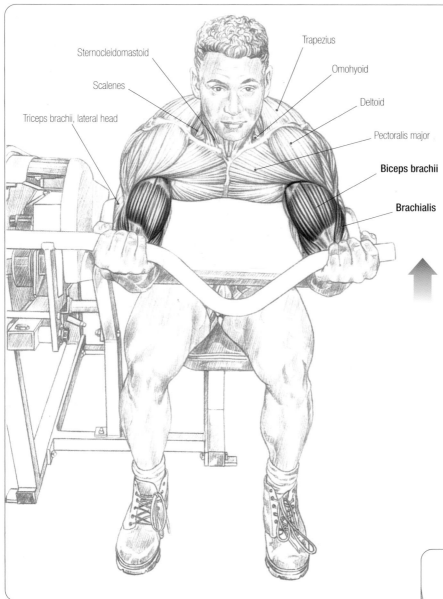

Sternocleidomastoid

Trapezius

Scalenes

Omohyoid

Triceps brachii, lateral head

Deltoid

Pectoralis major

Biceps brachii

Brachialis

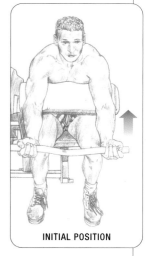

INITIAL POSITION

Sit at the machine and grasp the bar with an underhand grip, arms extended and resting on the support:

- Inhale and raise the forearms.
- Exhale at the end of the movement.

This is one of the best exercises for working the biceps brachii. Fixing the arms against the support makes it impossible to "cheat."

At the beginning, the muscle tension is intense, so be sure to warm up properly using light weights. To avoid the risk of tendonitis, do not completely extend the arm.

This movement also works the brachialis and, to a lesser extent, the brachioradialis and pronator teres.

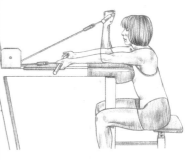

VARIATION
Performing the curl with an Atlas pulley
is a great way to pump up the muscle.

PREACHER CURLS 9

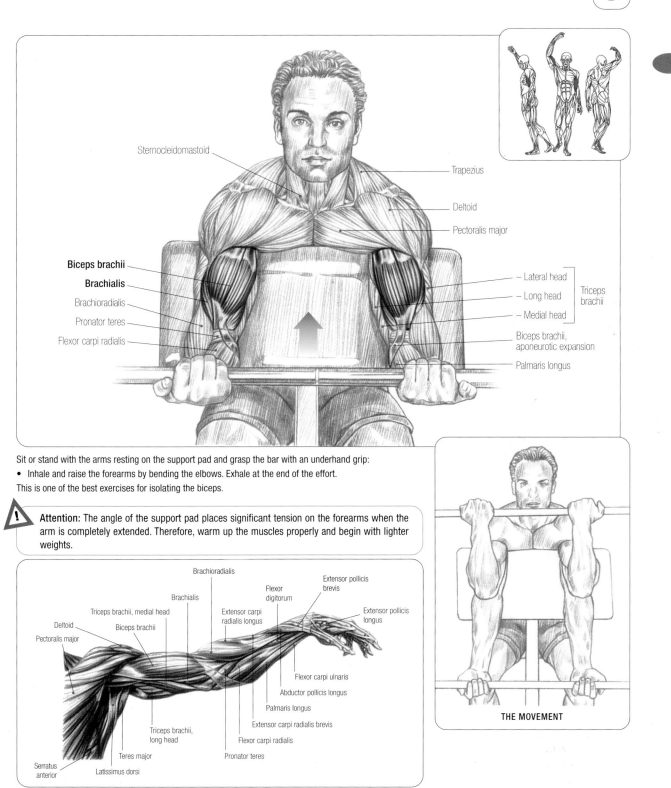

Sternocleidomastoid

Trapezius

Deltoid

Pectoralis major

Biceps brachii

Brachialis

Brachioradialis

Pronator teres

Flexor carpi radialis

– Lateral head
– Long head
– Medial head

Triceps brachii

Biceps brachii, aponeurotic expansion

Palmaris longus

Sit or stand with the arms resting on the support pad and grasp the bar with an underhand grip:
• Inhale and raise the forearms by bending the elbows. Exhale at the end of the effort.
This is one of the best exercises for isolating the biceps.

Attention: The angle of the support pad places significant tension on the forearms when the arm is completely extended. Therefore, warm up the muscles properly and begin with lighter weights.

Brachioradialis

Brachialis

Triceps brachii, medial head

Biceps brachii

Deltoid

Pectoralis major

Extensor carpi radialis longus

Flexor digitorum

Extensor pollicis brevis

Extensor pollicis longus

Flexor carpi ulnaris

Abductor pollicis longus

Palmaris longus

Extensor carpi radialis brevis

Flexor carpi radialis

Pronator teres

Triceps brachii, long head

Teres major

Latissimus dorsi

Serratus anterior

THE MOVEMENT

10 REVERSE WRIST CURLS

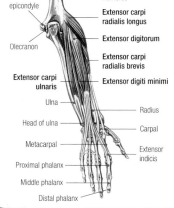

FINAL POSITION

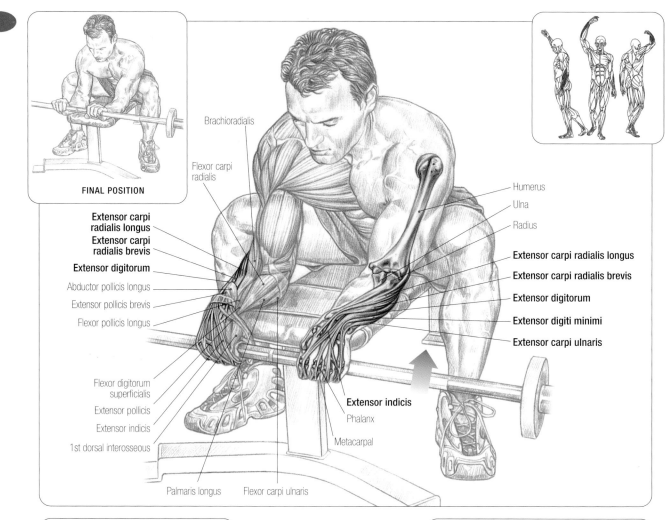

Brachioradialis

Flexor carpi radialis

Extensor carpi radialis longus

Extensor carpi radialis brevis

Extensor digitorum

Abductor pollicis longus

Extensor pollicis brevis

Flexor pollicis longus

Flexor digitorum superficialis

Extensor pollicis

Extensor indicis

1st dorsal interosseous

Palmaris longus

Flexor carpi ulnaris

Humerus

Ulna

Radius

Extensor carpi radialis longus

Extensor carpi radialis brevis

Extensor digitorum

Extensor digiti minimi

Extensor carpi ulnaris

Extensor indicis

Phalanx

Metacarpal

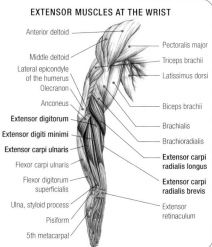

WRIST EXTENSORS

Medial epicondyle

Humerus

Extensor carpi radialis longus

Extensor digitorum

Olecranon

Extensor carpi radialis brevis

Extensor carpi ulnaris

Extensor digiti minimi

Ulna

Head of ulna

Radius

Metacarpal

Carpal

Extensor indicis

Proximal phalanx

Middle phalanx

Distal phalanx

Sit with the forearms resting on the thighs or on a bench and grasp the bar with an overhand grip and keep the wrists relaxed:

- Inhale and raise the hands by extending at the wrists.

This exercise contracts the extensor carpi radialis longus and brevis, extensor digitorum, extensor digiti minimi, and the extensor carpi ulnaris.

Comment: This exercise strengthens the wrists, which are often vulnerable because of weak wrist extensors.

EXTENSOR MUSCLES AT THE WRIST

Anterior deltoid

Middle deltoid

Lateral epicondyle of the humerus

Olecranon

Anconeus

Extensor digitorum

Extensor digiti minimi

Extensor carpi ulnaris

Flexor carpi ulnaris

Flexor digitorum superficialis

Ulna, styloid process

Pisiform

5th metacarpal

Pectoralis major

Triceps brachii

Latissimus dorsi

Biceps brachii

Brachialis

Brachioradialis

Extensor carpi radialis longus

Extensor carpi radialis brevis

Extensor retinaculum

WRIST CURLS 11

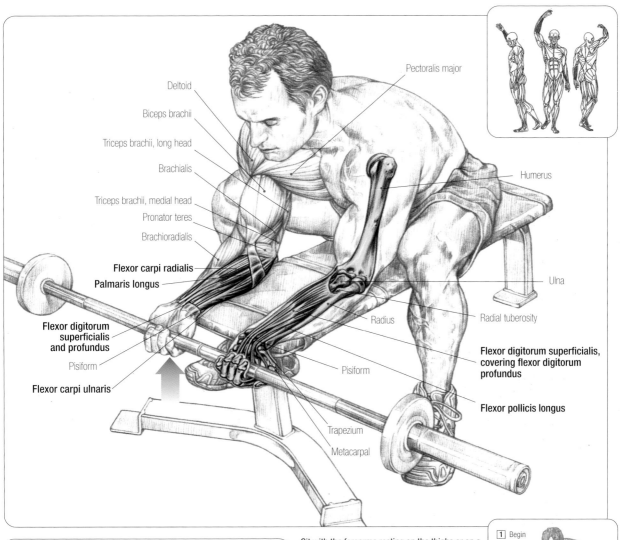

Pectoralis major

Deltoid

Biceps brachii

Triceps brachii, long head

Brachialis

Triceps brachii, medial head

Pronator teres

Brachioradialis

Flexor carpi radialis

Palmaris longus

Humerus

**Flexor digitorum
superficialis
and profundus**

Pisiform

Flexor carpi ulnaris

Ulna

Radial tuberosity

Radius

Pisiform

**Flexor digitorum superficialis,
covering flexor digitorum
profundus**

Flexor pollicis longus

Trapezium

Metacarpal

WRIST FLEXORS

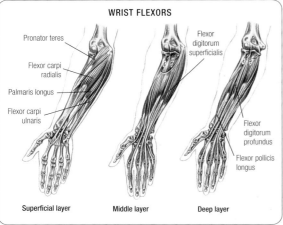

Pronator teres

Flexor carpi
radialis

Palmaris longus

Flexor carpi
ulnaris

Flexor
digitorum
superficialis

Flexor
digitorum
profundus

Flexor
pollicis
longus

Superficial layer   Middle layer   Deep layer

Sit with the forearms resting on the thighs or on a
bench and grasp the bar with an underhand grip
with wrists relaxed:

- Inhale and raise the hands by flexing at the
  wrists.

This exercise contracts the flexor carpi radialis,
palmaris longus, flexor carpi ulnaris, and the flexors
digitorum superficialis and profundus.

The latter two muscles, although located deep in
the wrist, make up most of the muscle mass of the
wrist flexors.

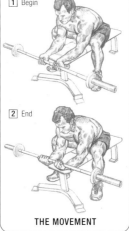

1 Begin

2 End

THE MOVEMENT

12 REVERSE BARBELL CURLS

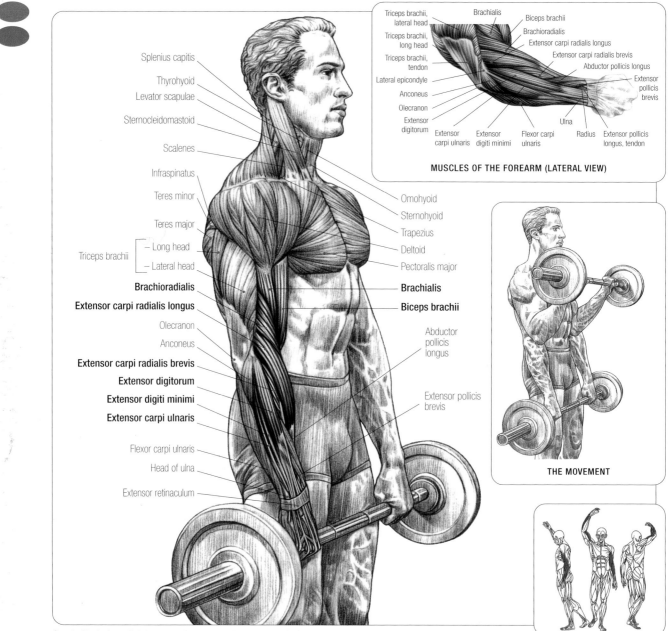

Splenius capitis

Thyrohyoid

Levator scapulae

Sternocleidomastoid

Scalenes

Infraspinatus

Teres minor

Teres major

Triceps brachii
— Long head
— Lateral head

Brachioradialis

Extensor carpi radialis longus

Olecranon

Anconeus

Extensor carpi radialis brevis

Extensor digitorum

Extensor digiti minimi

Extensor carpi ulnaris

Flexor carpi ulnaris

Head of ulna

Extensor retinaculum

Omohyoid

Sternohyoid

Trapezius

Deltoid

Pectoralis major

Brachialis

Biceps brachii

Abductor pollicis longus

Extensor pollicis brevis

Triceps brachii, lateral head

Triceps brachii, long head

Triceps brachii, tendon

Lateral epicondyle

Anconeus

Olecranon

Extensor digitorum

Extensor carpi ulnaris

Extensor digiti minimi

Flexor carpi ulnaris

Brachialis

Biceps brachii

Brachioradialis

Extensor carpi radialis longus

Extensor carpi radialis brevis

Abductor pollicis longus

Extensor pollicis brevis

Ulna

Radius

Extensor pollicis longus, tendon

MUSCLES OF THE FOREARM (LATERAL VIEW)

THE MOVEMENT

Stand with the legs slightly apart and arms extended and grasp the bar with an overhand grip (with the thumbs facing each other):

- Inhale and raise the forearms by bending the elbows.
- Exhale at the end of the movement.

This exercise works the extensor muscles of the wrist: extensor carpi radialis longus, extensor carpi radialis brevis, extensor digitorum, extensor digiti minimi, and extensor carpi ulnaris.

It also acts on the brachioradialis, brachialis, and, to a lesser degree, the biceps brachii.

Comment: This is an excellent exercise for strengthening the wrist, which is often weak because of an imbalance caused by using the wrist flexors rather than the wrist extensors. For this reason, many boxers include it in their training. Many bench press champions use it to keep their wrists from trembling under extreme weights.

STRETCHING THE FOREARM MUSCLES

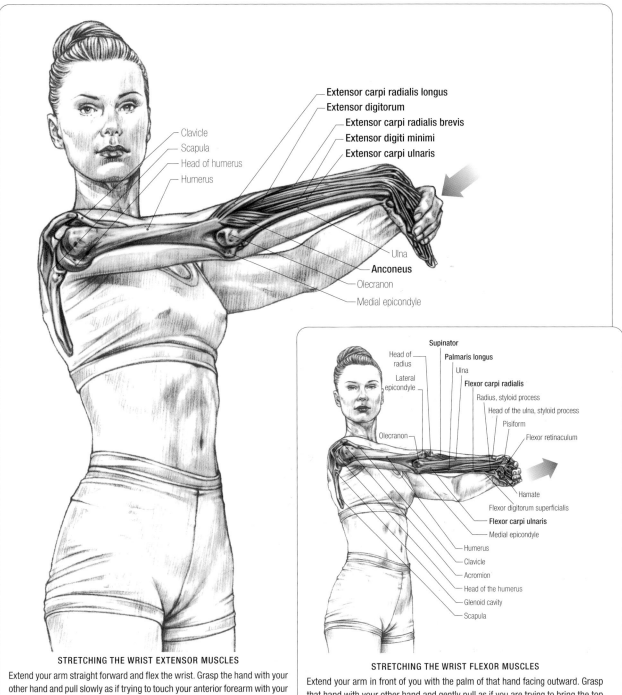

Clavicle
Scapula
Head of humerus
Humerus

Extensor carpi radialis longus
Extensor digitorum
Extensor carpi radialis brevis
Extensor digiti minimi
Extensor carpi ulnaris

Ulna
Anconeus
Olecranon
Medial epicondyle

Supinator
Head of radius
Palmaris longus
Lateral epicondyle
Ulna
Flexor carpi radialis
Radius, styloid process
Head of the ulna, styloid process
Pisiform
Flexor retinaculum
Olecranon
Hamate
Flexor digitorum superficialis
Flexor carpi ulnaris
Medial epicondyle
Humerus
Clavicle
Acromion
Head of the humerus
Glenoid cavity
Scapula

STRETCHING THE WRIST EXTENSOR MUSCLES

Extend your arm straight forward and flex the wrist. Grasp the hand with your other hand and pull slowly as if trying to touch your anterior forearm with your palm while extending at the elbow.

This exercise mainly stretches the extensor carpi radialis longus and brevis, extensor digitorum, extensor digiti minimi, extensor carpi ulnaris, and anconeus.

STRETCHING THE WRIST FLEXOR MUSCLES

Extend your arm in front of you with the palm of that hand facing outward. Grasp that hand with your other hand and gently pull as if you are trying to bring the top of your hand toward you while pushing the palm out. This exercise mainly stretches the palmaris longus, flexor carpi radialis, flexor carpi ulnaris, superficial and deep finger flexors, and supinator.

13 PUSH-DOWNS

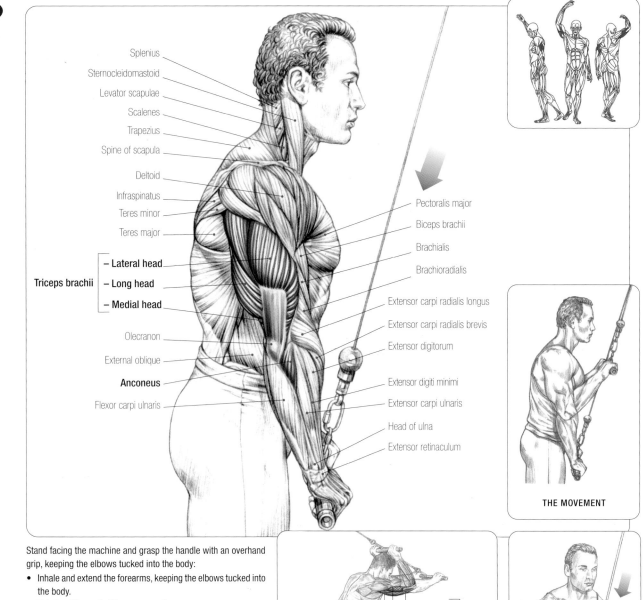

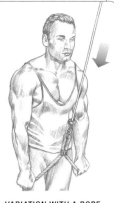

Splenius
Sternocleidomastoid
Levator scapulae
Scalenes
Trapezius
Spine of scapula
Deltoid
Infraspinatus
Teres minor
Teres major

Triceps brachii
– Lateral head
– Long head
– Medial head

Olecranon
External oblique
Anconeus
Flexor carpi ulnaris

Pectoralis major
Biceps brachii
Brachialis
Brachioradialis
Extensor carpi radialis longus
Extensor carpi radialis brevis
Extensor digitorum
Extensor digiti minimi
Extensor carpi ulnaris
Head of ulna
Extensor retinaculum

THE MOVEMENT

Stand facing the machine and grasp the handle with an overhand grip, keeping the elbows tucked into the body:

- Inhale and extend the forearms, keeping the elbows tucked into the body.
- Exhale at the end of the movement.

Comments: This exercise isolates the triceps and the anconeus.

The variation using a rope rather than a handle engages the lateral head of the triceps more intensely.

Performing the movement with an underhand grip requires more contribution from the medial head of the triceps.

Hold an isometric contraction for one or two seconds at the end of the movement to feel the effort more intensely.

When using heavy weights, lean forward with the torso.

Beginners can use this exercise to develop enough strength to move on to more difficult exercises.

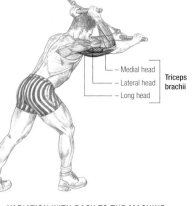

Triceps brachii
– Medial head
– Lateral head
– Long head

VARIATION WITH BACK TO THE MACHINE TO ISOLATE THE LONG HEAD OF THE TRICEPS

VARIATION WITH A ROPE TO ISOLATE THE LATERAL HEAD OF THE TRICEPS

REVERSE PUSH-DOWNS $\boxed{14}$

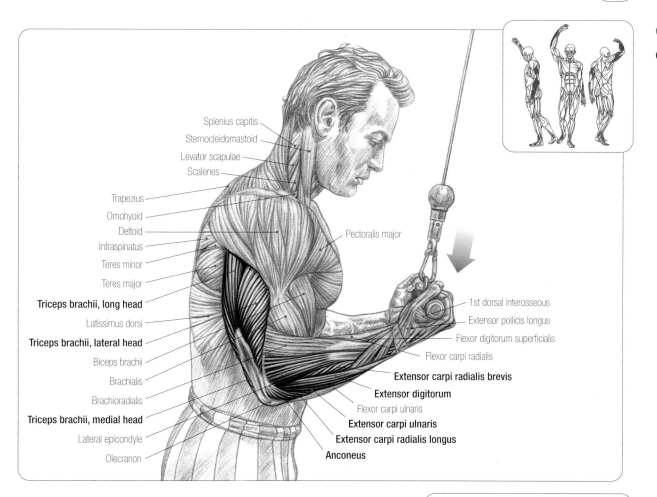

Splenius capitis
Sternocleidomastoid
Levator scapulae
Scalenes
Trapezius
Omohyoid
Deltoid
Infraspinatus
Teres minor
Teres major
Triceps brachii, long head
Latissimus dorsi
Triceps brachii, lateral head
Biceps brachii
Brachialis
Brachioradialis
Triceps brachii, medial head
Lateral epicondyle
Olecranon

Pectoralis major

1st dorsal interosseous
Extensor pollicis longus
Flexor digitorum superficialis
Flexor carpi radialis
Extensor carpi radialis brevis
Extensor digitorum
Flexor carpi ulnaris
Extensor carpi ulnaris
Extensor carpi radialis longus
Anconeus

Stand facing the machine with the arms next to the body and elbows bent and grasp the handle with an underhand grip:

- Inhale and extend the forearms by straightening the elbows, keeping them tucked into the body.
- Exhale at the end of the movement.

The underhand grip isolates the medial head of the triceps brachii and precludes working with heavy weights.

When extending the forearms, the anconeus and wrist extensors also contract.

The extensor carpi ulnaris, extensor digitorum, extensor digiti minimi, and extensors carpi radialis longus and brevis keep the wrist straight with isometric contraction during the exercise.

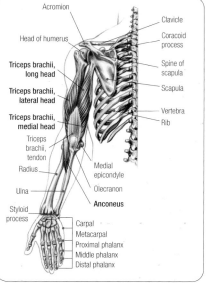

Acromion
Clavicle
Head of humerus
Coracoid process
Spine of scapula
Triceps brachii, long head
Scapula
Triceps brachii, lateral head
Vertebra
Rib
Triceps brachii, medial head
Triceps brachii, tendon
Radius
Medial epicondyle
Ulna
Olecranon
Styloid process
Anconeus
Carpal
Metacarpal
Proximal phalanx
Middle phalanx
Distal phalanx

15 ONE-ARM REVERSE PUSH-DOWNS

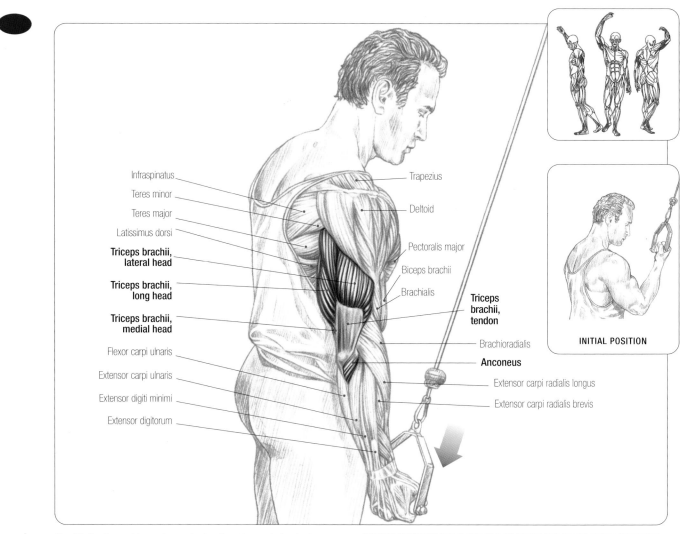

Infraspinatus
Teres minor
Teres major
Latissimus dorsi
Triceps brachii, lateral head
Triceps brachii, long head
Triceps brachii, medial head
Flexor carpi ulnaris
Extensor carpi ulnaris
Extensor digiti minimi
Extensor digitorum

Trapezius
Deltoid
Pectoralis major
Biceps brachii
Brachialis
Triceps brachii, tendon
Brachioradialis
Anconeus
Extensor carpi radialis longus
Extensor carpi radialis brevis

INITIAL POSITION

Stand facing the machine and grasp the handle with an underhand grip:

- Inhale and extend the forearm.
- Exhale at the end of the movement.

This exercise mainly works the lateral head of the triceps.

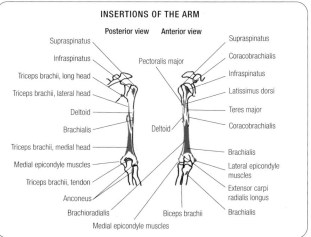

INSERTIONS OF THE ARM

Posterior view   Anterior view

Supraspinatus
Infraspinatus
Triceps brachii, long head
Triceps brachii, lateral head
Deltoid
Brachialis
Triceps brachii, medial head
Medial epicondyle muscles
Triceps brachii, tendon
Anconeus
Brachioradialis

Pectoralis major

Deltoid

Biceps brachii

Medial epicondyle muscles

Supraspinatus
Coracobrachialis
Infraspinatus
Latissimus dorsi
Teres major
Coracobrachialis
Brachialis
Lateral epicondyle muscles
Extensor carpi radialis longus
Brachialis

OVERHEAD CABLE TRICEPS EXTENSIONS 16

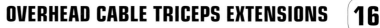

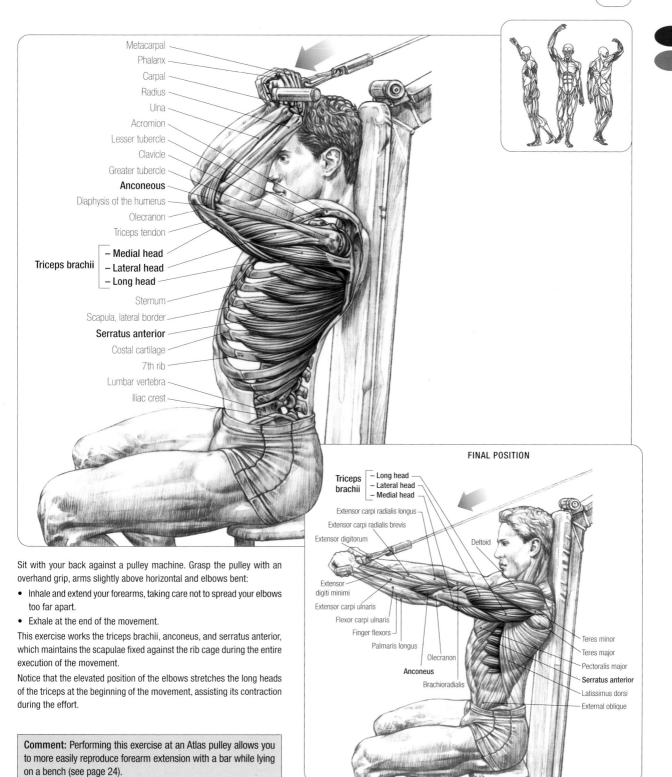

Metacarpal
Phalanx
Carpal
Radius
Ulna
Acromion
Lesser tubercle
Clavicle
Greater tubercle
Anconeous
Diaphysis of the humerus
Olecranon
Triceps tendon
Triceps brachii
– **Medial head**
– **Lateral head**
– **Long head**
Sternum
Scapula, lateral border
Serratus anterior
Costal cartilage
7th rib
Lumbar vertebra
Iliac crest

FINAL POSITION

Triceps brachii
– Long head
– Lateral head
– Medial head
Extensor carpi radialis longus
Extensor carpi radialis brevis
Extensor digitorum
Extensor digiti minimi
Extensor carpi ulnaris
Flexor carpi ulnaris
Finger flexors
Palmaris longus
Anconeus
Brachioradialis
Olecranon
Deltoid
Teres minor
Teres major
Pectoralis major
Serratus anterior
Latissimus dorsi
External oblique

Sit with your back against a pulley machine. Grasp the pulley with an overhand grip, arms slightly above horizontal and elbows bent:

- Inhale and extend your forearms, taking care not to spread your elbows too far apart.
- Exhale at the end of the movement.

This exercise works the triceps brachii, anconeus, and serratus anterior, which maintains the scapulae fixed against the rib cage during the entire execution of the movement.

Notice that the elevated position of the elbows stretches the long heads of the triceps at the beginning of the movement, assisting its contraction during the effort.

Comment: Performing this exercise at an Atlas pulley allows you to more easily reproduce forearm extension with a bar while lying on a bench (see page 24).

17 LYING TRICEPS EXTENSIONS

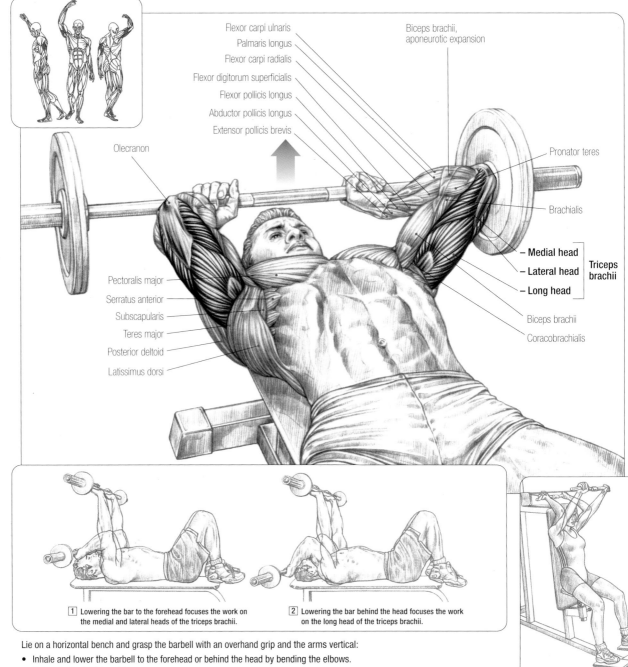

Flexor carpi ulnaris
Palmaris longus
Flexor carpi radialis
Flexor digitorum superficialis
Flexor pollicis longus
Abductor pollicis longus
Extensor pollicis brevis

Biceps brachii, aponeurotic expansion

Olecranon

Pronator teres

Brachialis

— Medial head
— Lateral head   Triceps brachii
— Long head

Pectoralis major
Serratus anterior
Subscapularis
Teres major
Posterior deltoid
Latissimus dorsi

Biceps brachii
Coracobrachialis

1 Lowering the bar to the forehead focuses the work on the medial and lateral heads of the triceps brachii.

2 Lowering the bar behind the head focuses the work on the long head of the triceps brachii.

Lie on a horizontal bench and grasp the barbell with an overhand grip and the arms vertical:

- Inhale and lower the barbell to the forehead or behind the head by bending the elbows.
- Return to the initial position.
- Exhale at the end of the effort.

Comments: Because of individual variations in shoulder width, valgus angle at the elbows, and wrist flexibility, the hands can be closer or farther apart on the bar and the elbow angle more or less open during the exercise. Using an E-Z bar helps prevent excessive strain at the wrists.

VARIATION ON A MACHINE

Performing this exercise at an Atlas triceps pulley simulates th movement with a barbell and ena you to isolate the long head of th triceps brachii.

LYING DUMBBELL TRICEPS EXTENSIONS 18

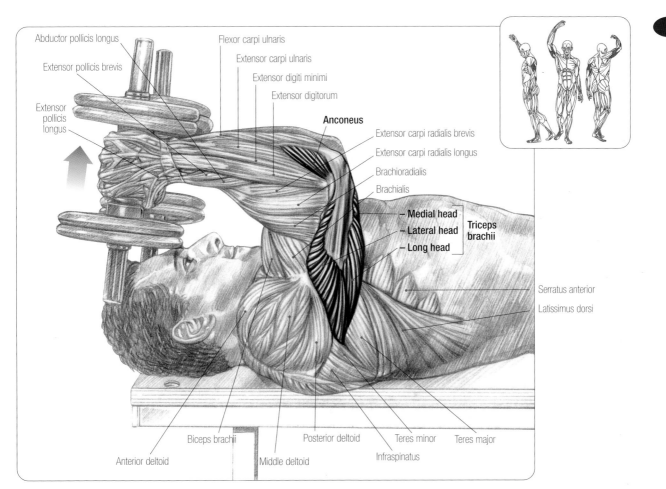

Abductor pollicis longus
Extensor pollicis brevis
Extensor pollicis longus
Flexor carpi ulnaris
Extensor carpi ulnaris
Extensor digiti minimi
Extensor digitorum
Anconeus
Extensor carpi radialis brevis
Extensor carpi radialis longus
Brachioradialis
Brachialis
— Medial head
— Lateral head **Triceps brachii**
— Long head
Serratus anterior
Latissimus dorsi
Biceps brachii
Posterior deltoid
Teres minor
Teres major
Anterior deltoid
Middle deltoid
Infraspinatus

Lie on a flat bench and grasp a dumbbell in each hand with the arms vertical:

- Inhale and lower the forearms by bending the elbow with a controlled movement.
- Return to the initial position.
- Exhale at the end of the effort.

This exercise works all three heads of the triceps brachii equally.

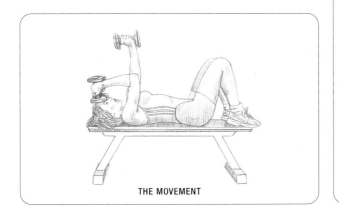

THE MOVEMENT

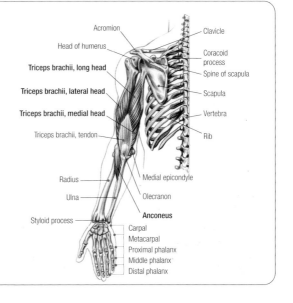

Acromion
Clavicle
Head of humerus
Coracoid process
Spine of scapula
Triceps brachii, long head
Triceps brachii, lateral head
Scapula
Triceps brachii, medial head
Vertebra
Triceps brachii, tendon
Rib
Radius
Medial epicondyle
Ulna
Olecranon
Anconeus
Styloid process
Carpal
Metacarpal
Proximal phalanx
Middle phalanx
Distal phalanx

19 ONE-ARM OVERHEAD DUMBBELL TRICEPS EXTENSIONS

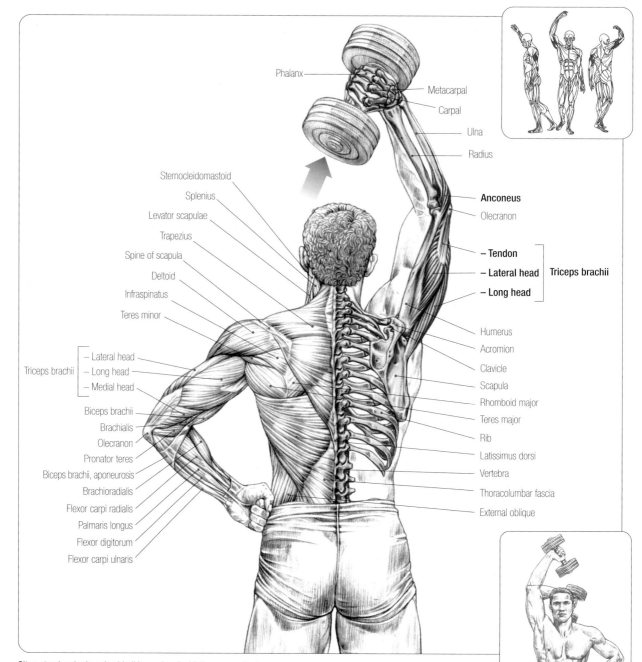

Phalanx

Metacarpal

Carpal

Ulna

Radius

Sternocleidomastoid

Splenius

Levator scapulae

Trapezius

Spine of scapula

Deltoid

Infraspinatus

Teres minor

Triceps brachii
– Lateral head
– Long head
– Medial head

Biceps brachii

Brachialis

Olecranon

Pronator teres

Biceps brachii, aponeurosis

Brachioradialis

Flexor carpi radialis

Palmaris longus

Flexor digitorum

Flexor carpi ulnaris

Anconeus
Olecranon

– Tendon
– Lateral head   Triceps brachii
– Long head

Humerus

Acromion

Clavicle

Scapula

Rhomboid major

Teres major

Rib

Latissimus dorsi

Vertebra

Thoracolumbar fascia

External oblique

Sit or stand and grip a dumbbell in one hand with the arm vertical:

• Inhale and bend the elbow to lower the dumbbell behind the head to the neck.
• Return to the initial position.
• Exhale at the end of the movement.

The vertical position of the arm stretches the long head of the triceps brachii, emphasizing its contraction while working.

Comment: Contract the abdominal core to prevent arching the low back. If possible use a bench with support for the low back.

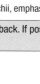

THE MOVEMENT

TRICEPS KICKBACKS 20

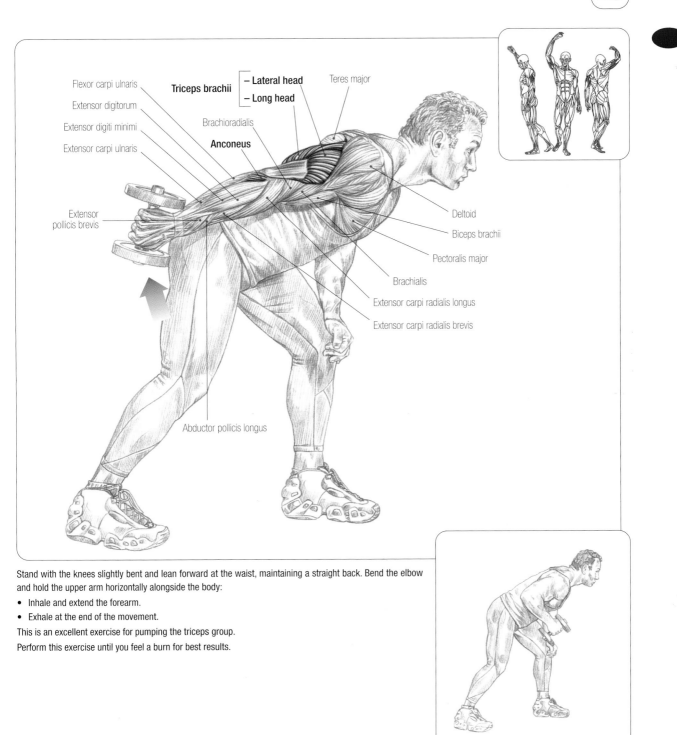

Flexor carpi ulnaris

Triceps brachii — **Lateral head** — **Long head**

Teres major

Extensor digitorum

Extensor digiti minimi

Brachioradialis

Extensor carpi ulnaris

Anconeus

Extensor pollicis brevis

Deltoid

Biceps brachii

Pectoralis major

Brachialis

Extensor carpi radialis longus

Extensor carpi radialis brevis

Abductor pollicis longus

INITIAL POSITION

Stand with the knees slightly bent and lean forward at the waist, maintaining a straight back. Bend the elbow and hold the upper arm horizontally alongside the body:

- Inhale and extend the forearm.
- Exhale at the end of the movement.

This is an excellent exercise for pumping the triceps group.

Perform this exercise until you feel a burn for best results.

21 SEATED DUMBBELL TRICEPS EXTENSIONS

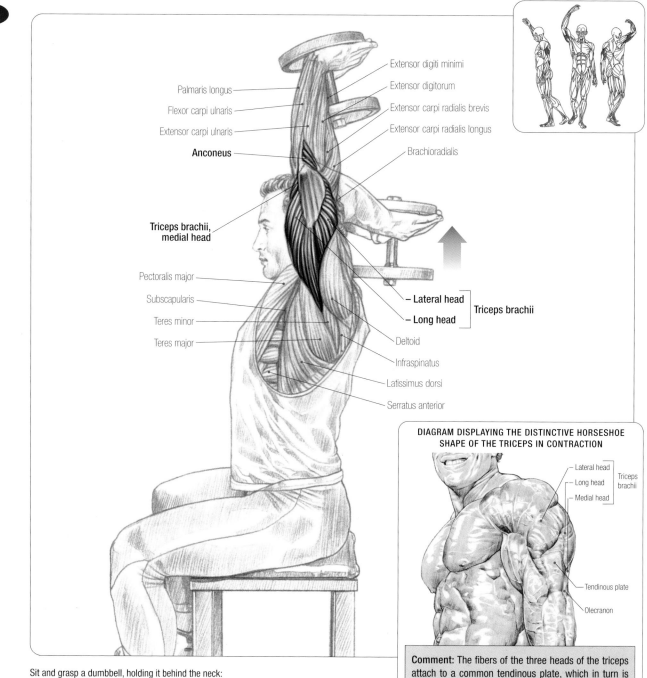

Palmaris longus

Flexor carpi ulnaris

Extensor carpi ulnaris

Anconeus

Triceps brachii, medial head

Pectoralis major

Subscapularis

Teres minor

Teres major

Extensor digiti minimi

Extensor digitorum

Extensor carpi radialis brevis

Extensor carpi radialis longus

Brachioradialis

– Lateral head

– Long head   **Triceps brachii**

Deltoid

Infraspinatus

Latissimus dorsi

Serratus anterior

DIAGRAM DISPLAYING THE DISTINCTIVE HORSESHOE SHAPE OF THE TRICEPS IN CONTRACTION

Lateral head

Long head   Triceps brachii

Medial head

Tendinous plate

Olecranon

Sit and grasp a dumbbell, holding it behind the neck:

- Inhale and extend the forearms.
- Exhale at the end of the movement.

The vertical position of the arms strongly stretches the long head of the triceps brachii, emphasizing its contraction while working.

Contract the abdominal core to prevent arching the low back. If possible use a bench with support for the low back.

Comment: The fibers of the three heads of the triceps attach to a common tendinous plate, which in turn is attached to the olecranon by a tendon. When the triceps contracts, the tendinous plate is drawn into the fibers of the heads of the triceps, much as a wooden plate drawn into butter. The contracted muscle bulges out from the plate, creating this characteristic horseshoe shape.

SEATED E-Z BAR TRICEPS EXTENSIONS 22

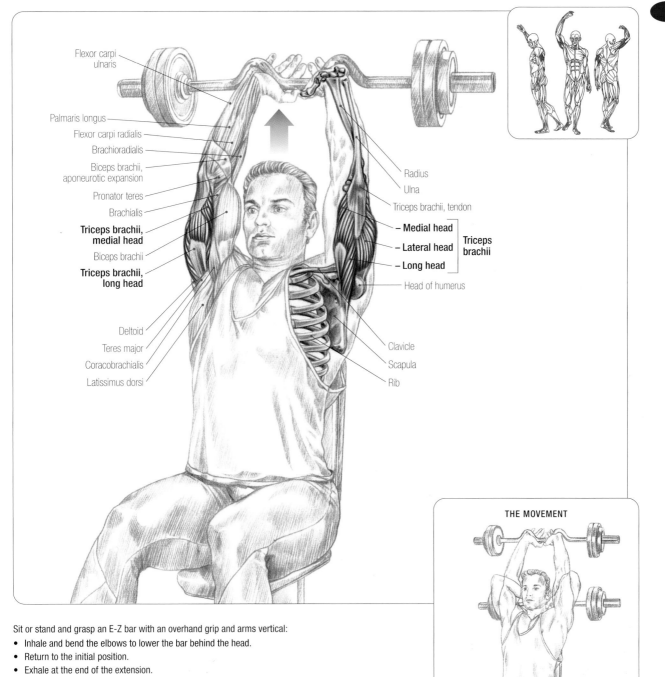

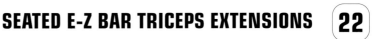

Flexor carpi ulnaris

Palmaris longus

Flexor carpi radialis

Brachioradialis

Biceps brachii, aponeurotic expansion

Pronator teres

Brachialis

Triceps brachii, medial head

Biceps brachii

Triceps brachii, long head

Deltoid

Teres major

Coracobrachialis

Latissimus dorsi

Radius

Ulna

Triceps brachii, tendon

– **Medial head**
– **Lateral head**   Triceps brachii
– **Long head**

Head of humerus

Clavicle

Scapula

Rib

THE MOVEMENT

Sit or stand and grasp an E-Z bar with an overhand grip and arms vertical:
• Inhale and bend the elbows to lower the bar behind the head.
• Return to the initial position.
• Exhale at the end of the extension.
The vertical position of the arms strongly stretches the long head of the triceps brachii, emphasizing its contraction while working.
An overhand grip isolates the lateral head of the triceps brachii.
Contract the abdominal muscles and avoid arching the low back. If possible use a bench with support for the low back.

23 TRICEPS DIPS

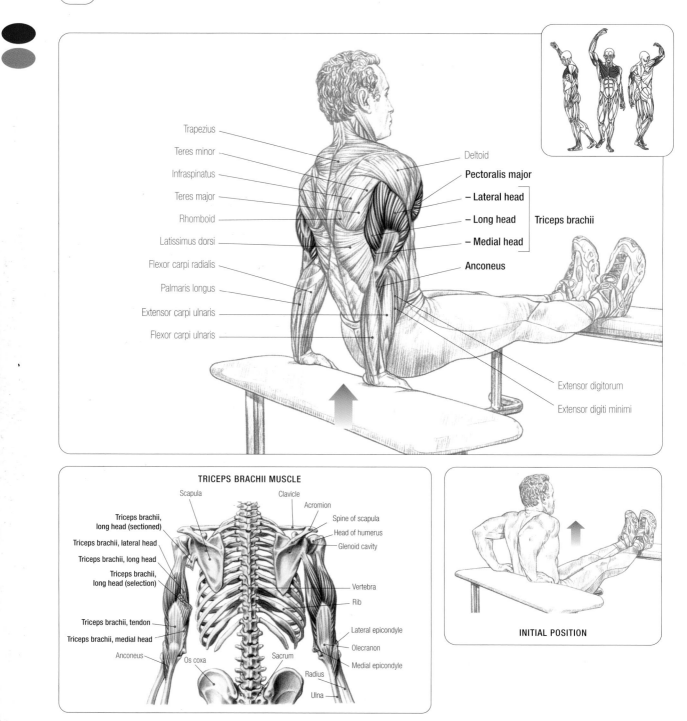

TRICEPS BRACHII MUSCLE

Suspend the body between two benches by placing the hands on the edge of one bench and the feet on the edge of the other bench:

• Inhale, then dip by bending the elbows and rise by extending the forearms.

• Exhale at the end of the movement.

This exercise works the triceps and pectorals as well as the anterior deltoid.

Resting weights on top of the thighs increases the difficulty and intensity of the dip.

STRETCHING THE TRICEPS

Stand or sit with a very straight back. Hold one arm vertical against the side of your head and bend the elbow to 90 degrees.

- Try to bring your elbow behind your head.
- Hold the stretch for a few seconds while breathing slowly.

This exercise mainly stretches the triceps, teres major, and latissimus dorsi.

Variation: To accentuate the stretch on the triceps, perform this exercise with the elbow flexed and the opposing hand slowly pulling the elbow down behind the head.

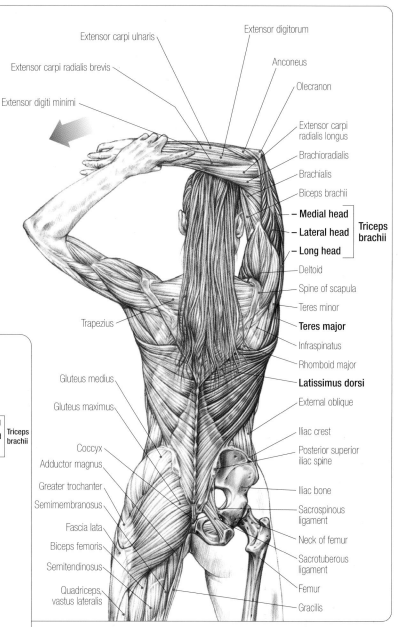

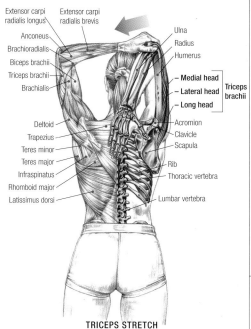

TRICEPS STRETCH

Stand or sit with your back straight and one arm raised vertically beside your head. Bend the arm at the elbow and touch the top of the back with your hand. With the other hand grasp the elbow and slowly try to pull it behind your head. This stretches the teres major, the long head of the triceps brachii, and, to a lesser extent, the latissimus dorsi.

Variation: Pull the hand rather than the elbow. For greater intensity, place the raised arm against a wall.

Comment: These stretching exercises for the triceps help avoid tears, which may occur with heavy lifting on the triceps, but also when executing heavy pullovers or heavy vertical pulls. Vertical pulls have a tendency to pull excessively on the long head of the triceps.

2 SHOULDERS

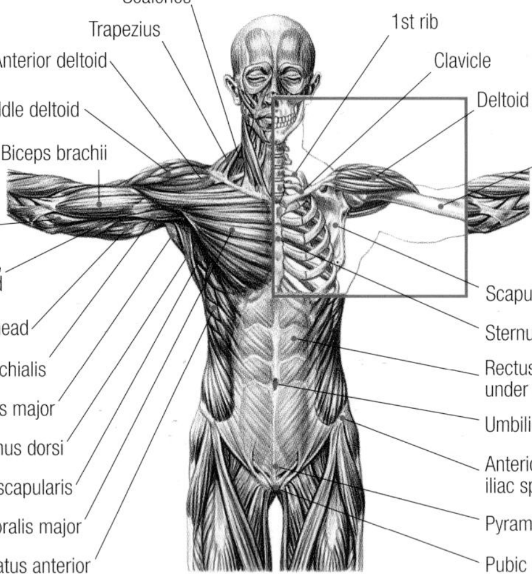

FRONT

Scalenes
Trapezius
Anterior deltoid
Middle deltoid
Biceps brachii
Brachialis
Triceps brachii, medial head
Triceps brachii, long head
Coracobrachialis
Teres major
Latissiumus dorsi
Subscapularis
Pectoralis major
Serratus anterior

1st rib
Clavicle
Deltoid
Humerus
Scapula
Sternum
Rectus abdominis, under the aponeurosis
Umbilicus
Anterior superior iliac spine
Pyramidalis
Pubic symphysis

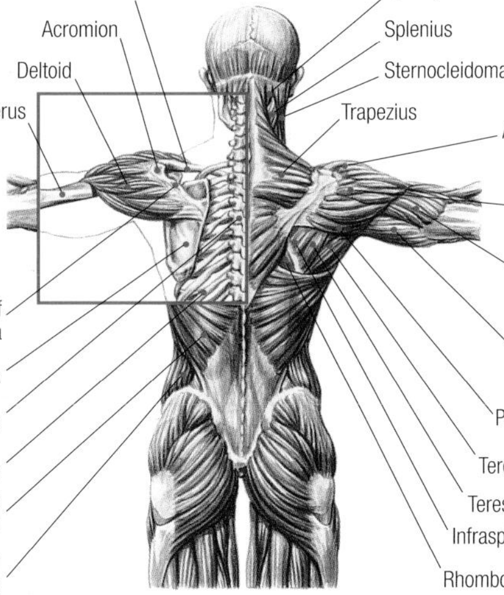

BACK

Clavicle
Acromion
Deltoid
Humerus
Spine of scapula
Scapula
Vertebra
Rib
Latissimus dorsi
External oblique

Semispinalis capitis
Splenius
Sternocleidomastoid
Trapezius
Anterior deltoid
Middle deltoid
Triceps brachii, lateral head
Triceps brachii, long head
Posterior deltoid
Teres major
Teres minor
Infraspinatus
Rhomboid

BACK PRESSES ① 1

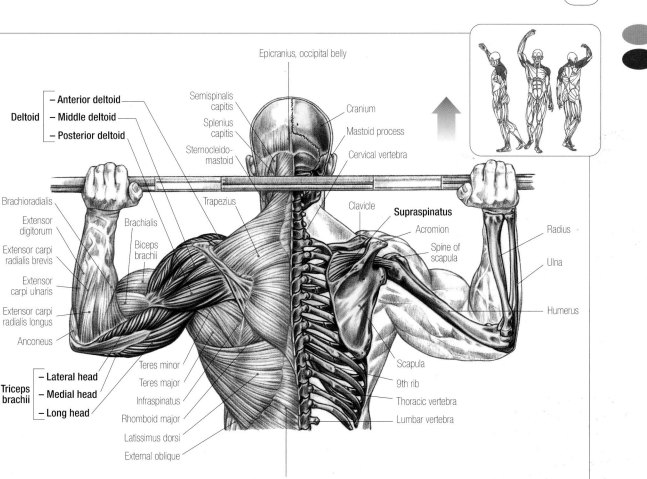

Deltoid
- Anterior deltoid
- Middle deltoid
- Posterior deltoid

Epicranius, occipital belly

Semispinalis capitis

Splenius capitis

Sternocleido-mastoid

Cranium

Mastoid process

Cervical vertebra

Brachioradialis

Extensor digitorum

Extensor carpi radialis brevis

Extensor carpi ulnaris

Extensor carpi radialis longus

Anconeus

Brachialis

Biceps brachii

Trapezius

Clavicle

Supraspinatus

Acromion

Spine of scapula

Radius

Ulna

Humerus

Triceps brachii
- Lateral head
- Medial head
- Long head

Teres minor

Teres major

Infraspinatus

Rhomboid major

Latissimus dorsi

External oblique

Scapula

9th rib

Thoracic vertebra

Lumbar vertebra

Thoracolumbar fascia

Sit with the back straight and hold the bar across the back of the neck with an overhand grip:

- Inhale and extend the bar straight up, keeping the low back as straight as possible.
- Exhale at the end of the effort.

This exercise uses the deltoid, mainly the middle and posterior fibers, as well as the trapezius, triceps brachii, and serratus anterior. Although not worked as intensely, the rhomboids, infraspinatus, teres minor, and, deeper in, the supraspinatus also contract. You can also perform this exercise while standing at a frame that guides the barbell. Various specific machines can help with the performance of this exercise.

Attention: To prevent injury to the shoulder joint, which is vulnerable, lower the bar only as far as your unique shoulder structure and flexibility allow you to do comfortably (see page 39).

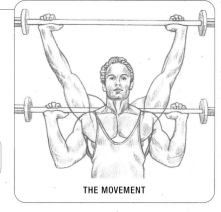

THE MOVEMENT

2 SEATED FRONT PRESSES

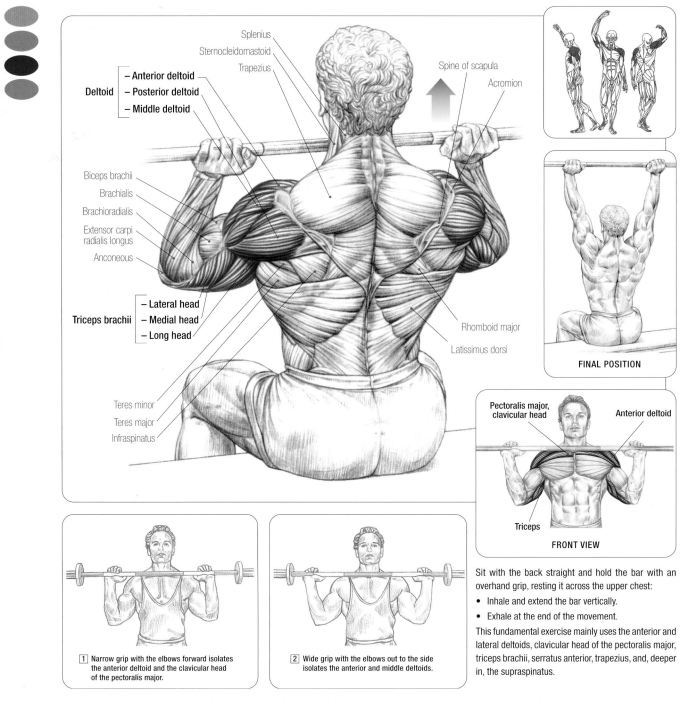

Splenius

Sternocleidomastoid

Trapezius

Spine of scapula

Acromion

Deltoid
— Anterior deltoid
— Posterior deltoid
— Middle deltoid

Biceps brachii

Brachialis

Brachioradialis

Extensor carpi radialis longus

Anconeous

Triceps brachii
— Lateral head
— Medial head
— Long head

Rhomboid major

Latissimus dorsi

Teres minor

Teres major

Infraspinatus

FINAL POSITION

Pectoralis major, clavicular head

Anterior deltoid

Triceps

FRONT VIEW

1 Narrow grip with the elbows forward isolates the anterior deltoid and the clavicular head of the pectoralis major.

2 Wide grip with the elbows out to the side isolates the anterior and middle deltoids.

Sit with the back straight and hold the bar with an overhand grip, resting it across the upper chest:

- Inhale and extend the bar vertically.
- Exhale at the end of the movement.

This fundamental exercise mainly uses the anterior and lateral deltoids, clavicular head of the pectoralis major, triceps brachii, serratus anterior, trapezius, and, deeper in, the supraspinatus.

You can also perform this exercise standing, as long as you keep the back straight, avoiding excessive curvature of the lumbar spine.

Extending the barbell with the elbows forward isolates the anterior deltoid. Extending the bar with the elbows spread apart isolates the middle deltoid.

You can use various machines for this exercise.

SEATED DUMBBELL PRESSES 3

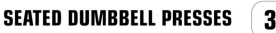

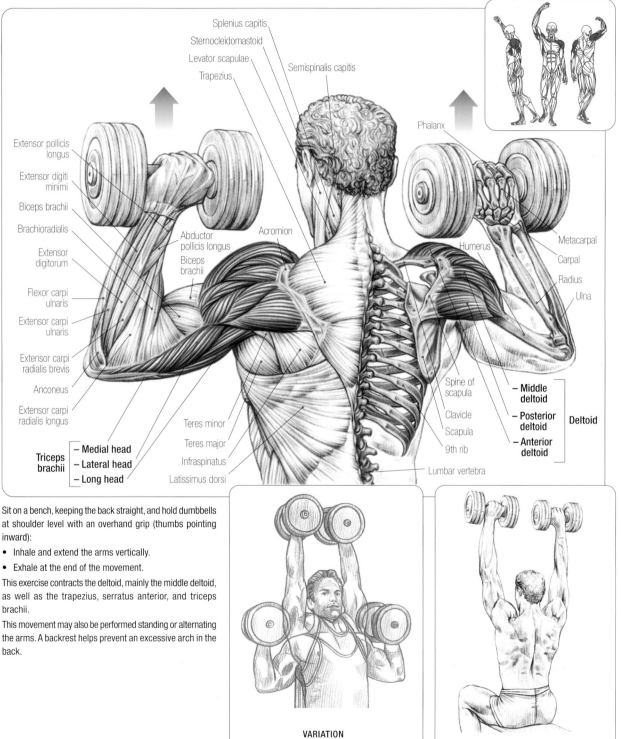

Splenius capitis
Sternocleidomastoid
Levator scapulae
Trapezius
Semispinalis capitis
Phalanx
Extensor pollicis longus
Extensor digiti minimi
Biceps brachii
Brachioradialis
Extensor digitorum
Abductor pollicis longus
Acromion
Biceps brachii
Flexor carpi ulnaris
Extensor carpi ulnaris
Extensor carpi radialis brevis
Anconeus
Extensor carpi radialis longus
Humerus
Metacarpal
Carpal
Radius
Ulna
Triceps brachii
— Medial head
— Lateral head
— Long head
Teres minor
Teres major
Infraspinatus
Latissimus dorsi
Spine of scapula
Clavicle
Scapula
9th rib
Lumbar vertebra
— Middle deltoid
— Posterior deltoid
— Anterior deltoid
Deltoid

Sit on a bench, keeping the back straight, and hold dumbbells at shoulder level with an overhand grip (thumbs pointing inward):

- Inhale and extend the arms vertically.
- Exhale at the end of the movement.

This exercise contracts the deltoid, mainly the middle deltoid, as well as the trapezius, serratus anterior, and triceps brachii.

This movement may also be performed standing or alternating the arms. A backrest helps prevent an excessive arch in the back.

**VARIATION
PALMS FACING EACH OTHER**

FINAL POSITION

✚ SHOULDER INJURIES

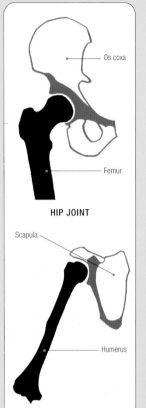

Os coxa

Femur

HIP JOINT

Scapula

Humerus

SHOULDER JOINT

Compared to the relatively
stable coxofemoral joint,
the shoulder joint is less
encased and is more mobile,
which makes it more
vulnerable to injury.

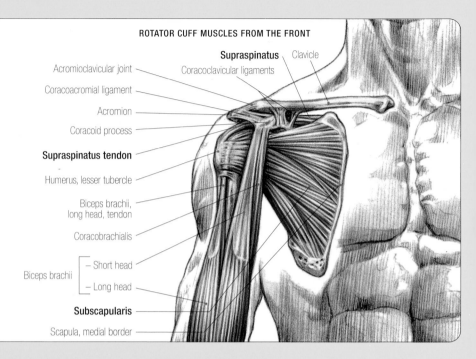

ROTATOR CUFF MUSCLES FROM THE FRONT

Supraspinatus
Clavicle
Acromioclavicular joint
Coracoclavicular ligaments
Coracoacromial ligament
Acromion
Coracoid process
Supraspinatus tendon
Humerus, lesser tubercle
Biceps brachii,
long head, tendon
Coracobrachialis
Biceps brachii — Short head
— Long head
Subscapularis
Scapula, medial border

Shoulder injuries occur frequently in weightlifting and especially in bodybuilding, where developing the entire deltoid group requires the athlete to perform a significant number of repetitions and variations in exercises, which multiplies the risk of injury.

Compared to the stability of the hip joint, where the head of the femur sits deep in the glenoid cavity of the pelvis, the shoulder joint, which is very mobile and allows the arm to move through a wide range of motion, is in fact much less contained and protected.

The shoulder is defined as a ball-and-socket joint because the head of the humerus is mainly held within the glenoid cavity of the scapula by a complex musculotendinous group.

Most weightlifting injuries occur when training the deltoids, and they rarely result in muscle pulls or tears. They are usually caused by poor technique or overuse of the tendons reinforcing the articular capsule.

In contrast to contact sports, such as football, where sudden arm movements can create serious injuries involving dislocation or even torn tendons, the most serious injury in weightlifting involves entrapment.

When some people perform exercises in which they raise the arms, such as extensions from the neck or lateral raises, the supraspinatus tendon is rubbed and compressed between the head of the humerus and the osteoligamentous ceiling created by the inferior surface of the acromion and the coracoacromial ligament.

Inflammation follows. This generally begins with the serous bursa, which normally protects the supraspinatus from excessive friction, and extends to the supraspinatus tendon itself, which, without treatment, ends up affecting the adjacent infraspinatus tendon posteriorly and the long head of the biceps brachii anteriorly. Raising the arm becomes extremely painful and

eventually can cause irreversible deterioration of the supraspinatus tendon through calcification and even tearing; however, this usually happens to people 40 years of age or older.

The space between the humerus and the osteoligamentous acromiocoracoid ceiling varies from person to person. Some athletes cannot raise their arms laterally without excessive friction. These people should avoid all extensions from the neck, lateral raises that go too high, and back presses.

All barbell extensions for the shoulders must be performed to the front with the elbows slightly forward. When doing lateral dumbbell raises, you'll need to determine the proper height to raise the arms to. The correct movement is the one you can perform without causing pain.

Not everyone responds the same way to the same shoulder injury. Some people may perform all sorts of arm raises that compress the tendon, sometimes even causing tendon degeneration, without initiating a painful inflammatory process. This is how a torn supraspinatus tendon can be discovered during assessment without that person ever having complained of pain.

Another cause of shoulder pain may be an imbalance in muscle tension around the articular capsule. Remember that the head of the humerus is solidly fixed against the glenoid fossa of the scapula by a group of muscle tendons adhering to or crossing over the articular capsule: In front, this is the subscapularis; a little more anterior is the long head of the biceps; superiorly, is the supraspinatus; and finally posteriorly, the infraspinatus and teres minor. Spasm, hypertonicity, or hypotonicity in one or more of these muscles can pull the shoulder joint into an incorrect position. This position can cause friction during arm movements, resulting in inflammation.

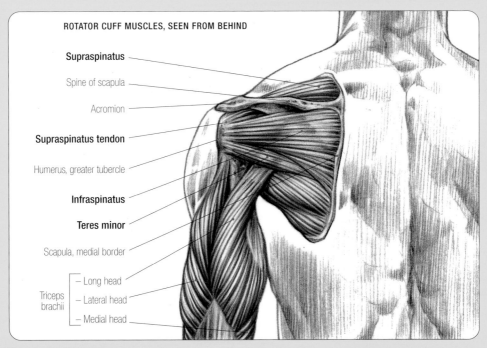

ROTATOR CUFF MUSCLES, SEEN FROM BEHIND

Supraspinatus

Spine of scapula

Acromion

Supraspinatus tendon

Humerus, greater tubercle

Infraspinatus

Teres minor

Scapula, medial border

Triceps brachii
- Long head
- Lateral head
- Medial head

Example: Shortening or spasm of the teres minor and the infraspinatus will pull the head of the humerus in external rotation, which will cause rubbing at the anterior shoulder joint during arm movement. Over time, this will injure the long head of the biceps brachii.

Balance the training of the shoulder muscles and avoid exercises that feel awkward or painful.

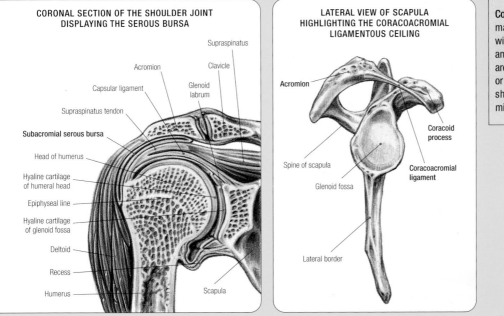

CORONAL SECTION OF THE SHOULDER JOINT
DISPLAYING THE SEROUS BURSA

Supraspinatus

Acromion

Clavicle

Capsular ligament

Glenoid labrum

Supraspinatus tendon

Subacromial serous bursa

Head of humerus

Hyaline cartilage of humeral head

Epiphyseal line

Hyaline cartilage of glenoid fossa

Deltoid

Recess

Humerus

Scapula

LATERAL VIEW OF SCAPULA
HIGHLIGHTING THE CORACOACROMIAL
LIGAMENTOUS CEILING

Acromion

Spine of scapula

Glenoid fossa

Coracoid process

Coracoacromial ligament

Lateral border

Comment: Massage, either manually or even better with an electric massager, and electrical stimulation are effective for decreasing or eliminating spasms and shortening of the teres minor and infraspinatus.

37

LYING DUMBBELL PRESSES

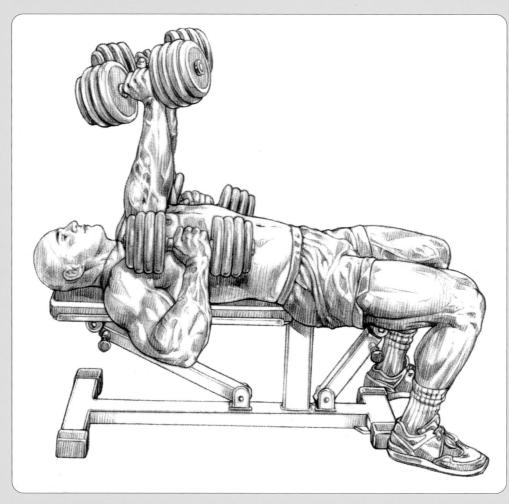

This is one of the rare exercises that may be performed by people suffering from the all-too-common entrapment syndrome.

Performing arm extensions with dumbbells while lying on a bench and keeping the elbows next to the body works the anterior deltoid and, to a lesser degree, the middle deltoid intensely while preventing excessive rubbing at the anterior shoulder.

When performed regularly, this maintains the size and tone of the deltoids despite the existence of injury. You can also use this exercise to reeducate the pectoralis major following tearing. Extending while keeping the elbows against the body reduces its stretch, thus reducing the risk of tearing the scarred area.

Performing the Exercise

Lie on a bench with the chest expanded, back slightly arched, feet flat on the ground, and the elbows bent next to the body, holding a dumbbell in each hand.

- Inhale and extend the arms vertically.
- Exhale at the end of the movement.
- Return to the initial position with a controlled movement.

HOW THE OSSEOUS MORPHOLOGY AFFECTS THE BACK PRESS

INFLUENCE OF THE LENGTH OF THE ARM ON LOWERING THE ELBOWS DURING THE BACK PRESS

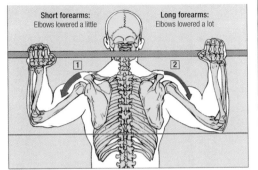

Short forearms: Elbows lowered a little

Long forearms: Elbows lowered a lot

1 Deltoid is stretched optimally, allowing for recruitment of the maximum number of muscle fibers during the initiation of the movement.
2 Deltoid is overstretched, which does not allow enough muscle fibers to be recruited for a powerful initiation of the movement.

INFLUENCE OF THE LENGTH OF THE CLAVICLES ON LOWERING THE BAR FROM THE BACK PRESS

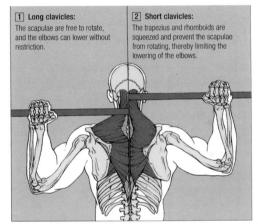

1 **Long clavicles:**
The scapulae are free to rotate, and the elbows can lower without restriction.

2 **Short clavicles:**
The trapezius and rhomboids are squeezed and prevent the scapulae from rotating, thereby limiting the lowering of the elbows.

It is important to take into account individual morphological differences when training the shoulders with the back press.

The length of the arms: The length of the arms, especially the forearms, plays a fundamental role in the execution of this exercise.

When lowering the bar below the ears, people with proportionately longer forearms bring their elbows down a lot lower than people with proportionately shorter forearms. This lower placement of the elbows strongly stretches the deltoid, putting it in an unfavorable position by not allowing the muscle to recruit the maximum number of fibers to initiate a powerful push.

To optimize training, people with proportionately longer arms should add heavier weights and not lower the bar too much below the ears. The most important issue is the intensity of feeling on the deltoids.

The length of the clavicles: The length of the clavicles has a considerable influence on the ability to lower the bar correctly behind the neck.

Short clavicles inevitably bring the shoulder blades toward the vertebral axis. During the extension from the neck, as both shoulder blades tilt to the center of the back (in adduction or external pendulum), the range of the shoulder blades is significantly reduced by the compression of the trapezius and rhomboid muscles in the middle of the back. This shortened range of the shoulder blades limits the ability to correctly lower the elbows in order to feel the deltoids working.

Furthermore, the greater the development of the muscles at the center of the back, the less the shoulder blades will be able to approach each other, which will further limit the lowering of the bar to the neck.

Comment: People with long forearms and short clavicles should avoid the back press in favor of better working the deltoids.

! Attention

1 When the humerus rotates externally with elevation of the arm, reduced space between the glenohumeral joint and the osteoligamentous coracoacromial ceiling may lead to excessive friction that, over time, can damage or even tear the supraspinatus tendon. Therefore, at the slightest sensation of unease accompanied by pain during the back press, change the movement in order to avoid developing degenerative tendinitis of the rotator cuff.

2 Raising the arm (as in lateral raises with dumbbells) causes the humerus to internally rotate. Too narrow a space between the glenohumeral joint and the osteoligamentous coracoacromial ceiling may lead to excessive friction that risks damaging the infraspinatus tendon.

ROTATOR CUFF INJURIES WITH RAISING OF THE ARM

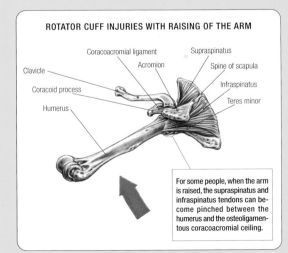

Coracoacromial ligament
Acromion
Clavicle
Coracoid process
Humerus
Supraspinatus
Spine of scapula
Infraspinatus
Teres minor

For some people, when the arm is raised, the supraspinatus and infraspinatus tendons can become pinched between the humerus and the osteoligamentous coracoacromial ceiling.

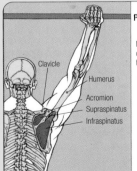

Clavicle
Humerus
Acromion
Supraspinatus
Infraspinatus

PINCHING OF THE SUPRASPINATUS WITH BACK PRESSES

During the back press, the supraspinatus tendon can get pinched between the acromion and the humerus.

4 ARNOLD PRESSES

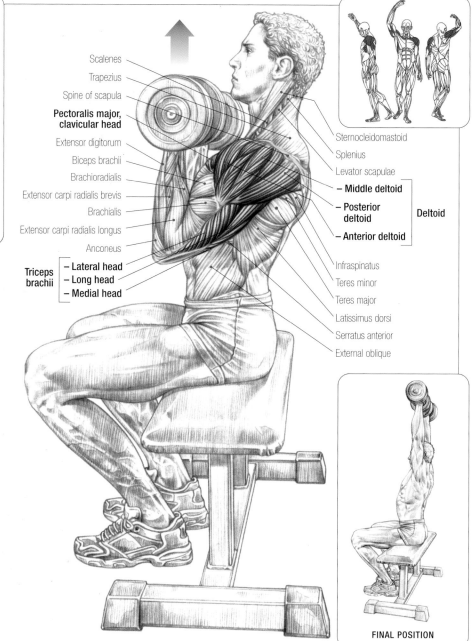

Pectoralis major, clavicular head

Anterior deltoid

Middle deltoid

Posterior deltoid

**VARIATION
WITH ALTERNATING EXTENSIONS**

Scalenes
Trapezius
Spine of scapula
**Pectoralis major,
clavicular head**
Extensor digitorum
Biceps brachii
Brachioradialis
Extensor carpi radialis brevis
Brachialis
Extensor carpi radialis longus
Anconeus

Triceps brachii
– Lateral head
– Long head
– Medial head

Sternocleidomastoid
Splenius
Levator scapulae
– **Middle deltoid**
– **Posterior deltoid**
– **Anterior deltoid**
Deltoid
Infraspinatus
Teres minor
Teres major
Latissimus dorsi
Serratus anterior
External oblique

FINAL POSITION

Sit on a bench, keeping the back straight. With elbows bent and pointing forward, hold the dumbbells at shoulder level with an underhand grip (thumbs pointing away from each other):

- Inhale and extend the arms vertically while rotating 180 degrees at the wrists, bringing them into an overhand grip (thumbs pointing toward each other).
- Exhale at the end of the movement.

This exercise solicits the deltoid, mainly the anterior deltoid, as well as the clavicular head of the pectoralis major, triceps brachii, trapezius, and serratus anterior.

Variations: This exercise may be performed seated against a backrest to help prevent an excessive arch in the back, standing, and alternating arms.

Comment: Working with the elbows pointing forward prevents excessive friction, which triggers inflammation in the shoulder that can eventually develop into a more serious injury.
This movement is recommended for people with weak shoulders and is meant to replace more intense exercises, such as classic dumbbell extensions with the elbows pointing to the sides or extensions from behind the neck.

BENT-OVER LATERAL RAISES 5

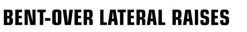

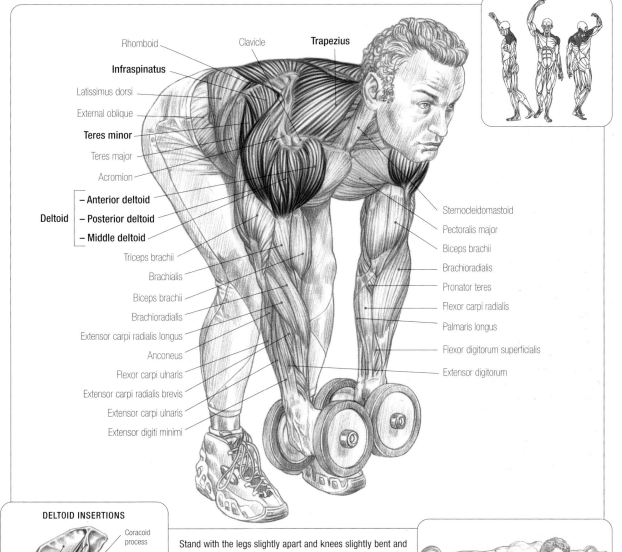

Rhomboid

Clavicle

Trapezius

Infraspinatus

Latissimus dorsi

External oblique

Teres minor

Teres major

Acromion

Deltoid

– **Anterior deltoid**

– **Posterior deltoid**

– **Middle deltoid**

Triceps brachii

Brachialis

Biceps brachii

Brachioradialis

Extensor carpi radialis longus

Anconeus

Flexor carpi ulnaris

Extensor carpi radialis brevis

Extensor carpi ulnaris

Extensor digiti minimi

Sternocleidomastoid

Pectoralis major

Biceps brachii

Brachioradialis

Pronator teres

Flexor carpi radialis

Palmaris longus

Flexor digitorum superficialis

Extensor digitorum

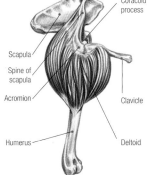

DELTOID INSERTIONS

Coracoid process

Scapula

Spine of scapula

Acromion

Clavicle

Humerus

Deltoid

Stand with the legs slightly apart and knees slightly bent and lean forward at the waist while keeping the back straight. With arms hanging down, grasp the dumbbells with the elbows slightly bent:

- Inhale and raise the arms to horizontal.
- Exhale at the end of the effort.

This exercise works the shoulder group, accenting the work of the posterior deltoid. Squeeze the shoulder blades together at the end of the movement to contract the middle and lower portions of the trapezius, rhomboids, teres minor, and infraspinatus.

Variation: The exercise may be performed facedown on an incline bench.

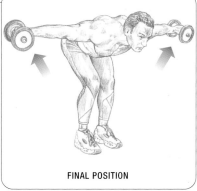

FINAL POSITION

6 LATERAL DUMBBELL RAISES

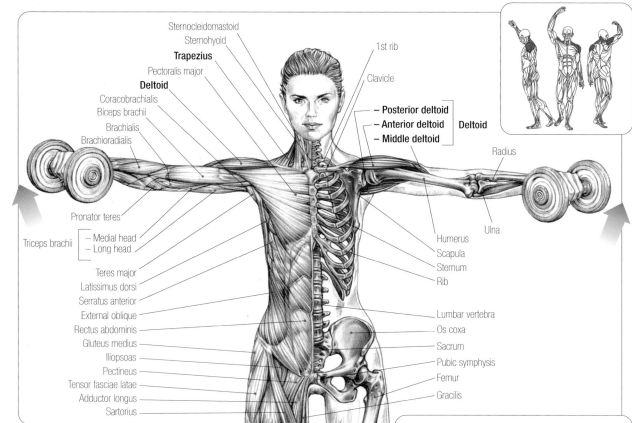

Sternocleidomastoid
Sternohyoid
Trapezius
Pectoralis major
Deltoid
Coracobrachialis
Biceps brachii
Brachialis
Brachioradialis
Pronator teres
Triceps brachii — Medial head
— Long head
Teres major
Latissimus dorsi
Serratus anterior
External oblique
Rectus abdominis
Gluteus medius
Iliopsoas
Pectineus
Tensor fasciae latae
Adductor longus
Sartorius

1st rib
Clavicle
— **Posterior deltoid**
— **Anterior deltoid**   Deltoid
— **Middle deltoid**
Radius
Humerus
Scapula
Sternum
Rib
Ulna
Lumbar vertebra
Os coxa
Sacrum
Pubic symphysis
Femur
Gracilis

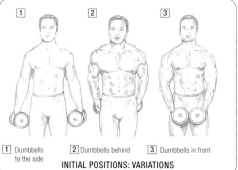

SUPRASPINATUS MUSCLE ACTION

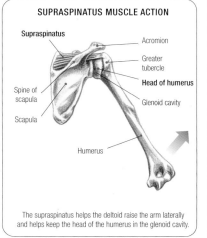

Supraspinatus
Acromion
Greater tubercle
Head of humerus
Spine of scapula
Glenoid cavity
Scapula
Humerus

The supraspinatus helps the deltoid raise the arm laterally and helps keep the head of the humerus in the glenoid cavity.

Stand with a straight back, with legs slightly apart, arms hanging next to the body, holding a barbell in each hand:

- Raise the arms to horizontal with the elbows slightly bent.
- Return to the initial position.

This exercise mainly uses the middle deltoid.

The three divisions of the deltoids create a multipennate muscle whose different fiber directions converge on the humerus. Their function is to support relatively heavy weight and to move the arm through its full range of motion with precision. Therefore, it is important to adapt training to the specifics of this muscle by varying the initial position of the movement (hands behind, to the side, or in front). This thoroughly works all the fibers of the middle deltoid. Because everyone's physical structure is different (length of the clavicle, shape of the acromion, and height of the insertion at the humerus), you must find the angle of the initial position that is best for you. Lateral raises contract the supraspinatus, although you can't see this because it is located deep in the supraspinatus fossa of the scapula (shoulder blade), where it attaches to the lesser tubercle of the humerus.

Raising the arm above horizontal contracts the upper part of the trapezius; however, many bodybuilders don't work above horizontal so that they isolate the lateral deltoid. This exercise should not be performed with heavy weights, but instead in sets of 10 to 25 reps, while varying the working angle without much recuperation time until you feel a burn. To increase the intensity, maintain an isometric contraction for a few seconds with the arm at horizontal between each repetition.

1 Dumbbells to the side   2 Dumbbells behind   3 Dumbbells in front

INITIAL POSITIONS: VARIATIONS

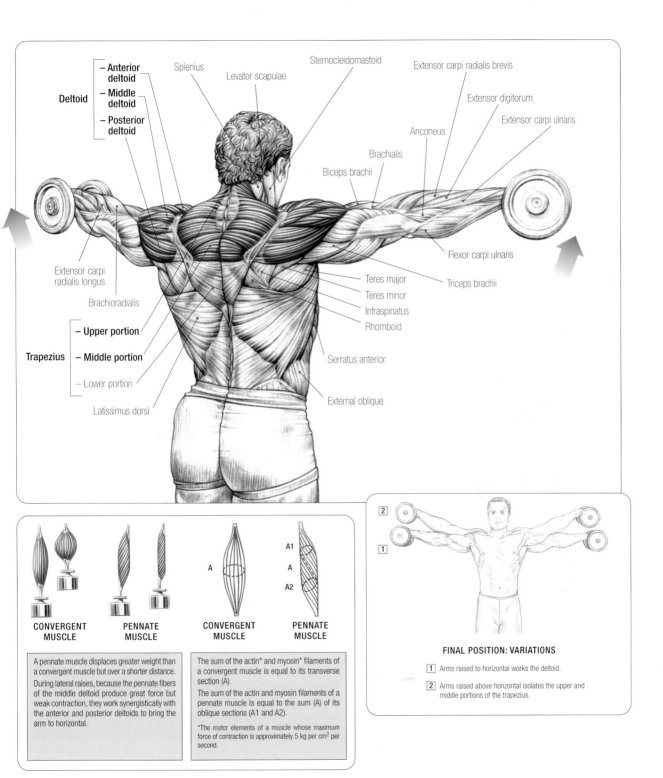

Deltoid
- Anterior deltoid
- Middle deltoid
- Posterior deltoid

Splenius

Levator scapulae

Sternocleidomastoid

Extensor carpi radialis brevis

Extensor digitorum

Extensor carpi ulnaris

Anconeus

Brachialis

Biceps brachii

Flexor carpi ulnaris

Triceps brachii

Extensor carpi radialis longus

Brachioradialis

Teres major

Teres minor

Infraspinatus

Rhomboid

Trapezius
- Upper portion
- Middle portion
- Lower portion

Serratus anterior

Latissimus dorsi

External oblique

CONVERGENT MUSCLE

PENNATE MUSCLE

CONVERGENT MUSCLE

A1
A
A2

A

PENNATE MUSCLE

A pennate muscle displaces greater weight than a convergent muscle but over a shorter distance.

During lateral raises, because the pennate fibers of the middle deltoid produce great force but weak contraction, they work synergistically with the anterior and posterior deltoids to bring the arm to horizontal.

The sum of the actin* and myosin* filaments of a convergent muscle is equal to its transverse section (A).

The sum of the actin and myosin filaments of a pennate muscle is equal to the sum (A) of its oblique sections (A1 and A2).

*The motor elements of a muscle whose maximum force of contraction is approximately 5 kg per cm^2 per second.

FINAL POSITION: VARIATIONS

1 Arms raised to horizontal works the deltoid.

2 Arms raised above horizontal isolates the upper and middle portions of the trapezius.

7 ALTERNATE FRONT ARM RAISES

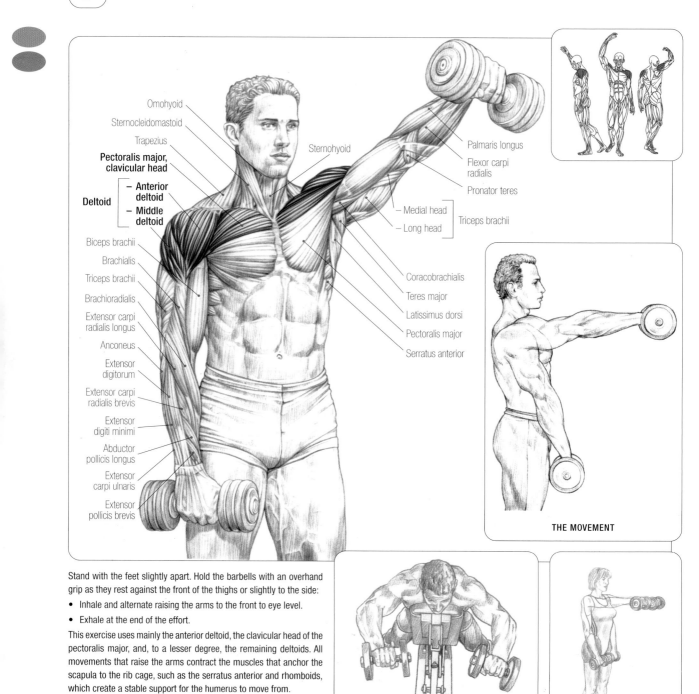

Omohyoid
Sternocleidomastoid
Trapezius
Pectoralis major, clavicular head
Sternohyoid
Deltoid
— **Anterior deltoid**
— **Middle deltoid**
Biceps brachii
Brachialis
Triceps brachii
Brachioradialis
Extensor carpi radialis longus
Anconeus
Extensor digitorum
Extensor carpi radialis brevis
Extensor digiti minimi
Abductor pollicis longus
Extensor carpi ulnaris
Extensor pollicis brevis

Palmaris longus
Flexor carpi radialis
Pronator teres
— Medial head
— Long head
Triceps brachii
Coracobrachialis
Teres major
Latissimus dorsi
Pectoralis major
Serratus anterior

THE MOVEMENT

Stand with the feet slightly apart. Hold the barbells with an overhand grip as they rest against the front of the thighs or slightly to the side:

- Inhale and alternate raising the arms to the front to eye level.
- Exhale at the end of the effort.

This exercise uses mainly the anterior deltoid, the clavicular head of the pectoralis major, and, to a lesser degree, the remaining deltoids. All movements that raise the arms contract the muscles that anchor the scapula to the rib cage, such as the serratus anterior and rhomboids, which create a stable support for the humerus to move from.

**VARIATION
LYING FACEDOWN ON AN INCLINE BENCH**

**VARIATION
RAISING TO THE FRONT
USING BOTH HANDS**

SIDE-LYING LATERAL RAISES 8

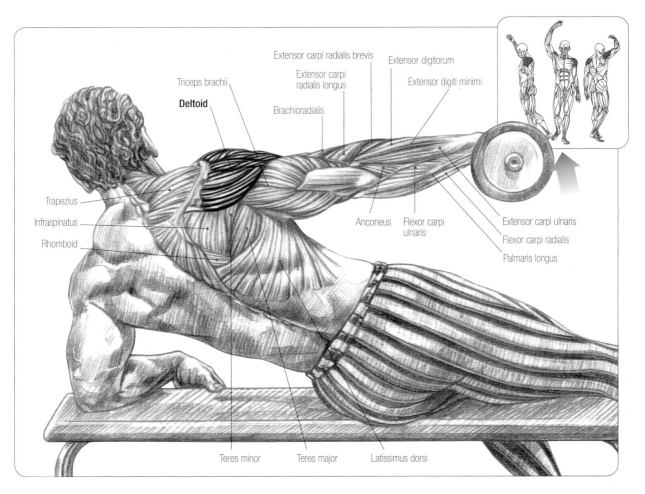

Extensor carpi radialis brevis
Extensor digitorum
Extensor carpi radialis longus
Extensor digiti minimi
Triceps brachii
Deltoid
Brachioradialis
Trapezius
Infraspinatus
Rhomboid
Anconeus
Flexor carpi ulnaris
Extensor carpi ulnaris
Flexor carpi radialis
Palmaris longus
Teres minor
Teres major
Latissimus dorsi

Lie on one side on the floor or on a bench holding a dumbbell with an overhand grip:

- Inhale and raise the arm to vertical.
- Exhale at the end of the movement.

Unlike standing raises, which progressively work the muscle to maximum intensity at the end of the movement (when the arm reaches horizontal), this exercise works the deltoid differently by focusing the effort at the beginning of the raise. Sets of 10 to 12 repetitions work best.

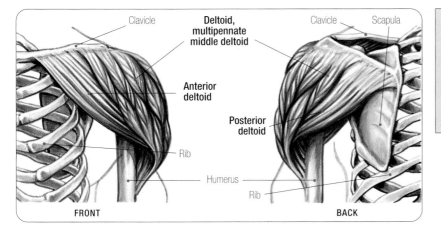

Clavicle
Deltoid, multipennate middle deltoid
Clavicle
Scapula
Anterior deltoid
Posterior deltoid
Rib
Humerus
Rib

FRONT

BACK

Comment: This movement contracts the supraspinatus, the muscle mainly responsible for initiating abduction. Varying the initial position (dumbbell in front of or behind the thigh) allows you to work all the deltoid fibers. To increase the intensity of the movement, perform this exercise with continuous tension without resting the dumbbell on the thigh.

9 LOW-PULLEY FRONT RAISES, OVERHAND GRIP

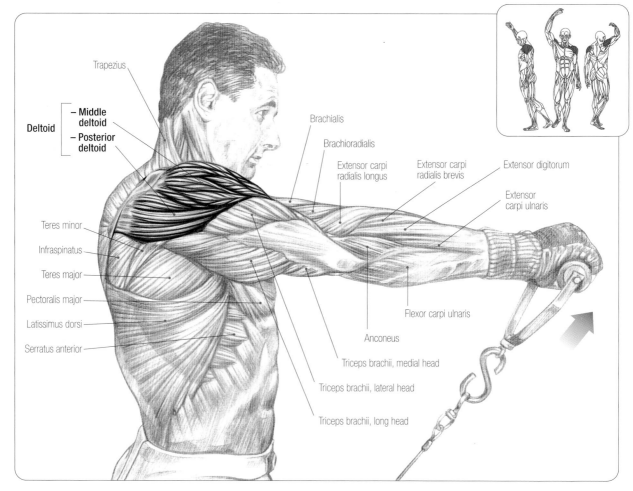

Trapezius

Deltoid
 – Middle deltoid
 – Posterior deltoid

Brachialis

Brachioradialis

Extensor carpi radialis longus

Extensor carpi radialis brevis

Extensor digitorum

Extensor carpi ulnaris

Teres minor

Infraspinatus

Teres major

Pectoralis major

Latissimus dorsi

Serratus anterior

Flexor carpi ulnaris

Anconeus

Triceps brachii, medial head

Triceps brachii, lateral head

Triceps brachii, long head

Stand with the feet slightly apart, arms next to the body. Grasp the handle with an overhand grip with one hand:

- Inhale and raise the arm up to eye level.
- Exhale at the end of the movement.

This exercise contracts the deltoid (mainly the anterior deltoid) as well as the clavicular head of the pectoralis major and, to a lesser degree, the short head of the biceps brachii.

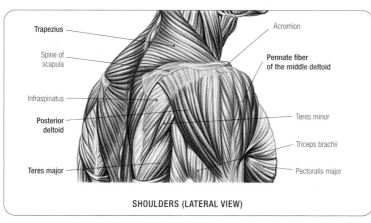

Trapezius

Spine of scapula

Infraspinatus

Posterior deltoid

Teres major

Acromion

Pennate fiber of the middle deltoid

Teres minor

Triceps brachii

Pectoralis major

SHOULDERS (LATERAL VIEW)

LOW-PULLEY FRONT RAISES, NEUTRAL GRIP 10

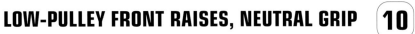

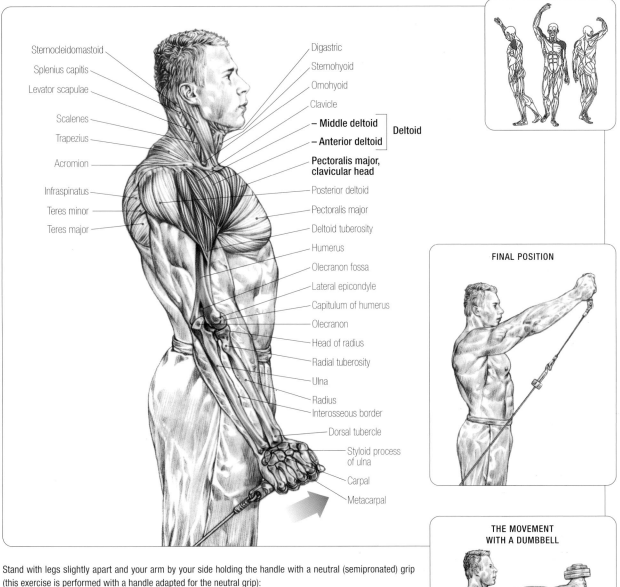

Sternocleidomastoid
Splenius capitis
Levator scapulae
Scalenes
Trapezius
Acromion
Infraspinatus
Teres minor
Teres major

Digastric
Sternohyoid
Omohyoid
Clavicle
– **Middle deltoid**   } Deltoid
– **Anterior deltoid**
Pectoralis major, clavicular head
Posterior deltoid
Pectoralis major
Deltoid tuberosity
Humerus
Olecranon fossa
Lateral epicondyle
Capitulum of humerus
Olecranon
Head of radius
Radial tuberosity
Ulna
Radius
Interosseous border
Dorsal tubercle
Styloid process of ulna
Carpal
Metacarpal

FINAL POSITION

THE MOVEMENT WITH A DUMBBELL

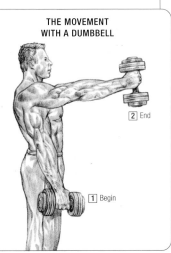

2 End

1 Begin

Stand with legs slightly apart and your arm by your side holding the handle with a neutral (semipronated) grip (this exercise is performed with a handle adapted for the neutral grip):

- Inhale and raise your arm forward up to eye level; exhale at the end of the raise.
- Slowly return to the initial position and repeat.

This exercise mainly works the anterior deltoid as well as the clavicular part of the pectoralis major and, to a lesser degree, the middle deltoid and the short head of the biceps.

It is preferable to work this movement in a long series.

Variation: Perform the exercise with a harness.

Comment: This exercise is excellent for people who have difficulty developing the anterior deltoid. The semipronated grip engages the humerus in external rotation, which at the beginning of the movement stretches the anterior fibers of the deltoid, allowing you to feel them working.

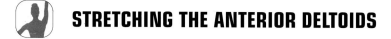

STRETCHING THE ANTERIOR DELTOIDS

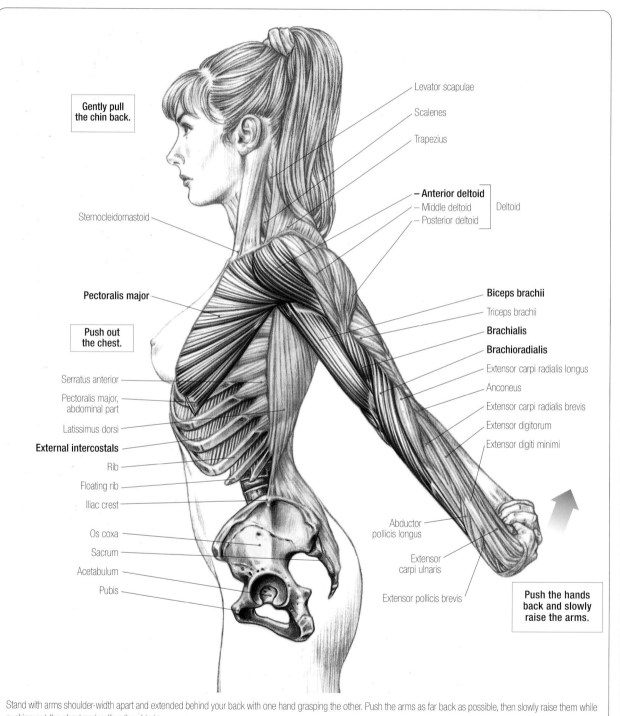

Gently pull
the chin back.

Sternocleidomastoid

Pectoralis major

Push out
the chest.

Serratus anterior

Pectoralis major,
abdominal part

Latissimus dorsi

External intercostals

Rib

Floating rib

Iliac crest

Os coxa

Sacrum

Acetabulum

Pubis

Levator scapulae

Scalenes

Trapezius

– **Anterior deltoid**   ⎤
– Middle deltoid   ⎬ Deltoid
– Posterior deltoid   ⎦

Biceps brachii

Triceps brachii

Brachialis

Brachioradialis

Extensor carpi radialis longus

Anconeus

Extensor carpi radialis brevis

Extensor digitorum

Extensor digiti minimi

Abductor
pollicis longus

Extensor
carpi ulnaris

Extensor pollicis brevis

Push the hands
back and slowly
raise the arms.

Stand with arms shoulder-width apart and extended behind your back with one hand grasping the other. Push the arms as far back as possible, then slowly raise them while pushing out the chest and pulling the chin in.

Hold this position for 10 seconds.

This exercise mainly stretches the anterior deltoid as well as the pectoralis major and biceps brachii.

The brachialis, brachioradialis, and extensor muscle group at the wrist are also recruited.

HIGH-PULLEY LATERAL EXTENSIONS 11

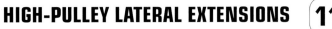

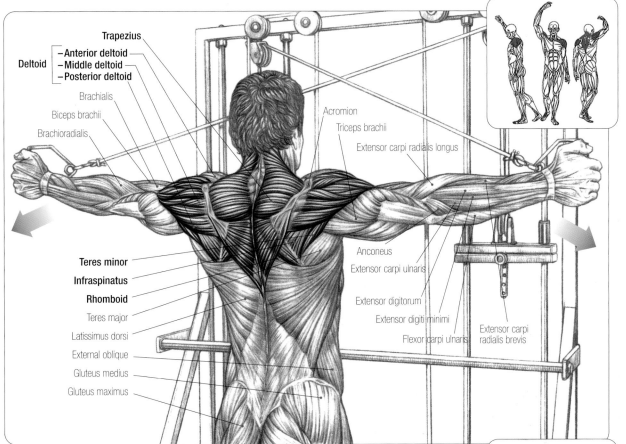

Trapezius

Deltoid
— Anterior deltoid
— Middle deltoid
— Posterior deltoid

Brachialis

Biceps brachii

Brachioradialis

Teres minor

Infraspinatus

Rhomboid

Teres major

Latissimus dorsi

External oblique

Gluteus medius

Gluteus maximus

Acromion

Triceps brachii

Extensor carpi radialis longus

Anconeus

Extensor carpi ulnaris

Extensor digitorum

Extensor digiti minimi

Flexor carpi ulnaris

Extensor carpi radialis brevis

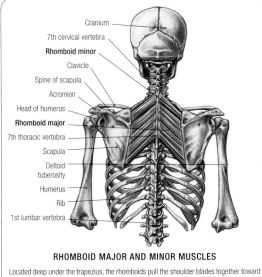

Cranium

7th cervical vertebra

Rhomboid minor

Clavicle

Spine of scapula

Acromion

Head of humerus

Rhomboid major

7th thoracic vertebra

Scapula

Deltoid tuberosity

Humerus

Rib

1st lumbar vertebra

RHOMBOID MAJOR AND MINOR MUSCLES

Located deep under the trapezius, the rhomboids pull the shoulder blades together toward the spine and press them against the rib cage.

In some people, the major and minor rhomboids are fused, creating one muscle.

Stand facing the pulleys with the arms extended to the front. Grip the right handle with the left hand and the left handle with the right hand:

• Inhale and extend the arms to the side and back.

• Exhale at the end of the movement.

• Return to the initial position with a controlled movement and begin again.

This exercise mainly contracts the posterior deltoid, infraspinatus, teres minor, and, at the end of the movement as the shoulder blades come together, the trapezius and, deeper in, the rhomboids.

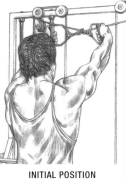

INITIAL POSITION

Comment: People who carry their shoulders forward because of chest muscle development can perform this exercise in addition to posterior shoulder work at a machine to help rebalance their posture.

To realign the shoulders where they belong, work with moderate weights and squeeze the shoulders back at the end of the movement.

12 EXTERNAL ARM ROTATIONS AT A PULLEY

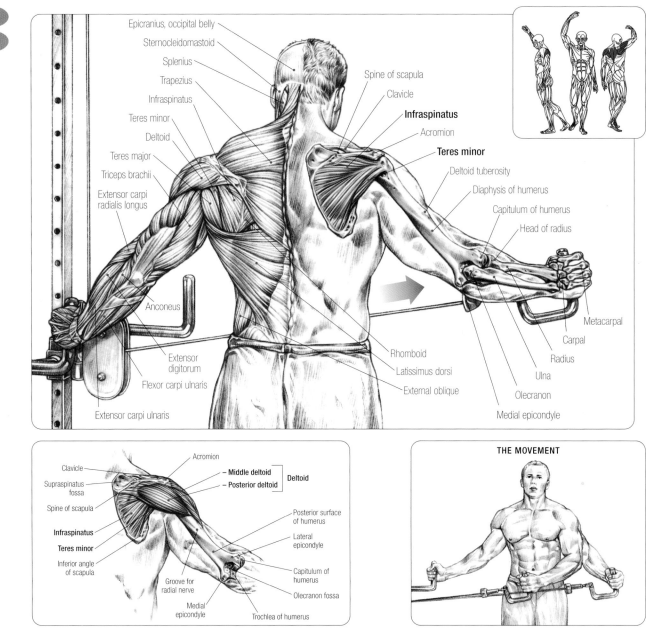

Epicranius, occipital belly
Sternocleidomastoid
Splenius
Trapezius
Infraspinatus
Teres minor
Deltoid
Teres major
Triceps brachii
Extensor carpi radialis longus
Anconeus
Extensor digitorum
Flexor carpi ulnaris
Extensor carpi ulnaris

Spine of scapula
Clavicle
Infraspinatus
Acromion
Teres minor
Deltoid tuberosity
Diaphysis of humerus
Capitulum of humerus
Head of radius
Metacarpal
Carpal
Radius
Ulna
Olecranon
Medial epicondyle

Rhomboid
Latissimus dorsi
External oblique

Clavicle
Supraspinatus fossa
Spine of scapula
Infraspinatus
Teres minor
Inferior angle of scapula
Groove for radial nerve
Medial epicondyle
Trochlea of humerus

Acromion
– Middle deltoid
– Posterior deltoid
Deltoid
Posterior surface of humerus
Lateral epicondyle
Capitulum of humerus
Olecranon fossa

THE MOVEMENT

Position the pulley at waist level and position your body in line with the apparatus. Grip the handle with your forearm in front of your body, your elbow bent, and your upper arm against your body:

• Externally rotate your arm, trying to keep the upper arm against your body with the elbow bent.

This exercise mainly works the infraspinatus and teres minor as well as the posterior deltoid. If at the end of the movement the scapula is brought to the center of the body, the rhomboids and the middle and inferior portions of the trapezius will be worked at the same time.

This movement is mainly used to strengthen the infraspinatus and prevent painful contractures and frequent injuries of this muscle.

External rotations of the arm at the pulley are often recommended during recovery from a tear or partial tear of the infraspinatus. Use very light weights initially.

Comment: Perform this exercise with the objective of working the posterior deltoid, which is often difficult to recruit. In this case, move your arm slightly away from the body and extend the elbow at the end of the movement.

LOW-PULLEY BENT-OVER LATERAL RAISES 13

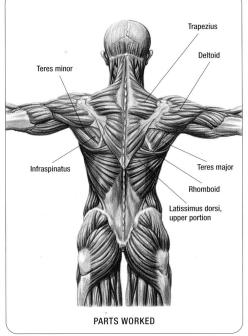

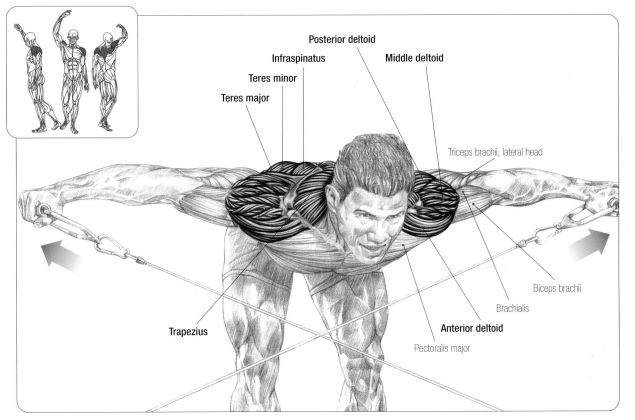

Posterior deltoid

Infraspinatus

Middle deltoid

Teres minor

Teres major

Triceps brachii, lateral head

Biceps brachii

Brachialis

Anterior deltoid

Pectoralis major

Trapezius

Stand with the feet apart and legs slightly bent. Lean forward from the waist, keeping a flat back. Grip a handle in each hand with the cables crossed:

- Inhale and raise the arms to the sides to horizontal.
- Exhale at the end of the effort.

This exercise mainly works the posterior deltoid. At the end of the movement, as the shoulder blades squeeze together, the trapezius (middle and lower portions) and the rhomboids contract.

Trapezius

Deltoid

Teres minor

Teres major

Infraspinatus

Rhomboid

Latissimus dorsi, upper portion

PARTS WORKED

14 LOW-PULLEY LATERAL RAISES

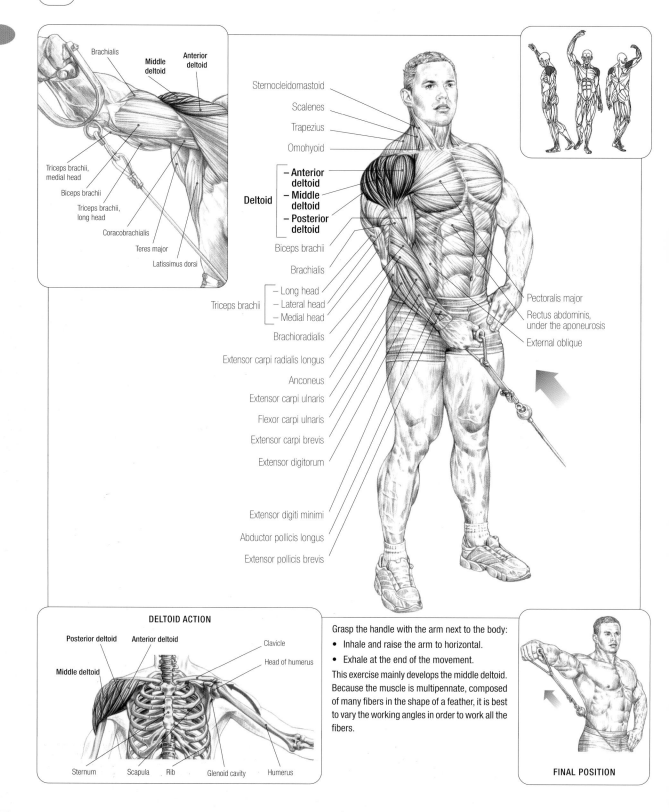

Brachialis

Middle deltoid

Anterior deltoid

Triceps brachii, medial head

Biceps brachii

Triceps brachii, long head

Coracobrachialis

Teres major

Latissimus dorsi

Sternocleidomastoid

Scalenes

Trapezius

Omohyoid

Deltoid
- Anterior deltoid
- Middle deltoid
- Posterior deltoid

Biceps brachii

Brachialis

Triceps brachii
- Long head
- Lateral head
- Medial head

Brachioradialis

Extensor carpi radialis longus

Anconeus

Extensor carpi ulnaris

Flexor carpi ulnaris

Extensor carpi brevis

Extensor digitorum

Extensor digiti minimi

Abductor pollicis longus

Extensor pollicis brevis

Pectoralis major

Rectus abdominis, under the aponeurosis

External oblique

DELTOID ACTION

Posterior deltoid

Anterior deltoid

Middle deltoid

Clavicle

Head of humerus

Sternum   Scapula   Rib   Glenoid cavity   Humerus

Grasp the handle with the arm next to the body:
- Inhale and raise the arm to horizontal.
- Exhale at the end of the movement.

This exercise mainly develops the middle deltoid. Because the muscle is multipennate, composed of many fibers in the shape of a feather, it is best to vary the working angles in order to work all the fibers.

FINAL POSITION

IMPORTANCE OF PULLING THE SHOULDERS BACK

MUSCLES ENGAGED WHILE PULLING THE SHOULDERS BACK

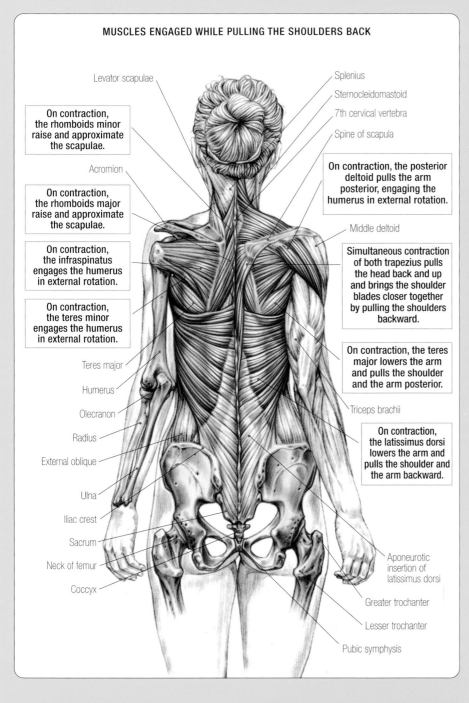

Levator scapulae

On contraction, the rhomboids minor raise and approximate the scapulae.

Acromion

On contraction, the rhomboids major raise and approximate the scapulae.

On contraction, the infraspinatus engages the humerus in external rotation.

On contraction, the teres minor engages the humerus in external rotation.

Teres major

Humerus

Olecranon

Radius

External oblique

Ulna

Iliac crest

Sacrum

Neck of femur

Coccyx

Splenius

Sternocleidomastoid

7th cervical vertebra

Spine of scapula

On contraction, the posterior deltoid pulls the arm posterior, engaging the humerus in external rotation.

Middle deltoid

Simultaneous contraction of both trapezius pulls the head back and up and brings the shoulder blades closer together by pulling the shoulders backward.

On contraction, the teres major lowers the arm and pulls the shoulder and the arm posterior.

Triceps brachii

On contraction, the latissimus dorsi lowers the arm and pulls the shoulder and the arm backward.

Aponeurotic insertion of latissimus dorsi

Greater trochanter

Lesser trochanter

Pubic symphysis

One of the major postural defects encountered most frequently in modern society, where we spend inordinate amounts of time in the sitting posture, is kyphosis (rounding of the upper thoracic spine).

This bad position of the upper body is most often due to the hypotonic state of the muscles approximating the shoulder blades and the external rotators of the arms, or, more frequently with men, the hypertonicity and predominance of the development of the chest muscles. In weight training, focusing extensively on the pectorals or overtraining in bench presses can also contribute to this postural defect.

It is important to perform postural rebalancing by practicing specific exercises to straighten the shoulders, such as the pec deck rear-delt laterals (page 58), external arm rotations at a pulley (page 50), or bent-over lateral raises (page 41).

Rounding the upper back during deadlifts limits the power of the lift. To avoid this rounding of the back, perform specific exercises to strengthen the muscles responsible for straightening the shoulders.

Comment: With powerlifting and heavy deadlifts, it is essential to avoid rounding of the shoulders to the front and excessive cantilevering, which can restrict the power of the lift. Always straighten the shoulders during the execution of the movement and use specific exercises to prepare for powerlifts and heavy deadlifts.

15 ONE-DUMBBELL FRONT RAISES

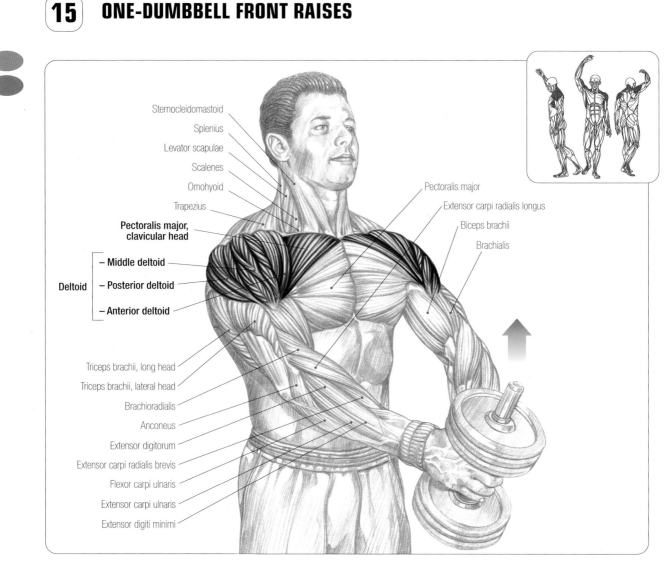

Sternocleidomastoid
Splenius
Levator scapulae
Scalenes
Omohyoid
Trapezius
Pectoralis major, clavicular head

Deltoid
– **Middle deltoid**
– **Posterior deltoid**
– **Anterior deltoid**

Triceps brachii, long head
Triceps brachii, lateral head
Brachioradialis
Anconeus
Extensor digitorum
Extensor carpi radialis brevis
Flexor carpi ulnaris
Extensor carpi ulnaris
Extensor digiti minimi

Pectoralis major
Extensor carpi radialis longus
Biceps brachii
Brachialis

Stand with the legs slightly apart, back straight, and the abdominal muscles contracted. With arms extended, grasp a dumbbell in both hands with fingers crossed over each other and rest it against the thighs:

- Inhale and raise the dumbbell to eye level.
- Lower gently, avoiding abrupt movements.
- Exhale at the end of the movement.

This exercise mainly contracts the anterior deltoid, the clavicular head of the pectoralis major, and the short head of the biceps.

Note that all the fixators of the scapula are used during the isometric contraction, which allows the humerus to move from a stable position.

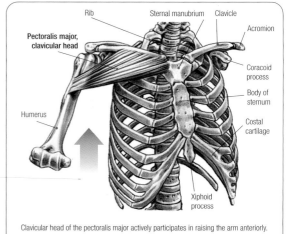

Rib
Sternal manubrium
Clavicle
Acromion
Pectoralis major, clavicular head
Coracoid process
Body of sternum
Costal cartilage
Humerus
Xiphoid process

Clavicular head of the pectoralis major actively participates in raising the arm anteriorly.

BARBELL FRONT RAISES 16

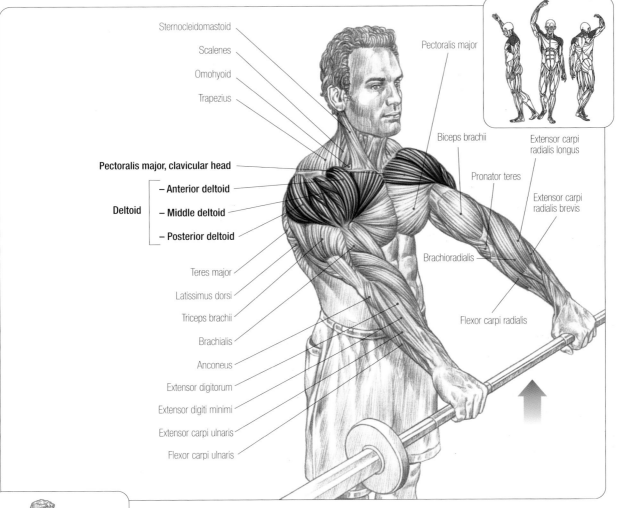

Sternocleidomastoid

Scalenes

Omohyoid

Trapezius

Pectoralis major, clavicular head

Deltoid
– Anterior deltoid
– Middle deltoid
– Posterior deltoid

Teres major

Latissimus dorsi

Triceps brachii

Brachialis

Anconeus

Extensor digitorum

Extensor digiti minimi

Extensor carpi ulnaris

Flexor carpi ulnaris

Pectoralis major

Biceps brachii

Pronator teres

Extensor carpi radialis longus

Extensor carpi radialis brevis

Brachioradialis

Flexor carpi radialis

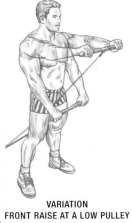

VARIATION
FRONT RAISE AT A LOW PULLEY

Stand with the legs slightly apart and the back straight, contracting the abdominal muscles. Hold the barbell with an overhand grip and rest it against the thighs:

- Inhale and raise the barbell with extended arms to eye level.
- Exhale at the end of the movement.

This exercise contracts the anterior deltoid, the clavicular head of the pectoralis major, the infraspinatus, and, to a lesser degree, the trapezius, serratus anterior, and short head of the biceps.

If you continue raising the arms, the posterior deltoid contracts, reinforcing the work of the other muscles and allowing you to raise the arms to vertical.

The exercise may also be performed with your back to a low pulley and the cable passing between the legs.

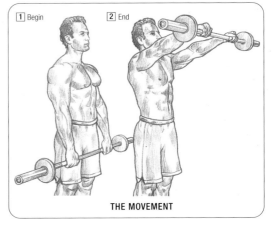

1 Begin   2 End

THE MOVEMENT

Comment: The biceps brachii participates to a lesser degree in all anterior arm raises.

17 UPRIGHT ROWS

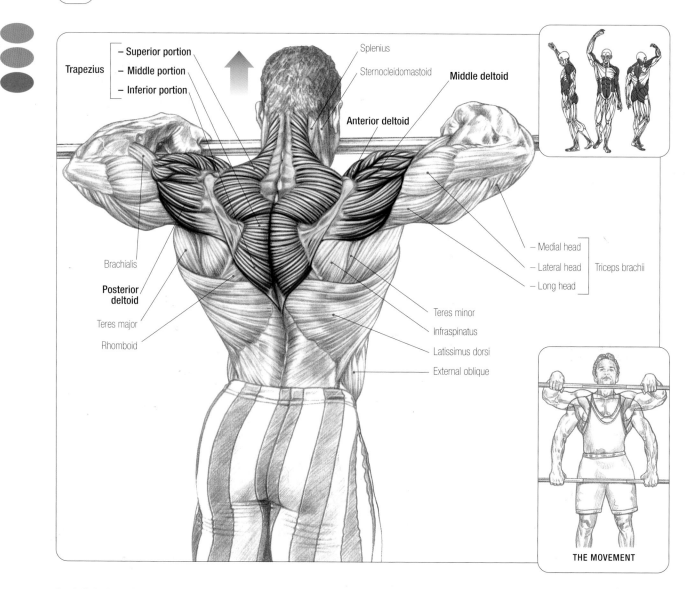

Trapezius
- Superior portion
- Middle portion
- Inferior portion

Splenius

Sternocleidomastoid

Middle deltoid

Anterior deltoid

Brachialis

Posterior deltoid

Teres major

Rhomboid

- Medial head
- Lateral head
- Long head

Triceps brachii

Teres minor

Infraspinatus

Latissimus dorsi

External oblique

THE MOVEMENT

Stand with the legs slightly apart and back straight. Grasp the barbell with an overhand grip slightly wider than shoulder width and rest it against the thighs:

- Inhale and pull the barbell up along the body to the chin, keeping the elbows as high as possible.
- Lower the bar in a controlled manner without abrupt movements.
- Exhale at the end of the effort.

This exercise mainly uses the deltoid, trapezius, and biceps, and, to a lesser degree, the muscles of the forearms, the gluteal muscles, the lumbosacralis group, and the abdominal muscles.

This is a fundamental exercise that is comprehensive and helps develop a "Hercules" physique.

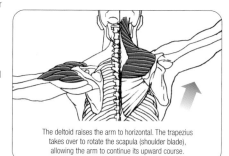

The deltoid raises the arm to horizontal. The trapezius takes over to rotate the scapula (shoulder blade), allowing the arm to continue its upward course.

MACHINE LATERAL RAISES 18

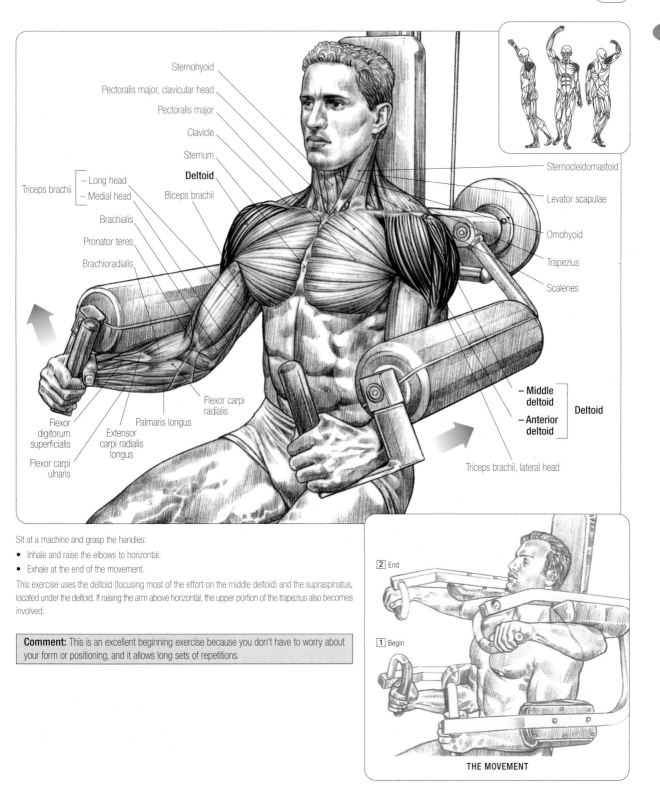

Sternohyoid

Pectoralis major, clavicular head

Pectoralis major

Clavicle

Sternum

Deltoid

Biceps brachii

Triceps brachii
— Long head
— Medial head

Brachialis

Pronator teres

Brachioradialis

Flexor carpi radialis

Flexor digitorum superficialis

Palmaris longus

Extensor carpi radialis longus

Flexor carpi ulnaris

Sternocleidomastoid

Levator scapulae

Omohyoid

Trapezius

Scalenes

— Middle deltoid
— Anterior deltoid
Deltoid

Triceps brachii, lateral head

Sit at a machine and grasp the handles:

- Inhale and raise the elbows to horizontal.
- Exhale at the end of the movement.

This exercise uses the deltoid (focusing most of the effort on the middle deltoid) and the supraspinatus, located under the deltoid. If raising the arm above horizontal, the upper portion of the trapezius also becomes involved.

Comment: This is an excellent beginning exercise because you don't have to worry about your form or positioning, and it allows long sets of repetitions.

2 End

1 Begin

THE MOVEMENT

19 PEC DECK REAR-DELT LATERALS

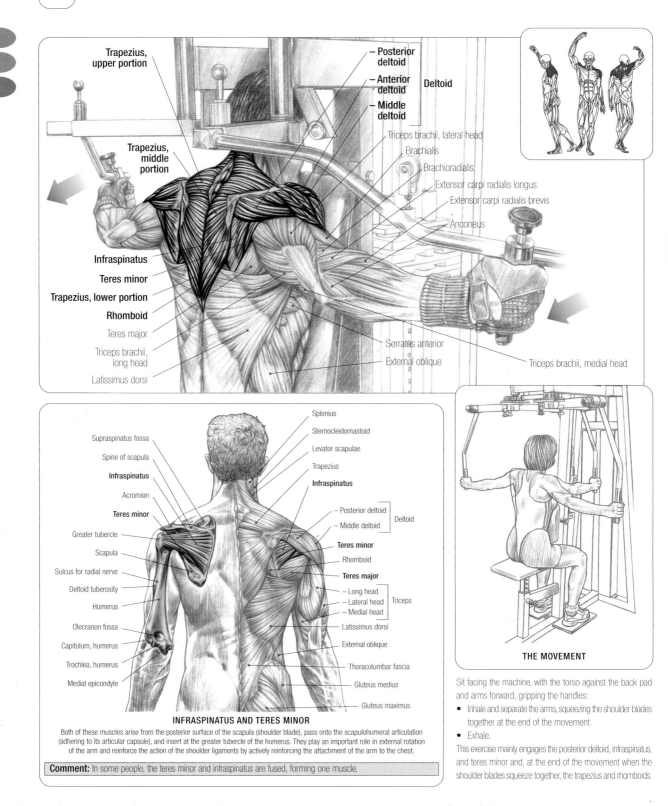

Trapezius, upper portion

Trapezius, middle portion

Infraspinatus

Teres minor

Trapezius, lower portion

Rhomboid

Teres major

Triceps brachii, long head

Latissimus dorsi

Posterior deltoid

Anterior deltoid

Middle deltoid

Deltoid

Triceps brachii, lateral head

Brachialis

Brachioradialis

Extensor carpi radialis longus

Extensor carpi radialis brevis

Anconeus

Serratus anterior

External oblique

Triceps brachii, medial head

Supraspinatus fossa

Spine of scapula

Infraspinatus

Acromion

Teres minor

Greater tubercle

Scapula

Sulcus for radial nerve

Deltoid tuberosity

Humerus

Olecranon fossa

Capitulum, humerus

Trochlea, humerus

Medial epicondyle

Splenius

Sternocleidomastoid

Levator scapulae

Trapezius

Infraspinatus

Posterior deltoid

Middle deltoid

Deltoid

Teres minor

Rhomboid

Teres major

Long head

Lateral head

Medial head

Triceps

Latissimus dorsi

External oblique

Thoracolumbar fascia

Gluteus medius

Gluteus maximus

INFRASPINATUS AND TERES MINOR

Both of these muscles arise from the posterior surface of the scapula (shoulder blade), pass onto the scapulohumeral articulation (adhering to its articular capsule), and insert at the greater tubercle of the humerus. They play an important role in external rotation of the arm and reinforce the action of the shoulder ligaments by actively reinforcing the attachment of the arm to the chest.

Comment: In some people, the teres minor and infraspinatus are fused, forming one muscle.

THE MOVEMENT

Sit facing the machine, with the torso against the back pad and arms forward, gripping the handles:

- Inhale and separate the arms, squeezing the shoulder blades together at the end of the movement.
- Exhale.

This exercise mainly engages the posterior deltoid, infraspinatus, and teres minor and, at the end of the movement when the shoulder blades squeeze together, the trapezius and rhomboids.

STRETCHING THE POSTERIOR ROTATOR CUFF MUSCLES

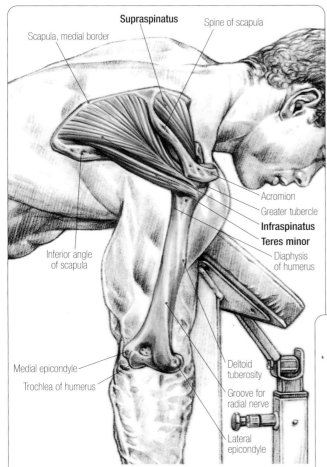

Scapula, medial border
Supraspinatus
Spine of scapula
Acromion
Greater tubercle
Infraspinatus
Teres minor
Diaphysis of humerus
Inferior angle of scapula
Medial epicondyle
Trochlea of humerus
Deltoid tuberosity
Groove for radial nerve
Lateral epicondyle

Stand with a dumbbell in your hand, with your torso cantilevered forward and resting on the machine (for example, the arm rest of a Larry Scott desk or on a bench with lumbar extensions).

With your arm released, let the dumbbell hang for a minute while trying to relax the shoulder.

This exercise allows you to stretch the infraspinatus, teres minor, and, to a lesser extent, the supraspinatus; these muscles attach to the posterior surface of the scapula. In weightlifting, these muscles are often the site of contractures and spasms that engage the shoulder in a bad position, which over time may lead to particularly incapacitating tendon overuse pathologies.

Comment: Contractures or spasms of the teres minor and infraspinatus will engage the humerus in external rotation. This creates excessive friction on the long head of the biceps at the front of the arm (in the bicipital groove). If not treated, this can lead to inflammation and tearing of the tendon. Therefore, at the slightest suspicion of a contracture, it is important to relax these muscles while performing this specific stretch.

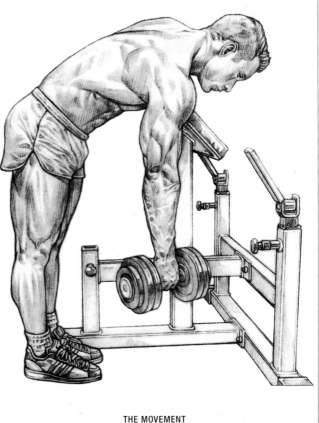

THE MOVEMENT

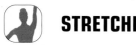

STRETCHING THE SHOULDER

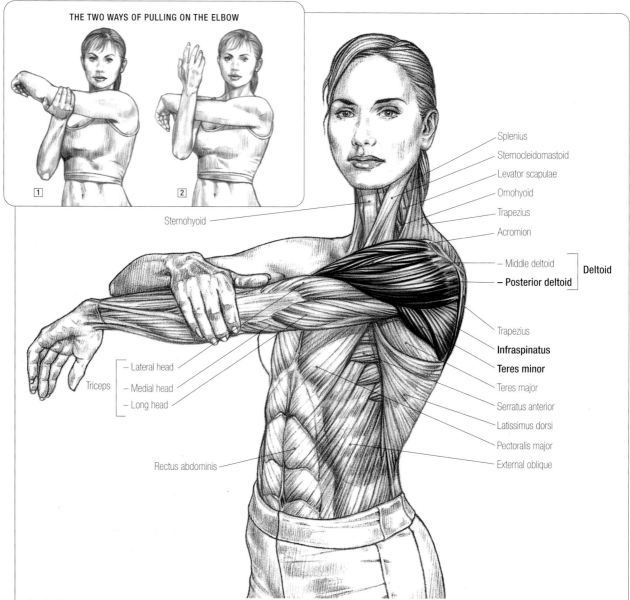

THE TWO WAYS OF PULLING ON THE ELBOW

1

2

Sternohyoid

Splenius

Sternocleidomastoid

Levator scapulae

Omohyoid

Trapezius

Acromion

— Middle deltoid

Deltoid

— **Posterior deltoid**

Trapezius

Infraspinatus

Teres minor

Teres major

Serratus anterior

Latissimus dorsi

Pectoralis major

External oblique

— Lateral head

— Medial head

— Long head

Triceps

Rectus abdominis

Stand with your head level and one arm horizontal. Grasp the elbow with the opposite hand and pull on the arm to slowly bring the elbow toward the opposite shoulder.

Maintain this position for 10 to 20 seconds, the time it takes to properly feel the stretch.

This exercise mainly works the posterior fascicle of the middle deltoid and the teres minor and infraspinatus. These small external rotator muscles of the humerus are frequently the site of contractures, which can lead to functional disequilibrium of the shoulder (such as excessive friction of the tendon of the long head of the biceps in the bicipital groove of the humerus) and may result in pathological inflammation.

The middle and inferior portions of the trapezius muscle and the rhomboid major are also stretched.

Variation: Pull the elbow with the opposite arm passing underneath.

Comment: For some people with very well-developed muscles, adduction of the arm can be hindered by compression of the biceps brachii against the pectoralis major, which will limit the stretch at the posterior part of the shoulder.

3
CHEST

1 INCLINE BENCH PRESSES

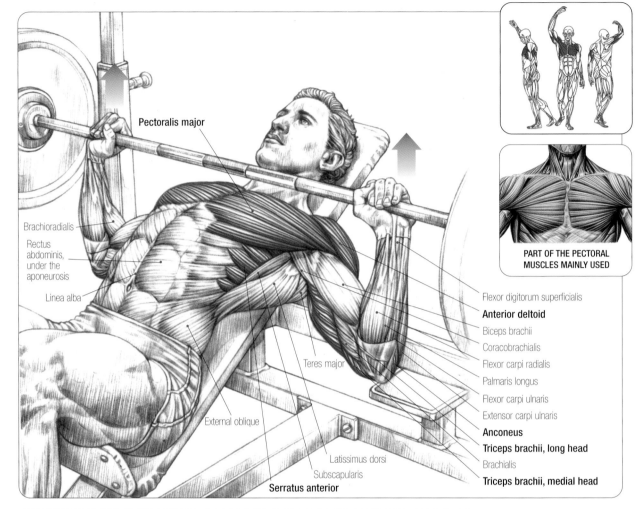

Pectoralis major

Brachioradialis

Rectus abdominis, under the aponeurosis

Linea alba

External oblique

Teres major

Latissimus dorsi

Subscapularis

Serratus anterior

Flexor digitorum superficialis

Anterior deltoid

Biceps brachii

Coracobrachialis

Flexor carpi radialis

Palmaris longus

Flexor carpi ulnaris

Extensor carpi ulnaris

Anconeus

Triceps brachii, long head

Brachialis

Triceps brachii, medial head

PART OF THE PECTORAL MUSCLES MAINLY USED

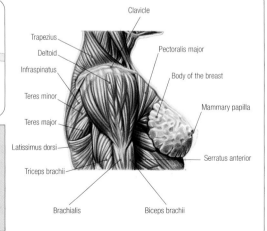

Clavicle

Trapezius

Deltoid

Infraspinatus

Teres minor

Teres major

Latissimus dorsi

Triceps brachii

Brachialis

Biceps brachii

Pectoralis major

Body of the breast

Mammary papilla

Serratus anterior

Comment: Contrary to popular lore, the incline press does not tone the breasts and in no way prevents their sagging. Breasts are composed of adipose tissue containing the mammary glands, all of which is contained in a net of connective tissue that rests on top of the pectoralis major.

Sit on an incline bench angled at 45 to 60 degrees and grasp the barbell with an overhand grip wider than shoulder width:

- Inhale and lower the barbell to the sternal notch.
- Extend the arms.
- Exhale at the end of the movement.

This exercise mainly solicits the clavicular head of the pectoralis major, anterior deltoid, triceps brachii, serratus anterior, and pectoralis minor. This exercise may be done at a frame that guides the bar.

STRETCHING THE PECTORALIS MAJOR

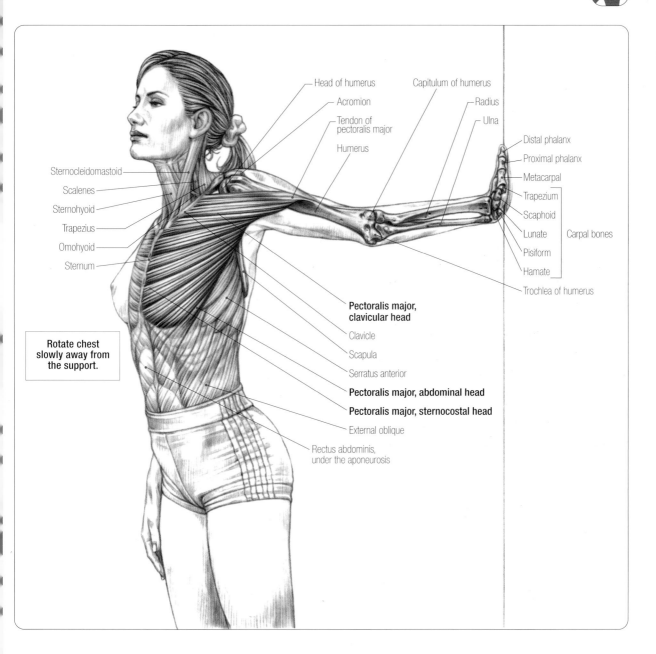

Head of humerus

Acromion

Tendon of pectoralis major

Humerus

Capitulum of humerus

Radius

Ulna

Distal phalanx

Proximal phalanx

Metacarpal

Trapezium

Scaphoid

Lunate — Carpal bones

Pisiform

Hamate

Trochlea of humerus

Sternocleidomastoid

Scalenes

Sternohyoid

Trapezius

Omohyoid

Sternum

Pectoralis major, clavicular head

Clavicle

Scapula

Serratus anterior

Pectoralis major, abdominal head

Pectoralis major, sternocostal head

External oblique

Rectus abdominis, under the aponeurosis

Rotate chest slowly away from the support.

Stand with your arm extended. Grip a support with your hand and slowly rotate your chest to the opposite side, away from the support.

This exercise mainly stretches the pectoralis major, anterior deltoid, and biceps brachii.

Variation: Position your hand at various levels in order to stretch all the fascicles of pectoralis major.

Comment: This is an excellent stretch for the bench press in weightlifting and all throwing sports, including tennis, volleyball, and handball.

2 BENCH PRESSES

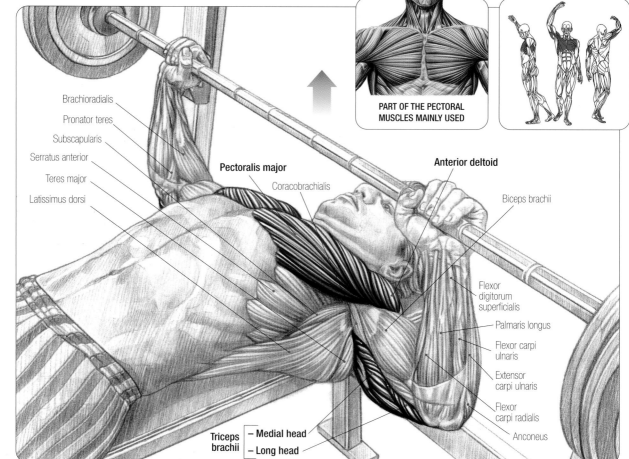

Brachioradialis
Pronator teres
Subscapularis
Serratus anterior
Teres major
Latissimus dorsi

Pectoralis major
Coracobrachialis

PART OF THE PECTORAL MUSCLES MAINLY USED

Anterior deltoid
Biceps brachii

Flexor digitorum superficialis
Palmaris longus
Flexor carpi ulnaris
Extensor carpi ulnaris
Flexor carpi radialis
Anconeus

Triceps brachii — Medial head
— Long head

Lie faceup on a horizontal bench, with buttocks on the bench and feet flat on the ground:
- Grasp the barbell with an overhand grip wider than shoulder width.
- Inhale and lower the bar to the chest with a controlled movement.
- Extend the arms and exhale at the end of the effort.

This exercise engages the complete pectoralis major muscle, pectoralis minor, anterior deltoid, serratus anterior, and coracobrachialis.

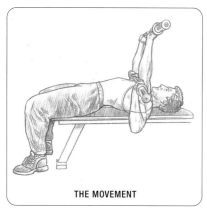

THE MOVEMENT

Variations
1. This movement may be performed while arching the back powerlifter style. This position brings the more powerful lower part of the pectoral muscle into play, allowing you to lift heavier weights.
2. Executing the extension with the elbows next to the body concentrates the work onto the anterior deltoid.
3. Varying the width of the hands isolates different parts of the muscle:
   - Hands closer together isolates the central part of the pectorals.
   - Hands wider apart isolates the lateral part of the pectorals.
4. Varying the angle of the barbell isolates different parts of the muscle:
   - Lowering the bar to the chondrocostal border of the rib cage isolates the lower part of the pectorals.
   - Lowering the barbell onto the middle part of the pectorals isolates the midline fibers.
   - Lowering the bar onto the sternal notch isolates the clavicular head of the muscle.
5. If you have back problems or want to isolate the pectorals, perform the extension with the legs raised.
6. Perform the extension at a frame that guides the bar.

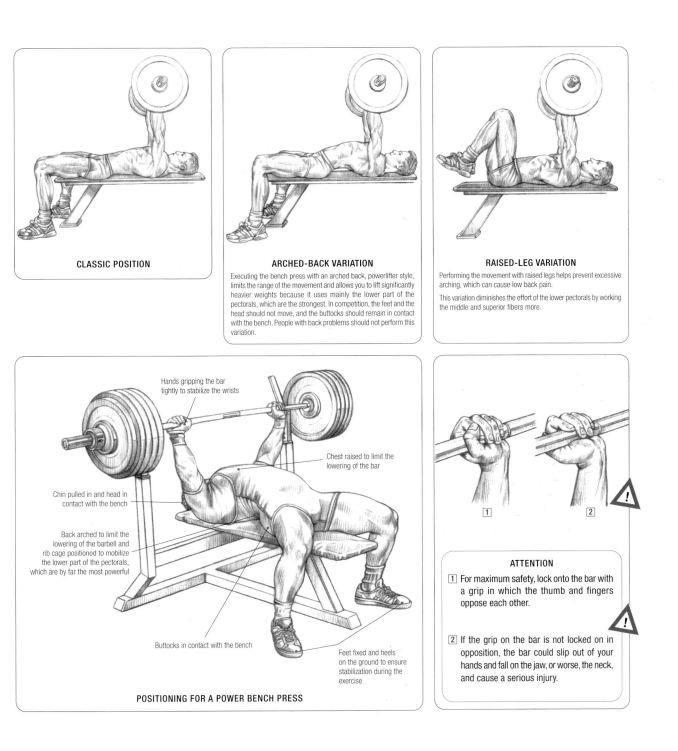

CLASSIC POSITION

ARCHED-BACK VARIATION

Executing the bench press with an arched back, powerlifter style, limits the range of the movement and allows you to lift significantly heavier weights because it uses mainly the lower part of the pectorals, which are the strongest. In competition, the feet and the head should not move, and the buttocks should remain in contact with the bench. People with back problems should not perform this variation.

RAISED-LEG VARIATION

Performing the movement with raised legs helps prevent excessive arching, which can cause low back pain.

This variation diminishes the effort of the lower pectorals by working the middle and superior fibers more.

Hands gripping the bar tightly to stabilize the wrists

Chest raised to limit the lowering of the bar

Chin pulled in and head in contact with the bench

Back arched to limit the lowering of the barbell and rib cage positioned to mobilize the lower part of the pectorals, which are by far the most powerful

Buttocks in contact with the bench

Feet fixed and heels on the ground to ensure stabilization during the exercise

POSITIONING FOR A POWER BENCH PRESS

ATTENTION

1 For maximum safety, lock onto the bar with a grip in which the thumb and fingers oppose each other.

2 If the grip on the bar is not locked on in opposition, the bar could slip out of your hands and fall on the jaw, or worse, the neck, and cause a serious injury.

✚ ACROMIOCLAVICULAR PROBLEMS

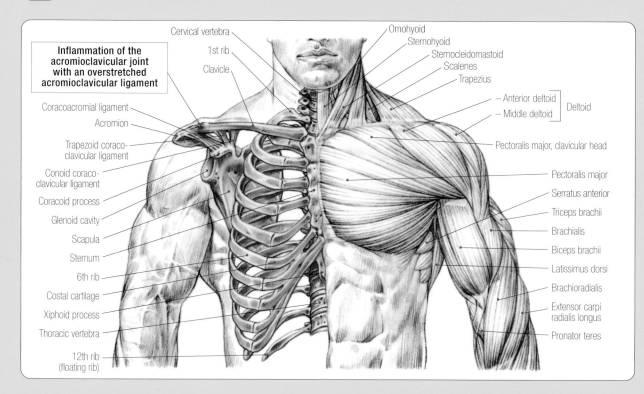

Inflammation of the acromioclavicular joint with an overstretched acromioclavicular ligament

Cervical vertebra
1st rib
Clavicle
Coracoacromial ligament
Acromion
Trapezoid coraco-clavicular ligament
Conoid coraco-clavicular ligament
Coracoid process
Glenoid cavity
Scapula
Sternum
6th rib
Costal cartilage
Xiphoid process
Thoracic vertebra
12th rib (floating rib)

Omohyoid
Sternohyoid
Sternocleidomastoid
Scalenes
Trapezius
Anterior deltoid
Middle deltoid
Deltoid
Pectoralis major, clavicular head
Pectoralis major
Serratus anterior
Triceps brachii
Brachialis
Biceps brachii
Latissimus dorsi
Brachioradialis
Extensor carpi radialis longus
Pronator teres

Acromioclavicular injuries are common in weightlifting. Most dedicated weightlifters encounter this problem.

Unlike other sports (such as rugby, football, and riding) and combat sports with throws (wrestling and judo) where the shoulder joint can become severely injured with violent contact or a fall involving acromioclavicular dislocation with ligament tearing, in weightlifting, acromioclavicular pathologies are mainly due to microtraumas resulting from excessive and repetitive stress and poor control of the shoulder articulation.

Pain develops progressively. Although pain is easily tolerated at the beginning, it gradually disturbs the practice of weightlifting until it finally hinders the ability to perform a great number of exercises such as bench presses and dips. All downward propulsions become painful, and leaning on the elbows might also be painful.

Examination of the acromioclavicular articulation reveals slight swelling and pain on palpation. Although not really serious, this type of injury generally takes a long time to heal. It also takes a long time for the inflammation to subside and the articular capsule with the stretched acromioclavicular ligaments to revert to their normal size and allow for normal joint play.

When this injury occurs, training of the upper body must stop for two weeks.

CROSS SECTION OF THE ACROMIOCLAVICULAR JOINT

Acromioclavicular ligament* with a traumatic inflammation

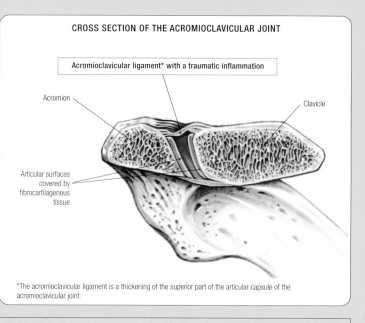

Acromion
Clavicle
Articular surfaces covered by fibrocartilagenous tissue

*The acromioclavicular ligament is a thickening of the superior part of the articular capsule of the acromioclavicular joint.

Comment: At the osseous level, the upper extremity is attached to the chest by the clavicle, which extends from the sternum to the shoulder blade. Although not very mobile, the clavicular articulations are often overused and subject to inflammatory wear pathologies.

THE SHOULDER GIRDLE

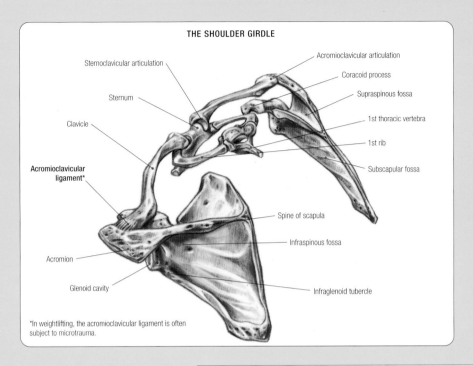

Sternoclavicular articulation

Sternum

Clavicle

Acromioclavicular ligament*

Acromion

Glenoid cavity

Acromioclavicular articulation

Coracoid process

Supraspinous fossa

1st thoracic vertebra

1st rib

Subscapular fossa

Spine of scapula

Infraspinous fossa

Infraglenoid tubercle

*In weightlifting, the acromioclavicular ligament is often subject to microtrauma.

On resuming training of the upper body, avoid for at least two months the bench press and all movements that involve pushing down, such as decline presses and dips, since they risk stretching the acromioclavicular ligaments all over again. On the other hand, all movements that involve pushing up, such as incline presses or presses for the shoulders with barbells and dumbbells, can be performed without risk because they tend to stabilize the acromioclavicular articulation, which limits the risk of stretching the ligaments.

Disregarding this advice will cause the articular inflammation to continue and, in certain people, will lead to intra-articular calcifications and may seriously compromise an athletic career.

Prevention: In weightlifting, acromioclavicular inflammations most often appear after overtraining of the bench press with series that are too long or poorly controlled (rapid lowering, jerking, and bouncing on the chest). Powerlifters who perform the bench press are also susceptible to tension generated on the acromioclavicular ligament that initiates inflammatory pathologies.

As soon as you feel any pain, stop these traumatizing techniques for some time and replace them with exercises for the pectorals, such as standing spreads at the pulley in conjunction with movements using dumbbells. Always work with a certain degree of incline on the bench.

MOBILITY OF THE INJURED ACROMIOCLAVICULAR ARTICULATION RELATIVE TO THE DIFFERENT KINDS OF PUSHES

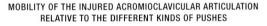
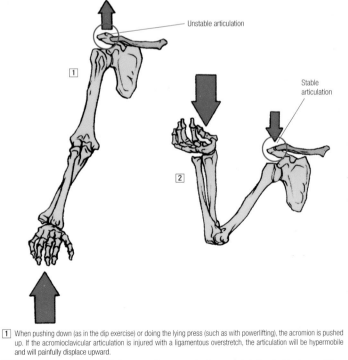

Unstable articulation

Stable articulation

1 When pushing down (as in the dip exercise) or doing the lying press (such as with powerlifting), the acromion is pushed up. If the acromioclavicular articulation is injured with a ligamentous overstretch, the articulation will be hypermobile and will painfully displace upward.

2 With upward presses, such as the incline press or the press on a bar, the acromioclavicular articulation is pressed down and stabilized.

✚ PECTORALIS MAJOR TEAR

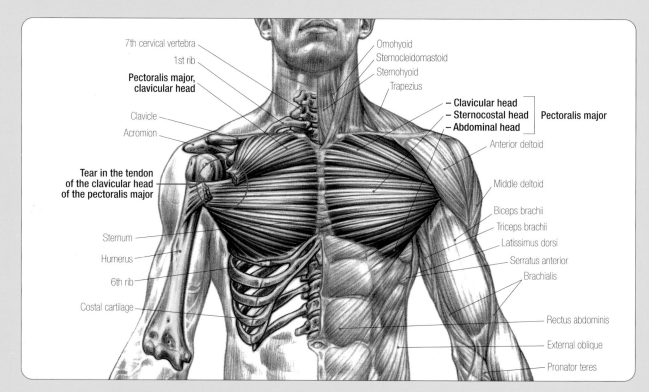

- 7th cervical vertebra
- 1st rib
- **Pectoralis major, clavicular head**
- Clavicle
- Acromion
- **Tear in the tendon of the clavicular head of the pectoralis major**
- Sternum
- Humerus
- 6th rib
- Costal cartilage

- Omohyoid
- Sternocleidomastoid
- Sternohyoid
- Trapezius
- **− Clavicular head**
- **− Sternocostal head** } Pectoralis major
- **− Abdominal head**
- Anterior deltoid
- Middle deltoid
- Biceps brachii
- Triceps brachii
- Latissimus dorsi
- Serratus anterior
- Brachialis
- Rectus abdominis
- External oblique
- Pronator teres

The pectoralis major originates at the anterior surface of the rib cage and inserts at the anterior surface of the upper end of the humerus.

It is a powerful muscle whose main function is to bring the arms together in front of the rib cage. (It is the hugging muscle.)

Unlike most sports, where pectoralis major injuries are rare, weightlifting, especially the bench press, can lead to small tears and even partial rupture of its tendon.

This ultimate injury is seen only in relatively powerful athletes using abnormally rapid force before the tendon has had time to strengthen. Sometimes it is associated with a low-calorie diet aimed at increased muscle definition. (These diets tend to weaken the muscles, tendons, and joints.)

The injury, which always occurs during heavy bench-pressing, generally affects only the tendon of the clavicular head of the pectoralis major.

A torn tendon is extremely painful, and the athlete may faint. Swelling and bruising often appear on the anterior surface of the arm, and retraction of the clavicular head leads to a hollow that is medial to the anterior deltoid.

The problem with this injury is that doctors often misdiagnose it. This mistake is unfortunately common but is understandable because during the post-traumatic examination the injured party is able to perform all the movements that indicate full motor function of the pectoralis major. Therefore, the injury appears to be a simple muscle tear rather than the more serious tear of the tendinous insertion.

For example, despite a tear of the clavicular head of the pectoralis major, anterior elevation of the arm, which is part of its function, is compensated for by the anterior deltoid. And abduction is performed by the sternal and abdominal heads of the pectoralis major.

If the tendon of the clavicular head of the pectoralis major is torn, it must be surgically reinserted onto the humerus as soon as possible. If this is not done promptly, retraction and fibrosis of the muscle occurs, and the operation will no longer be possible.

Although you can move your arm through its full range of motion without the superior head of the pectoralis major, you will never recover your initial strength and will be at a serious disadvantage if you want to continue heavy weight training.

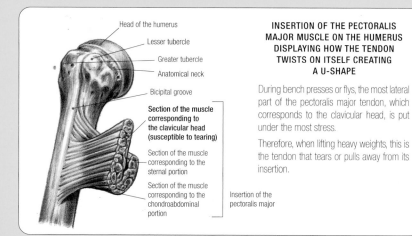

- Head of the humerus
- Lesser tubercle
- Greater tubercle
- Anatomical neck
- Bicipital groove
- Section of the muscle corresponding to the clavicular head (susceptible to tearing)
- Section of the muscle corresponding to the sternal portion
- Section of the muscle corresponding to the chondroabdominal portion

Insertion of the pectoralis major

INSERTION OF THE PECTORALIS MAJOR MUSCLE ON THE HUMERUS DISPLAYING HOW THE TENDON TWISTS ON ITSELF CREATING A U-SHAPE

During bench presses or flys, the most lateral part of the pectoralis major tendon, which corresponds to the clavicular head, is put under the most stress.

Therefore, when lifting heavy weights, this is the tendon that tears or pulls away from its insertion.

CLOSE-GRIP BENCH PRESSES [3]

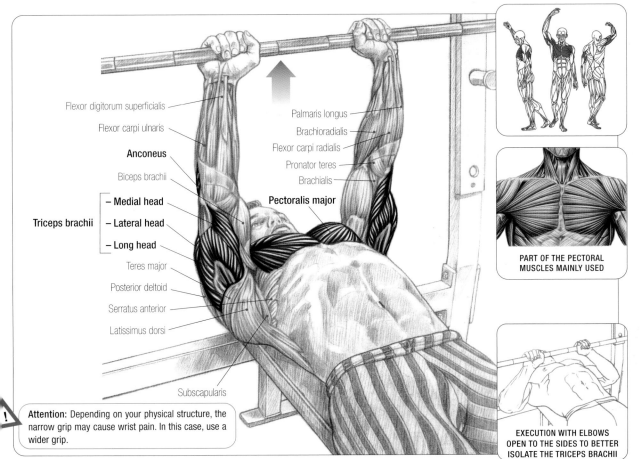

Flexor digitorum superficialis

Flexor carpi ulnaris

Anconeus

Biceps brachii

Triceps brachii
- **Medial head**
- **Lateral head**
- **Long head**

Teres major

Posterior deltoid

Serratus anterior

Latissimus dorsi

Subscapularis

Palmaris longus

Brachioradialis

Flexor carpi radialis

Pronator teres

Brachialis

Pectoralis major

PART OF THE PECTORAL MUSCLES MAINLY USED

EXECUTION WITH ELBOWS OPEN TO THE SIDES TO BETTER ISOLATE THE TRICEPS BRACHII

Attention: Depending on your physical structure, the narrow grip may cause wrist pain. In this case, use a wider grip.

Lie on a horizontal bench with the buttocks on the bench and the feet on the ground. Grip the barbell with an overhand grip and wrists 4 to 15 inches apart, depending on the flexibility of the wrists:
- Inhale and lower the bar with a controlled movement to the chest, with the elbows out to the sides.
- Extend and exhale at the end of the effort.

This exercise develops the pectoral muscles at the sternal notch and the triceps brachii. (With this in mind, it may be included in a program for the arms.) By extending and keeping the elbows next to the body, a greater part of the work is performed by the anterior deltoid. This movement may be performed at a frame that guides the bar.

Bench Presses and Elbow Pain

Elbow pain most often develops after bench pressing. This overuse injury is generally related to excessive training with long sets. In bench pressing, locking the extended arms at the end of the movement subjects the elbow to rubbing and microtrauma, which over time may lead to inflammation.

Comment: Occasionally, this condition can lead to intra-articular calcifications, which are particularly crippling. In this case, surgery is often the only solution for regaining complete arm extension.

At the first sign of elbow pain, avoid for several days exercises that involve arm extension in order to prevent serious injury.

When you resume exercises that include arm extension, avoid completely extending the forearms at the end of the movement until the pain has completely disappeared.

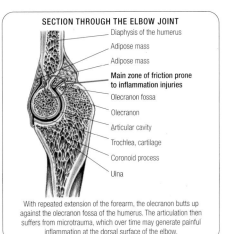

SECTION THROUGH THE ELBOW JOINT

Diaphysis of the humerus

Adipose mass

Adipose mass

Main zone of friction prone to inflammation injuries

Olecranon fossa

Olecranon

Articular cavity

Trochlea, cartilage

Coronoid process

Ulna

With repeated extension of the forearm, the olecranon butts up against the olecranon fossa of the humerus. The articulation then suffers from microtrauma, which over time may generate painful inflammation at the dorsal surface of the elbow.

✚ BENCH PRESSES AND MORPHOLOGY

The bench press is by far the most-used exercise in weightlifting. It is also the exercise that causes the most injuries. Therefore, to perform this movement correctly and to reduce risk, you must learn the basics of individual morphological differences.

Arm Length

Besides wear-and-tear pathologies, most injuries are muscle tears or tendon tears of the pectoralis major. These occur most often during the negative phase of the movement—that is, while lowering the barbell.

In lowering the barbell to the chest, the pectoralis major, which inserts onto the humerus, becomes increasingly stretched and vulnerable as the arm is lowered.

But the lowering of the arm and the stretch of the pectoralis major vary significantly depending on the individual. The longer the arm and especially the forearm, the lower the humerus will go down, and the more the pectoralis major will be dangerously stretched. Therefore, it is not surprising that most injuries occur in people with relatively longer arms.

Thickness of Rib Cage

The thicker the rib cage, the more the lowering of the barbell and by extension the stretching of the pectoralis major will be restricted.

People with a thick rib cage will theoretically perform the bench press without much risk of injury to the pectoralis major. It is therefore not surprising that most of the great bench press champions are shorter-limbed people (that is, people with proportionately shorter extremities and barrel chests). These two details allow them to achieve their records relatively safely.

Remember that injury is what often limits athletes' progress. In addition to training methods, nutrition, and mental state, individual morphology plays a fundamental role in success in sports. It is therefore essential to adapt your training to your morphology and to understand that what is good for one person may not be as good for another.

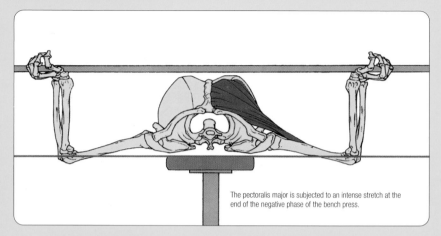

The pectoralis major is subjected to an intense stretch at the end of the negative phase of the bench press.

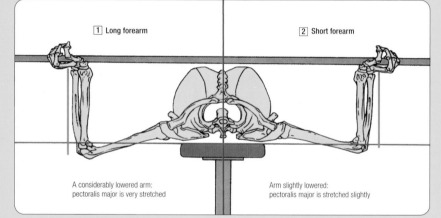

1 Long forearm

2 Short forearm

A considerably lowered arm: pectoralis major is very stretched

Arm slightly lowered: pectoralis major is stretched slightly

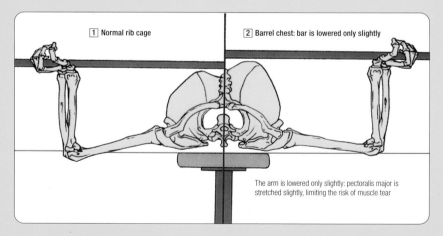

1 Normal rib cage

2 Barrel chest: bar is lowered only slightly

The arm is lowered only slightly: pectoralis major is stretched slightly, limiting the risk of muscle tear

Limiting the Risk of Injury

It is possible to perform the bench press by bringing the hands closer together. Because this variation limits the lowering of the arms, it reduces the stretch of the pectoralis major and limits the risk of injury.

Although the amplitude of the movement is greater, the work on the biceps is more intense, and the performance is reduced, this low-risk variation is sometimes used by certain long-limbed champions of the bench press.

To avoid excessive stretching of the pectoralis muscles, it is possible to partially perform the bench press by shortening the lowering phase of the bar so that it does not touch the chest.

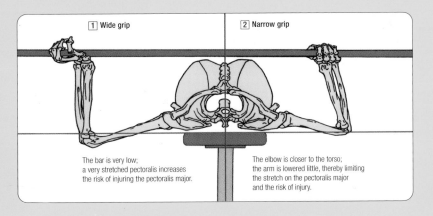

1 Wide grip   2 Narrow grip

The bar is very low;
a very stretched pectoralis increases
the risk of injuring the pectoralis major.

The elbow is closer to the torso;
the arm is lowered little, thereby limiting
the stretch on the pectoralis major
and the risk of injury.

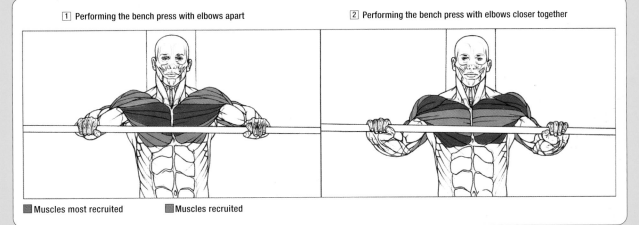

1 Performing the bench press with elbows apart   2 Performing the bench press with elbows closer together

■ Muscles most recruited   ■ Muscles recruited

Muscle Prominence

Note that there are two ways of performing the bench press according to the strong features of individual muscles.

The bench press can be performed with the elbows apart. This technique directs most of the effort onto the pectoralis major.

The bench press can also be performed with the elbows closer together, closing the angle of the arm and chest. People who have deltoids that are stronger than the pectoralis major will instinctively use this technique.

Aside from the morphology, both of these types of bench presses can be used to direct the work onto the pectoralis major (elbows spread) or onto the deltoids (elbows closer together).

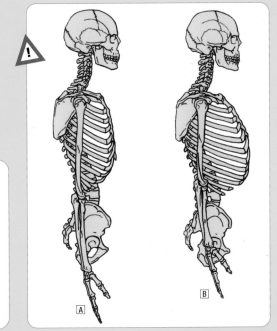

⚠ **Attention:** In the supine bench press, it is important to take the individual morphology into account.

A: A small rib cage combined with long arms increases the excursion of the bar, making the movement painful while at the same time limiting the strength developed. Furthermore, when the bar approaches the chest, the pectoralis major is dangerously stretched. When heavier weights are used, it increases the risk of muscular tears and tendinous disruptions.

B: A barrel chest coupled with short arms allows for safe performance of a supine bench press by limiting the amplitude of the movement and the stretch of the pectoralis major at the end of the descent of the bar (when the bar touches the chest). It is not surprising that the greatest champions of the supine bench press have this type of morphology.

4 DECLINE BENCH PRESSES

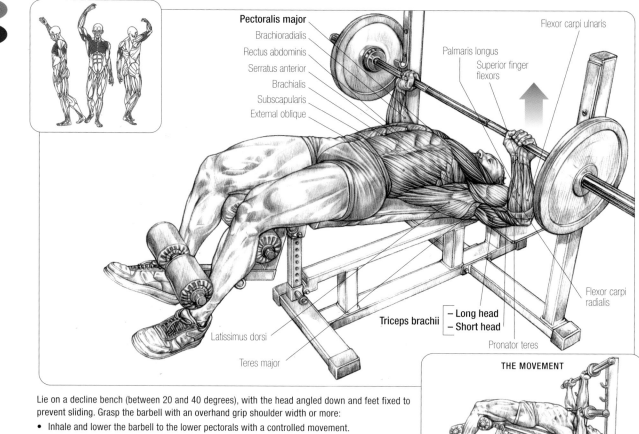

Pectoralis major
Brachioradialis
Rectus abdominis
Serratus anterior
Brachialis
Subscapularis
External oblique

Flexor carpi ulnaris
Palmaris longus
Superior finger flexors
Flexor carpi radialis
Pronator teres

Triceps brachii
— Long head
— Short head

Latissimus dorsi
Teres major

THE MOVEMENT

Lie on a decline bench (between 20 and 40 degrees), with the head angled down and feet fixed to prevent sliding. Grasp the barbell with an overhand grip shoulder width or more:

- Inhale and lower the barbell to the lower pectorals with a controlled movement.
- Extend the arms and exhale at the end of the movement.

This exercise contracts the pectoralis major (mainly its inferior fibers), triceps brachii, and the anterior deltoid.

This exercise is useful for outlining the inferior groove of the pectorals. Using light weights and lowering the bar to the neck stretches the pectoralis major correctly. The decline press may be performed at a frame that guides the bar.

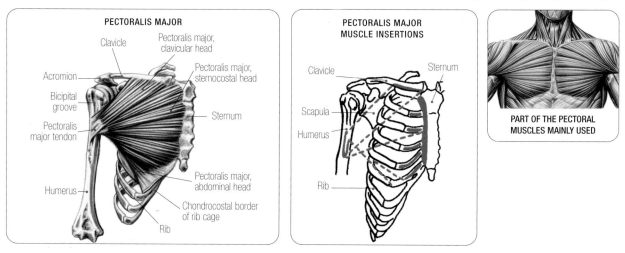

PECTORALIS MAJOR

Clavicle
Pectoralis major, clavicular head
Acromion
Pectoralis major, sternocostal head
Bicipital groove
Sternum
Pectoralis major tendon
Humerus
Pectoralis major, abdominal head
Chondrocostal border of rib cage
Rib

PECTORALIS MAJOR MUSCLE INSERTIONS

Clavicle
Sternum
Scapula
Humerus
Rib

PART OF THE PECTORAL MUSCLES MAINLY USED

MACHINE BENCH PRESSES ⑤

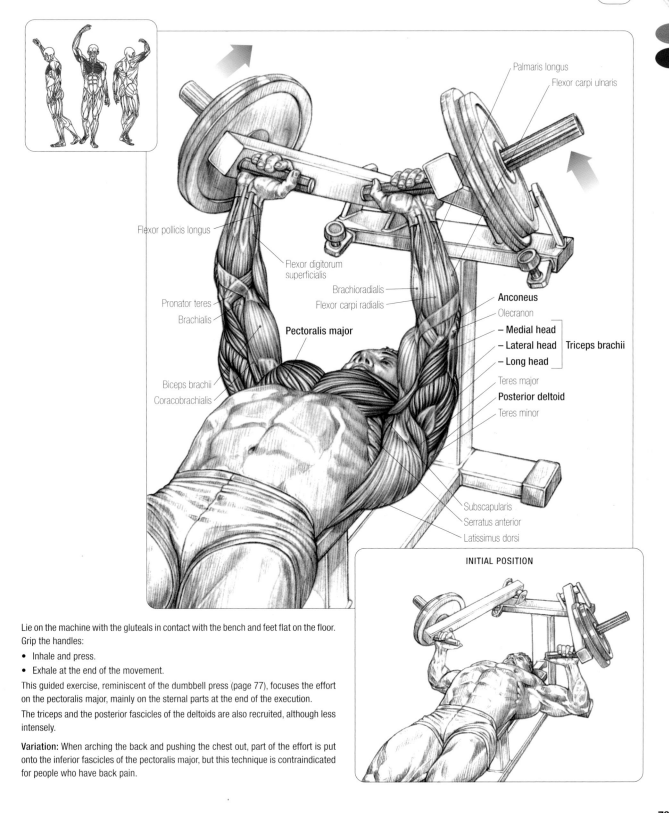

Palmaris longus
Flexor carpi ulnaris
Flexor pollicis longus
Flexor digitorum superficialis
Pronator teres
Brachioradialis
Brachialis
Flexor carpi radialis
Anconeus
Olecranon
Pectoralis major
– Medial head
– Lateral head } Triceps brachii
– Long head
Biceps brachii
Teres major
Coracobrachialis
Posterior deltoid
Teres minor
Subscapularis
Serratus anterior
Latissimus dorsi

INITIAL POSITION

Lie on the machine with the gluteals in contact with the bench and feet flat on the floor. Grip the handles:

- Inhale and press.
- Exhale at the end of the movement.

This guided exercise, reminiscent of the dumbbell press (page 77), focuses the effort on the pectoralis major, mainly on the sternal parts at the end of the execution.

The triceps and the posterior fascicles of the deltoids are also recruited, although less intensely.

Variation: When arching the back and pushing the chest out, part of the effort is put onto the inferior fascicles of the pectoralis major, but this technique is contraindicated for people who have back pain.

6 PARALLEL BAR DIPS

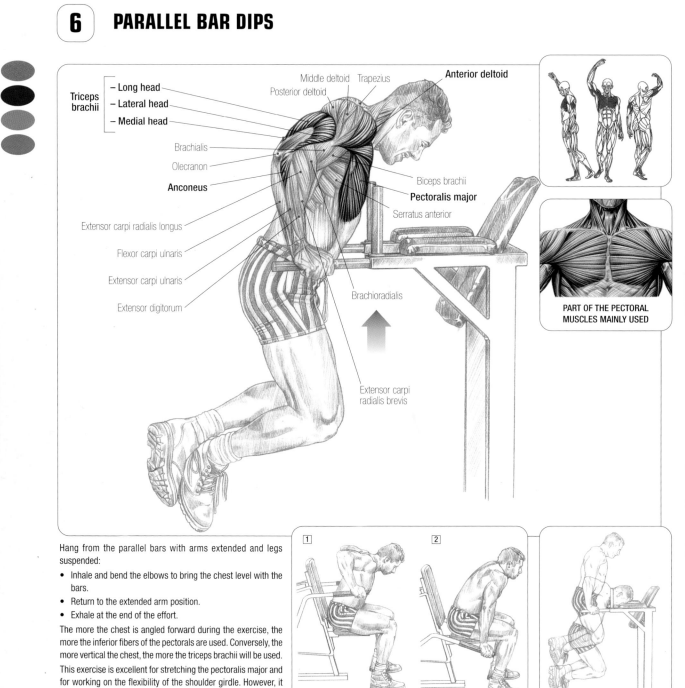

Triceps brachii
— Long head
— Lateral head
— Medial head

Brachialis

Olecranon

Anconeus

Extensor carpi radialis longus

Flexor carpi ulnaris

Extensor carpi ulnaris

Extensor digitorum

Middle deltoid   Trapezius

Posterior deltoid

Anterior deltoid

Biceps brachii

Pectoralis major

Serratus anterior

Brachioradialis

Extensor carpi radialis brevis

PART OF THE PECTORAL MUSCLES MAINLY USED

Hang from the parallel bars with arms extended and legs suspended:

- Inhale and bend the elbows to bring the chest level with the bars.
- Return to the extended arm position.
- Exhale at the end of the effort.

The more the chest is angled forward during the exercise, the more the inferior fibers of the pectorals are used. Conversely, the more vertical the chest, the more the triceps brachii will be used.

This exercise is excellent for stretching the pectoralis major and for working on the flexibility of the shoulder girdle. However, it is not recommended for beginners because it requires a certain amount of initial strength.

If you are a beginner, use a dips machine to familiarize yourself with the movement.

Sets of 10 to 20 repetitions provide the best results.

For developing more strength and also more size, athletes used to this movement may use a weight belt, or hang a weight from their legs.

EXECUTING DIPS AT A MACHINE

1 Initial position
2 Final position

THE MOVEMENT

Comment: Execute the dips with caution to prevent shoulder trauma.

PAY ATTENTION TO THE NECK POSITION! ✚

DIAGRAM OF THE NERVES OF THE UPPER EXTREMITY

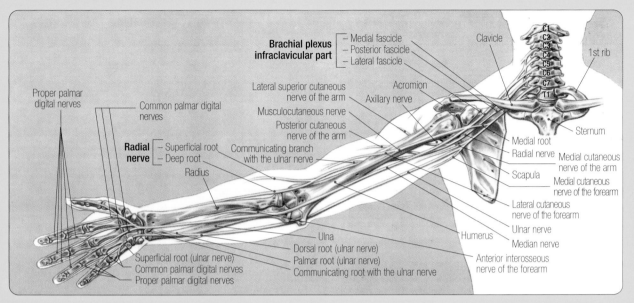

In weightlifting, a faulty position of the neck during certain exercises may lead to bothersome and incapacitating neuralgia in people predisposed to the condition.

These neuralgias manifest as numbness in the arm accompanied by the sensation of pins and needles and sometimes local insensitivity.

These symptoms most often appear in the days after the execution of dips (page 74), pec deck rear-delt laterals (page 58), squats (page 126), and deadlifts (page 104) when these movements are done with the neck in extension and the head thrown back.

In fact, throwing the head back can initiate spasms and contractions of the deep muscles of the neck, leading to compression of the spinal nerves as they exit from the cervical vertebrae.

This compression involves a neuralgia that most often affects the brachial plexus at the vertebral levels of C4, C5, C6, C7, C8, and T1 (C stands for cervical and T for thoracic).

To find out where the involved nerve exits the spine, you need only look at the diagram, then follow the nerve from its pins and needles and numbness and ascend to its vertebra.

To avoid these types of neuralgia, perform dips or reverse push-ups at a machine by bringing the head forward while at the same time bringing the chin to the chest.

With the squat or deadlift, perform the exercise while keeping the neck very straight and looking forward.

If neuralgia has manifested, stop performing the exercise with the head thrown backward and the neck in extension.

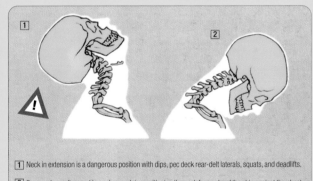

1 Neck in extension is a dangerous position with dips, pec deck rear-delt laterals, squats, and deadlifts.

2 For people predisposed to neck neuralgia, positioning the neck forward and the chin against the chest is recommended for dips and reverse push-ups at a machine.

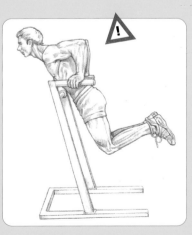

Attention: Executing dips with the neck in extension can cause neuralgia in some people.

7 PUSH-UPS

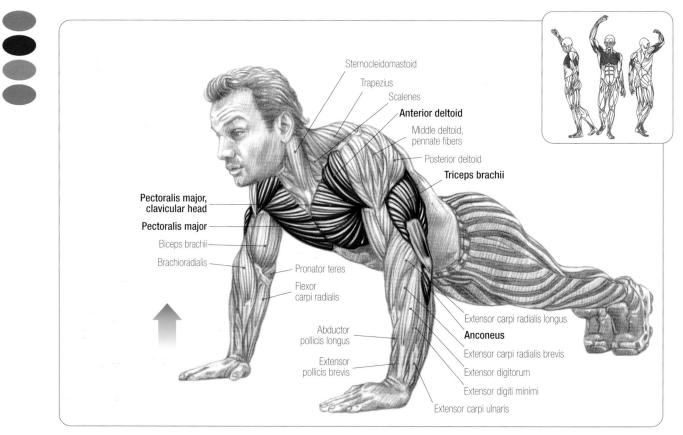

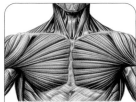

Sternocleidomastoid

Trapezius

Scalenes

Anterior deltoid

Middle deltoid, pennate fibers

Posterior deltoid

Triceps brachii

Pectoralis major, clavicular head

Pectoralis major

Biceps brachii

Brachioradialis

Pronator teres

Flexor carpi radialis

Abductor pollicis longus

Extensor pollicis brevis

Extensor carpi radialis longus

Anconeus

Extensor carpi radialis brevis

Extensor digitorum

Extensor digiti minimi

Extensor carpi ulnaris

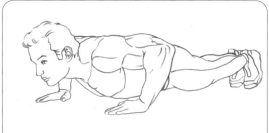

INITIAL POSITION

Support yourself facedown on the ground, with arms extended, hands shoulder-width (or more) apart, and feet touching or slightly apart:

- Inhale and bend the elbows to bring the rib cage close to the ground without arching the low back excessively.
- Push back up to complete arm extension.
- Exhale at the end of the movement.

This movement is excellent for the pectoralis major and the triceps brachii.

PART OF THE PECTORAL MUSCLES MAINLY USED

Variations

Varying the tilt of the chest focuses the work on different parts of the pectorals:

- Feet higher isolates the clavicular head of the pectoralis major.
- Chest higher isolates the inferior part of the pectoralis major.

Varying the width of the hands focuses the work on different parts of the pectorals:

- Hands wider isolates the lateral part of the pectoralis major.
- Hands closer together isolates the sternal head of the pectoralis major.

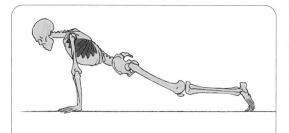

While performing push-ups the serratus anterior contracts to maintain the scapula against the rib cage, locking the arms onto the torso.

DUMBBELL PRESSES 8

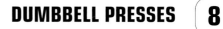

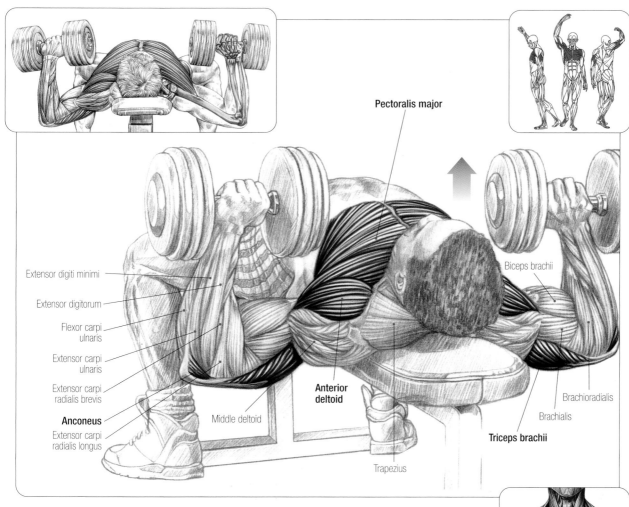

Pectoralis major

Extensor digiti minimi

Extensor digitorum

Flexor carpi ulnaris

Extensor carpi ulnaris

Extensor carpi radialis brevis

Anconeus

Extensor carpi radialis longus

Middle deltoid

Anterior deltoid

Trapezius

Biceps brachii

Brachioradialis

Brachialis

Triceps brachii

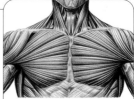

PART OF THE PECTORAL MUSCLES MAINLY USED

Lie faceup on a horizontal bench, with feet flat on the ground for stability and elbows bent. Hold the dumbbells with an overhand grip at chest level:

- Inhale and extend the arms vertically while rotating the forearms so that the palms face each other.
- Once the hands face each other, perform an isometric contraction to focus the effort on the sternal head of the pectoralis major.
- Exhale at the end of the movement.

This exercise is similar to the bench press, but with its greater range of motion, it stretches the pectoralis muscles.

Although not contracted as intensely, the triceps brachii and anterior deltoid are also used.

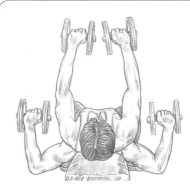

**VARIATION
EXECUTING THE EXERCISE
WITHOUT ROTATING THE FOREARMS**

CHEST

9 DUMBBELL FLYS

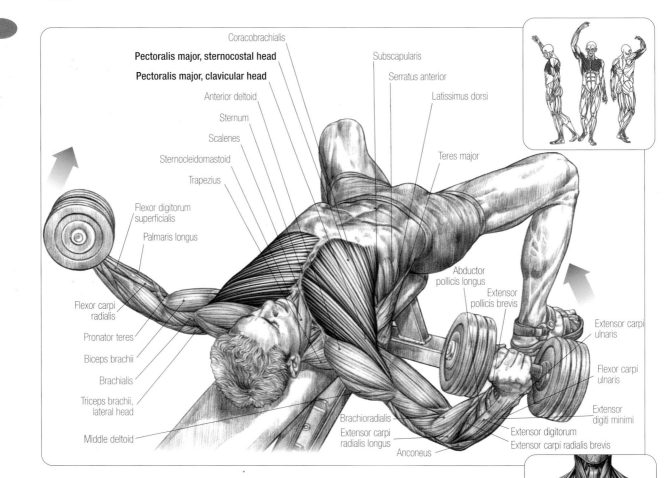

- Coracobrachialis
- **Pectoralis major, sternocostal head**
- **Pectoralis major, clavicular head**
- Anterior deltoid
- Sternum
- Scalenes
- Sternocleidomastoid
- Trapezius
- Flexor digitorum superficialis
- Palmaris longus
- Flexor carpi radialis
- Pronator teres
- Biceps brachii
- Brachialis
- Triceps brachii, lateral head
- Middle deltoid
- Subscapularis
- Serratus anterior
- Latissimus dorsi
- Teres major
- Abductor pollicis longus
- Extensor pollicis brevis
- Extensor carpi ulnaris
- Flexor carpi ulnaris
- Extensor digiti minimi
- Extensor digitorum
- Extensor carpi radialis brevis
- Brachioradialis
- Extensor carpi radialis longus
- Anconeus

Lie on a narrow bench that won't interfere with the shoulder movement and hold a dumbbell in each hand with arms extended or slightly bent to relieve stress on the joint:

- Inhale and open the arms to horizontal.
- Raise the arms to vertical while exhaling.
- Perform a small isometric contraction at the end of the movement to emphasize the work on the sternal head of the pectoralis major.

This exercise is never performed with heavy weights.

This exercise focuses the work on the pectoralis major. It serves as a basic exercise to increase thoracic expansion, which contributes to increased pulmonary capacity. It also develops muscle flexibility.

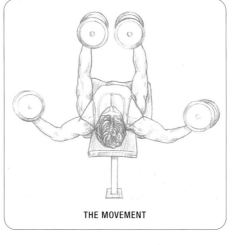

THE MOVEMENT

PART OF THE PECTORAL MUSCLES MAINLY USED

 Attention: To avoid the risk of tearing the pectoral muscles, perform the exercise with extreme caution when using heavier weights.

INCLINE DUMBBELL PRESSES 10

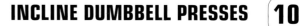

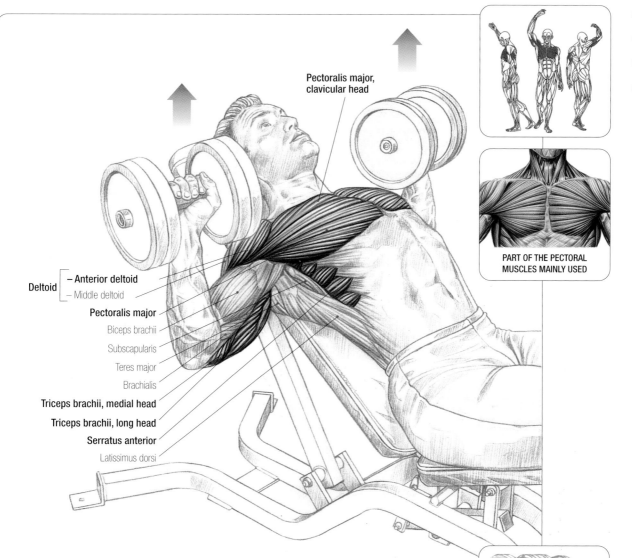

Pectoralis major, clavicular head

Deltoid
— Anterior deltoid
— Middle deltoid

Pectoralis major

Biceps brachii

Subscapularis

Teres major

Brachialis

Triceps brachii, medial head

Triceps brachii, long head

Serratus anterior

Latissimus dorsi

PART OF THE PECTORAL MUSCLES MAINLY USED

Sit on a bench with an angle of no more than 60 degrees (to prevent too much work with the deltoid), with elbows bent. Grasp the dumbbells with an overhand grip:

- Inhale and extend the arms vertically, bringing the dumbbells together.
- Exhale at the end of the movement.

This exercise, which is midway between an incline press and incline dumbbell fly, works the pectorals (mainly the clavicular head) and increases their flexibility. It also contracts the anterior deltoid, the serratus anterior, and the pectoralis minor (these last two muscles are fixators of the scapula, which stabilize the arm at the torso). It also uses the triceps brachii, but not as intensely as the barbell press does.

Variation: Beginning the press with the hands in an overhand grip and rotating the wrists halfway through the movement so that the dumbbells face each other focuses the effort on the sternal head of the pectoralis major.

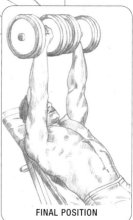

FINAL POSITION

11 INCLINE DUMBBELL FLYS

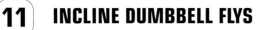

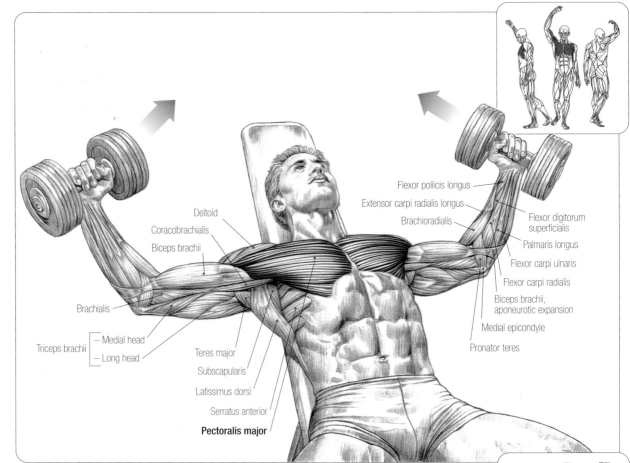

Deltoid
Coracobrachialis
Biceps brachii
Brachialis
Triceps brachii
— Medial head
— Long head
Teres major
Subscapularis
Latissimus dorsi
Serratus anterior
Pectoralis major

Flexor pollicis longus
Extensor carpi radialis longus
Brachioradialis
Flexor digitorum superficialis
Palmaris longus
Flexor carpi ulnaris
Flexor carpi radialis
Biceps brachii, aponeurotic expansion
Medial epicondyle
Pronator teres

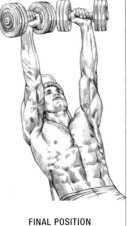

FINAL POSITION

Sit on a bench angled between 45 and 60 degrees, dumbbells in hand and arms extended vertically or slightly bent to ease stress when bringing the arms together:

• Inhale and extend the arms to horizontal.

• Raise the arms to vertical while exhaling.

This movement should not be performed with heavy weights. It focuses the effort mainly on the clavicular head of the pectoralis major. Along with the pullover, it is a fundamental exercise for developing thoracic expansion.

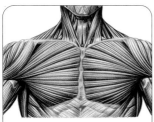

PART OF THE PECTORAL MUSCLES MAINLY USED

PEC DECK FLYS 12

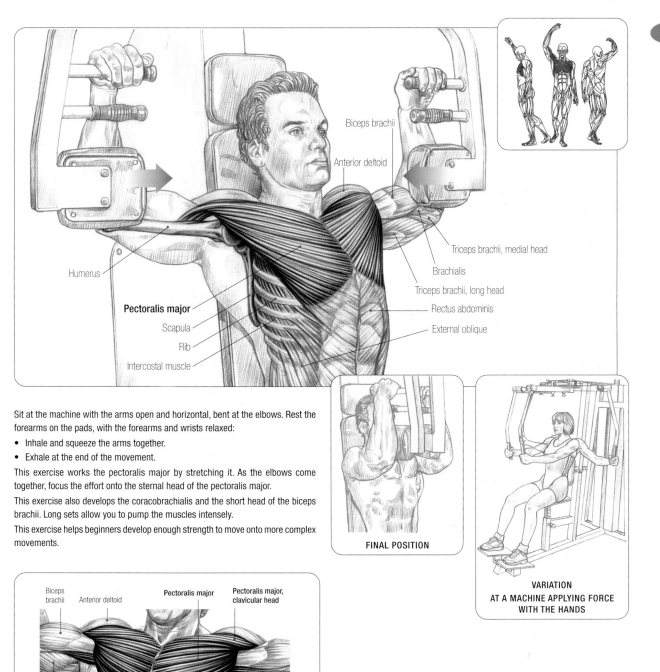

Biceps brachii

Anterior deltoid

Triceps brachii, medial head

Brachialis

Triceps brachii, long head

Rectus abdominis

External oblique

Humerus

Pectoralis major

Scapula

Rib

Intercostal muscle

Sit at the machine with the arms open and horizontal, bent at the elbows. Rest the forearms on the pads, with the forearms and wrists relaxed:

- Inhale and squeeze the arms together.
- Exhale at the end of the movement.

This exercise works the pectoralis major by stretching it. As the elbows come together, focus the effort onto the sternal head of the pectoralis major.

This exercise also develops the coracobrachialis and the short head of the biceps brachii. Long sets allow you to pump the muscles intensely.

This exercise helps beginners develop enough strength to move onto more complex movements.

FINAL POSITION

**VARIATION
AT A MACHINE APPLYING FORCE
WITH THE HANDS**

Biceps brachii

Anterior deltoid

Pectoralis major

Pectoralis major, clavicular head

Triceps brachii, long head

Coracobrachialis

Coracobrachialis

Teres major

Latissimus dorsi

Sternum

Serratus anterior

Subscapularis

13 CABLE CROSSOVER FLYS

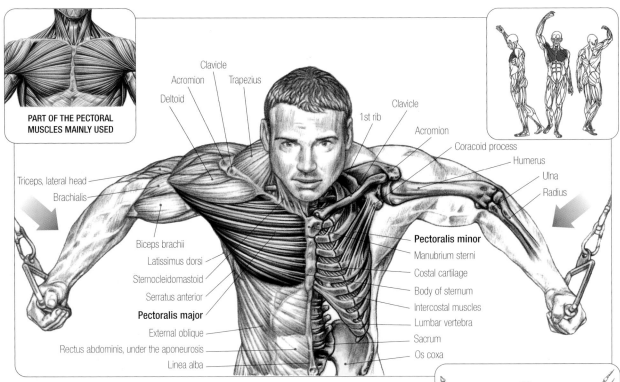

PART OF THE PECTORAL MUSCLES MAINLY USED

Clavicle
Acromion
Trapezius
Deltoid
Clavicle
1st rib
Acromion
Coracoid process
Humerus
Ulna
Radius
Triceps, lateral head
Brachialis
Biceps brachii
Latissimus dorsi
Sternocleidomastoid
Serratus anterior
Pectoralis major
External oblique
Rectus abdominis, under the aponeurosis
Linea alba
Pectoralis minor
Manubrium sterni
Costal cartilage
Body of sternum
Intercostal muscles
Lumbar vertebra
Sacrum
Os coxa

Stand with the legs slightly apart and lean the torso forward a bit, with the arms spread apart and elbows slightly bent:

- Inhale and squeeze the arms together until the wrists touch.
- Exhale at the end of the contraction.
- Return without jerking to the initial position and repeat.

This is an excellent exercise for working the pectoralis major muscles. Sets with a lot of reps allow you to pump the muscle well. You can work all the fibers of the pectoralis major by varying the angle of the chest and the working angle of the arms (squeezing the arms at various heights).

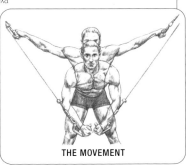

THE MOVEMENT

Comment: Cable crossover flys also contract the pectoralis minor, which is located deeper than the pectoralis major. Besides stabilizing the scapula (shoulder blade), this muscle also pulls it forward.

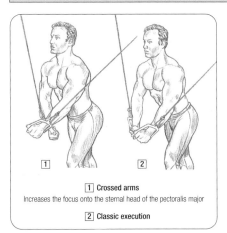

1 **Crossed arms**
Increases the focus onto the sternal head of the pectoralis major

2 **Classic execution**

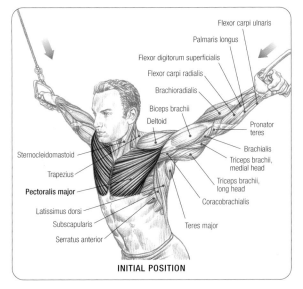

Flexor carpi ulnaris
Palmaris longus
Flexor digitorum superficialis
Flexor carpi radialis
Brachioradialis
Biceps brachii
Deltoid
Pronator teres
Brachialis
Triceps brachii, medial head
Triceps brachii, long head
Coracobrachialis
Teres major
Sternocleidomastoid
Trapezius
Pectoralis major
Latissimus dorsi
Subscapularis
Serratus anterior

INITIAL POSITION

DUMBBELL PULLOVERS 14

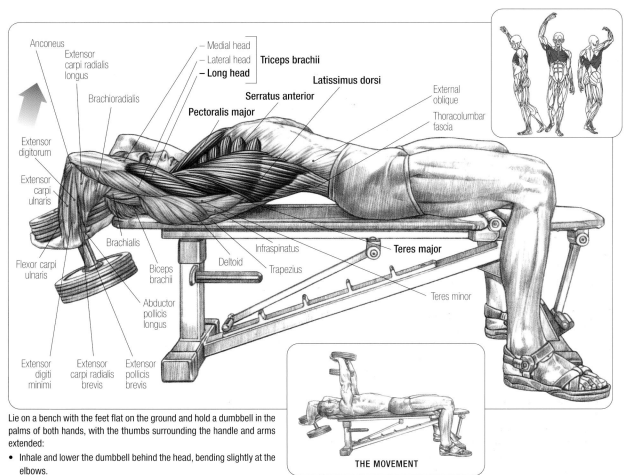

Anconeus
Extensor carpi radialis longus
Brachioradialis
Extensor digitorum
Extensor carpi ulnaris
Brachialis
Flexor carpi ulnaris
Biceps brachii
Abductor pollicis longus
Extensor digiti minimi
Extensor carpi radialis brevis
Extensor pollicis brevis

— Medial head
— Lateral head
— Long head
Triceps brachii
Pectoralis major
Serratus anterior
Latissimus dorsi
External oblique
Thoracolumbar fascia
Infraspinatus
Deltoid
Trapezius
Teres major
Teres minor

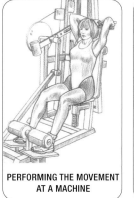

THE MOVEMENT

Lie on a bench with the feet flat on the ground and hold a dumbbell in the palms of both hands, with the thumbs surrounding the handle and arms extended:

- Inhale and lower the dumbbell behind the head, bending slightly at the elbows.
- Exhale and return to the initial position.

This exercise develops the bulk of the pectoralis major, long head of the triceps brachii, teres major, latissimus dorsi, serratus anterior, rhomboids, and pectoralis minor. The last three muscles stabilize the scapula so that the humerus can move from a stable base.

STABILIZERS OF THE SHOULDER BLADES

Cranium
Vertebra
Levator scapulae
Levator scapulae
Clavicle
Spine of scapula
Acromion
Rhomboid minor
Pectoralis minor
Sternum
Rhomboid major
Serratus anterior
Rib
Serratus anterior
Costal cartilage

BACK
FRONT

Trapezius

If you use this exercise to open the rib cage, you must work with light weights and avoid bending too much at the elbows. If possible, use a convex bench or place yourself across a horizontal bench and position the pelvis lower than the shoulder girdle. Take in a deep breath at the beginning of the movement and breathe out only at the end of the execution.

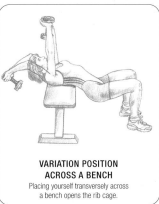

PERFORMING THE MOVEMENT AT A MACHINE

VARIATION POSITION ACROSS A BENCH
Placing yourself transversely across a bench opens the rib cage.

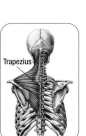

15 BARBELL PULLOVERS

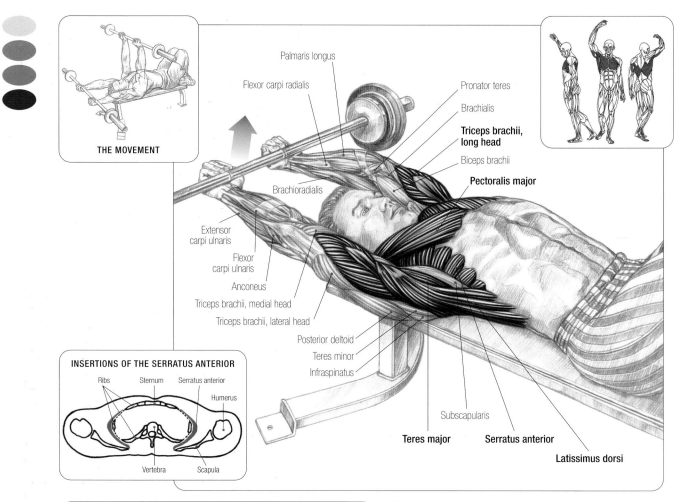

THE MOVEMENT

Palmaris longus

Flexor carpi radialis

Pronator teres

Brachialis

Triceps brachii, long head

Biceps brachii

Pectoralis major

Brachioradialis

Extensor carpi ulnaris

Flexor carpi ulnaris

Anconeus

Triceps brachii, medial head

Triceps brachii, lateral head

Posterior deltoid

Teres minor

Infraspinatus

Subscapularis

Teres major   **Serratus anterior**

Latissimus dorsi

INSERTIONS OF THE SERRATUS ANTERIOR

Ribs   Sternum   Serratus anterior

Humerus

Vertebra   Scapula

SERRATUS ANTERIOR MUSCLE

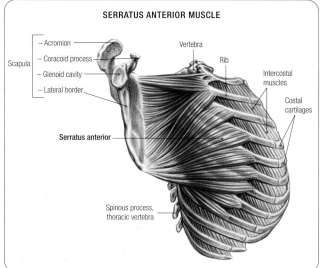

Scapula
– Acromion
– Coracoid process
– Glenoid cavity
– Lateral border

Vertebra

Rib

Intercostal muscles

Costal cartilages

Serratus anterior

Spinous process, thoracic vertebra

With arms extended, hold the barbell with an overhand grip and hands shoulder-width apart:

- Inhale and expand the chest as much as possible, lowering the barbell behind the head while bending slightly at the elbows.
- Exhale while returning to the initial position.

This exercise develops the pectoralis major, long head of the triceps brachii, teres major, latissimus dorsi, serratus anterior, rhomboids, and pectoralis minor.

This is an excellent movement for developing the flexibility and expansion of the rib cage. It should be performed with light weights using proper form and breathing.

4
BACK

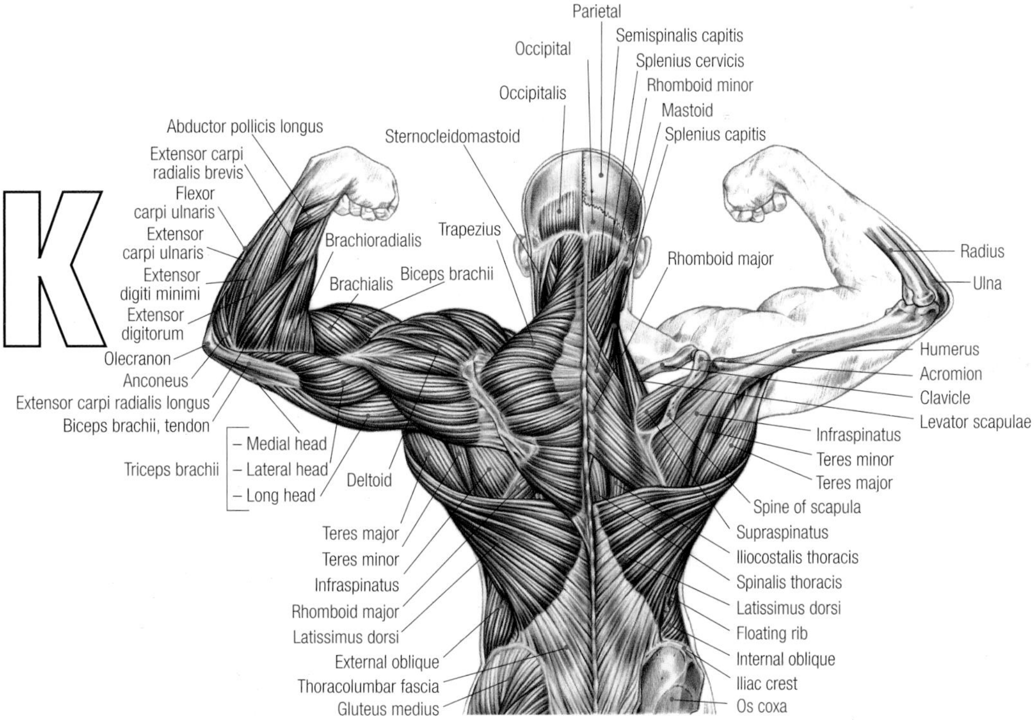

Parietal
Occipital
Semispinalis capitis
Occipitalis
Splenius cervicis
Rhomboid minor
Mastoid
Splenius capitis
Abductor pollicis longus
Sternocleidomastoid
Extensor carpi radialis brevis
Flexor carpi ulnaris
Trapezius
Rhomboid major
Extensor carpi ulnaris
Brachioradialis
Biceps brachii
Radius
Extensor digiti minimi
Brachialis
Ulna
Extensor digitorum
Humerus
Olecranon
Acromion
Anconeus
Clavicle
Extensor carpi radialis longus
Levator scapulae
Biceps brachii, tendon
Infraspinatus
Teres minor
– Medial head
Teres major
Triceps brachii
– Lateral head
Spine of scapula
– Long head
Deltoid
Supraspinatus
Teres major
Iliocostalis thoracis
Teres minor
Spinalis thoracis
Infraspinatus
Latissimus dorsi
Rhomboid major
Floating rib
Latissimus dorsi
Internal oblique
External oblique
Iliac crest
Thoracolumbar fascia
Os coxa
Gluteus medius

1 CHIN-UPS

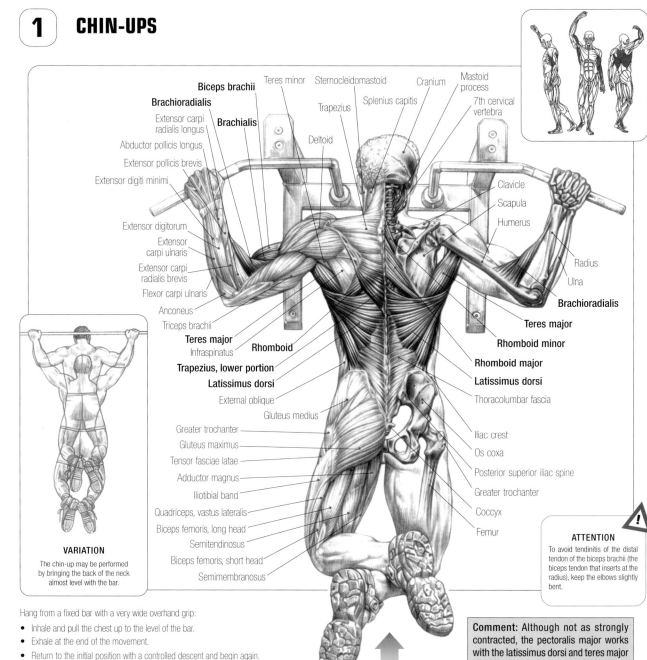

Biceps brachii
Brachioradialis
Extensor carpi
radialis longus
Brachialis
Abductor pollicis longus
Extensor pollicis brevis
Extensor digiti minimi
Extensor digitorum
Extensor
carpi ulnaris
Extensor carpi
radialis brevis
Flexor carpi ulnaris
Anconeus
Triceps brachii
Teres major
Infraspinatus
Rhomboid
Trapezius, lower portion
Latissimus dorsi
External oblique
Gluteus medius
Greater trochanter
Gluteus maximus
Tensor fasciae latae
Adductor magnus
Iliotibial band
Quadriceps, vastus lateralis
Biceps femoris, long head
Semitendinosus
Biceps femoris, short head
Semimembranosus

Teres minor
Sternocleidomastoid
Trapezius
Splenius capitis
Deltoid
Cranium
Mastoid
process
7th cervical
vertebra
Clavicle
Scapula
Humerus
Radius
Ulna
Brachioradialis
Teres major
Rhomboid minor
Rhomboid major
Latissimus dorsi
Thoracolumbar fascia
Iliac crest
Os coxa
Posterior superior iliac spine
Greater trochanter
Coccyx
Femur

VARIATION

The chin-up may be performed
by bringing the back of the neck
almost level with the bar.

⚠ ATTENTION

To avoid tendinitis of the distal
tendon of the biceps brachii (the
biceps tendon that inserts at the
radius), keep the elbows slightly
bent.

Hang from a fixed bar with a very wide overhand grip:

- Inhale and pull the chest up to the level of the bar.
- Exhale at the end of the movement.
- Return to the initial position with a controlled descent and begin again.

This exercise takes a certain amount of strength and is excellent for developing the latissimus dorsi and teres major and, when the shoulder blades come together at the top of the chin-up, the rhomboids and middle and lower portions of the trapezius. It also works the biceps brachii, brachialis, and brachioradialis.

Comment: Although not as strongly contracted, the pectoralis major works with the latissimus dorsi and teres major to create the angle between the arm and the trunk.

Variations: If you stick out your chest, you can pull yourself up so the bar touches your chin. To increase the intensity, wear a weight belt. Keeping the elbows in next to the body during the movement contracts mainly the lateral fibers of the latissimus dorsi and develops the width of the back.

Bringing the elbows back and the chest out as you raise the chin to the bar mainly solicits the upper and central fibers of the latissimus dorsi and those of the teres major. This exercise develops the bulk of the back when the shoulder blades come together and the rhomboids and the upper and lower portions of the trapezius are used equally.

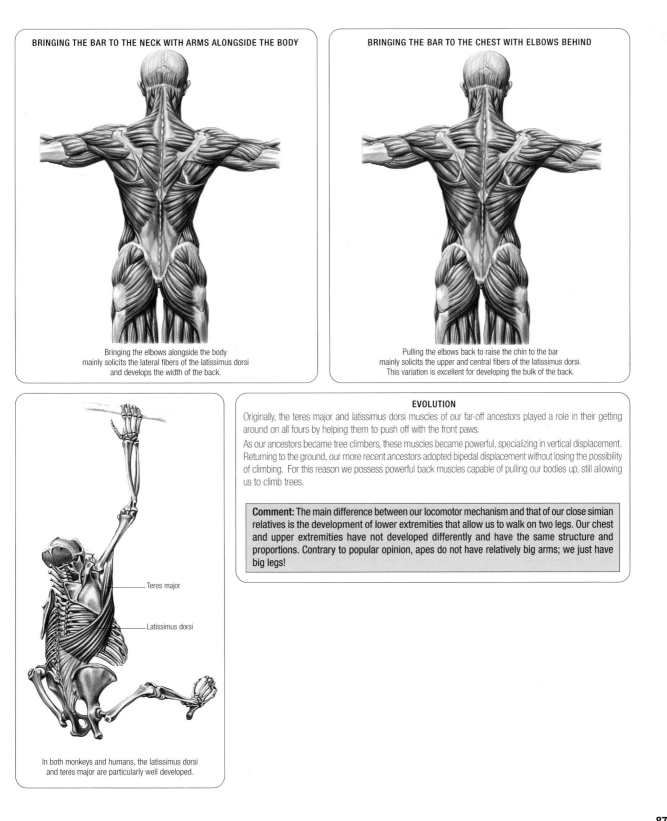

BRINGING THE BAR TO THE NECK WITH ARMS ALONGSIDE THE BODY

Bringing the elbows alongside the body
mainly solicits the lateral fibers of the latissimus dorsi
and develops the width of the back.

BRINGING THE BAR TO THE CHEST WITH ELBOWS BEHIND

Pulling the elbows back to raise the chin to the bar
mainly solicits the upper and central fibers of the latissimus dorsi.
This variation is excellent for developing the bulk of the back.

Teres major

Latissimus dorsi

In both monkeys and humans, the latissimus dorsi
and teres major are particularly well developed.

EVOLUTION

Originally, the teres major and latissimus dorsi muscles of our far-off ancestors played a role in their getting around on all fours by helping them to push off with the front paws.

As our ancestors became tree climbers, these muscles became powerful, specializing in vertical displacement. Returning to the ground, our more recent ancestors adopted bipedal displacement without losing the possibility of climbing. For this reason we possess powerful back muscles capable of pulling our bodies up, still allowing us to climb trees.

Comment: The main difference between our locomotor mechanism and that of our close simian relatives is the development of lower extremities that allow us to walk on two legs. Our chest and upper extremities have not developed differently and have the same structure and proportions. Contrary to popular opinion, apes do not have relatively big arms; we just have big legs!

2 REVERSE CHIN-UPS

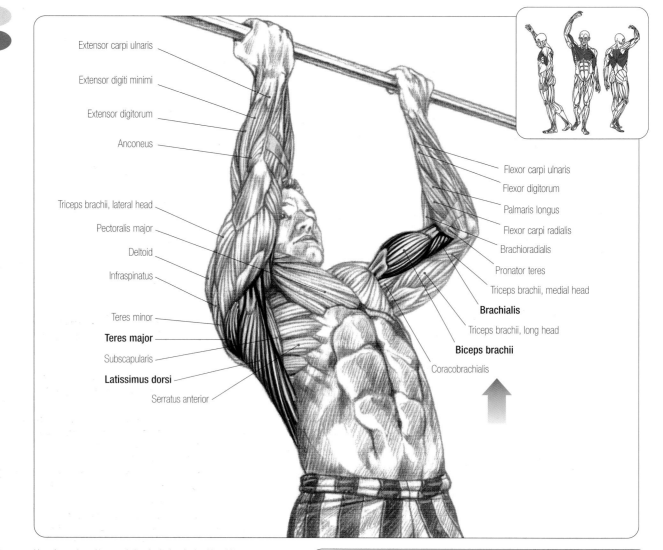

Extensor carpi ulnaris

Extensor digiti minimi

Extensor digitorum

Anconeus

Triceps brachii, lateral head

Pectoralis major

Deltoid

Infraspinatus

Teres minor

Teres major

Subscapularis

Latissimus dorsi

Serratus anterior

Flexor carpi ulnaris

Flexor digitorum

Palmaris longus

Flexor carpi radialis

Brachioradialis

Pronator teres

Triceps brachii, medial head

Brachialis

Triceps brachii, long head

Biceps brachii

Coracobrachialis

Hang from a bar with an underhand grip, hands shoulder-width apart:

- Inhale and push out the chest as you raise the chin to the bar.
- Exhale at the end of the movement.

This movement develops the latissimus dorsi and teres major and is associated with the intense work of the biceps brachii and brachialis.

Therefore, it could be included in an arm workout program.

This exercise also contracts the middle and lower portions of the trapezius, the rhomboids, and the pectorals.

Performing this exercise takes a certain amount of strength; use a high pulley to make it easier.

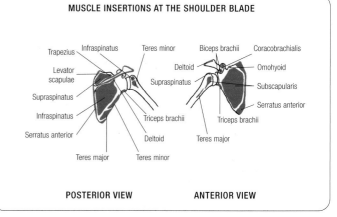

MUSCLE INSERTIONS AT THE SHOULDER BLADE

Trapezius

Infraspinatus

Teres minor

Biceps brachii

Coracobrachialis

Levator scapulae

Deltoid

Omohyoid

Supraspinatus

Subscapularis

Supraspinatus

Infraspinatus

Serratus anterior

Serratus anterior

Triceps brachii

Triceps brachii

Teres major

Teres major

Teres minor

Deltoid

POSTERIOR VIEW

ANTERIOR VIEW

STRETCHING THE LATISSIMUS DORSI AND TERES MAJOR

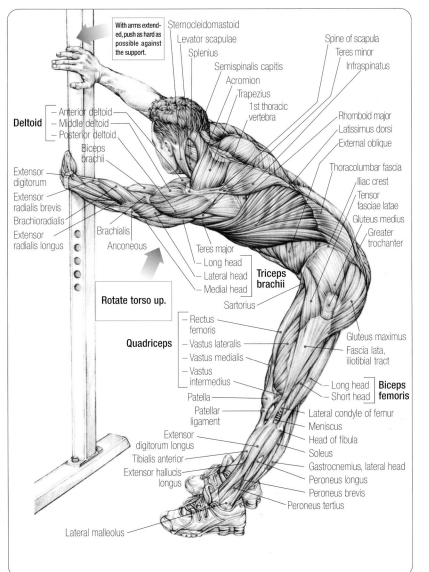

With arms extended, push as hard as possible against the support.

Sternocleidomastoid
Levator scapulae
Splenius
Semispinalis capitis
Acromion
Trapezius
1st thoracic vertebra

Spine of scapula
Teres minor
Infraspinatus

Rhomboid major
Latissimus dorsi
External oblique

Thoracolumbar fascia
Iliac crest
Tensor fasciae latae
Gluteus medius
Greater trochanter

Deltoid
— Anterior deltoid
— Middle deltoid
— Posterior deltoid

Biceps brachii

Extensor digitorum
Extensor radialis brevis
Brachioradialis
Extensor radialis longus

Brachialis
Anconeous

Teres major
— Long head
— Lateral head
— Medial head

Triceps brachii

Sartorius

Rotate torso up.

Quadriceps
— Rectus femoris
— Vastus lateralis
— Vastus medialis
— Vastus intermedius

Patella
Patellar ligament
Extensor digitorum longus
Tibialis anterior
Extensor hallucis longus

Lateral malleolus

Gluteus maximus
Fascia lata, iliotibial tract

— Long head
— Short head

Biceps femoris

Lateral condyle of femur
Meniscus
Head of fibula
Soleus
Gastrocnemius, lateral head
Peroneus longus
Peroneus brevis
Peroneus tertius

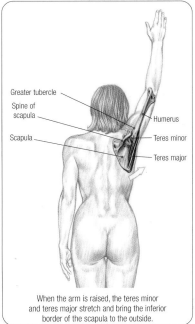

Greater tubercle
Spine of scapula
Scapula

Humerus
Teres minor
Teres major

When the arm is raised, the teres minor and teres major stretch and bring the inferior border of the scapula to the outside.

Stand with your legs slightly apart:

- Lean forward with the chest. With the arm extended, grasp a stable support such as a weightlifting machine or the frame of a squat cage.

- Place the palm of the other hand higher up on the support. With the arm extended, apply an increasingly powerful push against the machine while at the same time pulling with the other arm.

To accentuate the stretch of the latissimus dorsi and teres major, rotate the chest while trying to slowly raise the other shoulder.

When practiced regularly and incorporated into the first series of back-specific training, this stretch helps prevent tearing of the latissimus dorsi and teres major, which can occur during the execution of heavyweight pulls at the high pulley or tractions at the fixed bar with weight.

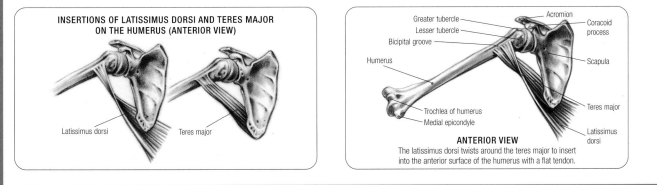

INSERTIONS OF LATISSIMUS DORSI AND TERES MAJOR ON THE HUMERUS (ANTERIOR VIEW)

Latissimus dorsi

Teres major

Greater tubercle
Lesser tubercle
Bicipital groove
Humerus

Acromion
Coracoid process
Scapula

Trochlea of humerus
Medial epicondyle

Teres major
Latissimus dorsi

ANTERIOR VIEW
The latissimus dorsi twists around the teres major to insert into the anterior surface of the humerus with a flat tendon.

3 LAT PULL-DOWNS

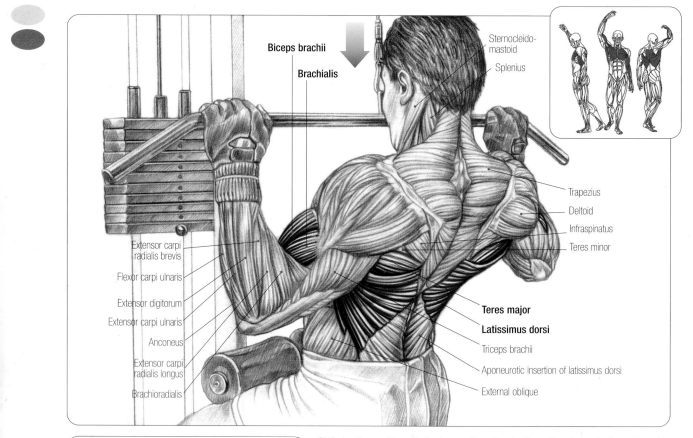

Biceps brachii

Brachialis

Sternocleido-mastoid

Splenius

Trapezius

Deltoid

Infraspinatus

Teres minor

Extensor carpi radialis brevis

Flexor carpi ulnaris

Extensor digitorum

Extensor carpi ulnaris

Anconeus

Extensor carpi radialis longus

Brachioradialis

Teres major

Latissimus dorsi

Triceps brachii

Aponeurotic insertion of latissimus dorsi

External oblique

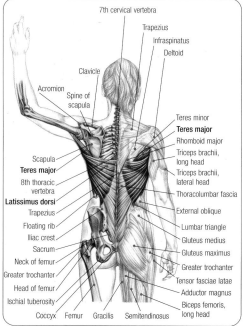

7th cervical vertebra

Trapezius

Infraspinatus

Deltoid

Clavicle

Acromion

Spine of scapula

Scapula

Teres major

8th thoracic vertebra

Latissimus dorsi

Trapezius

Floating rib

Iliac crest

Sacrum

Neck of femur

Greater trochanter

Head of femur

Ischial tuberosity

Coccyx Femur Gracilis Semitendinosus

Teres minor

Teres major

Rhomboid major

Triceps brachii, long head

Triceps brachii, lateral head

Thoracolumbar fascia

External oblique

Lumbar triangle

Gluteus medius

Gluteus maximus

Greater trochanter

Tensor fasciae latae

Adductor magnus

Biceps femoris, long head

Sit facing the machine with the legs positioned under the pads, gripping the bar with a wide overhand grip: Inhale and pull the bar down to the sternal notch while puffing out the chest and pulling the elbows back. Exhale at the end of the movement.

This exercise develops the bulk of the back. It mainly works the upper and central fibers of the latissimus dorsi. The middle and lower portions of the trapezius, the rhomboids, the biceps brachii, the brachialis, and, to a lesser extent, the pectorals also contract.

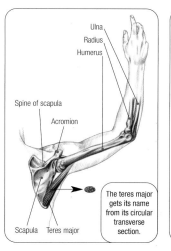

Ulna

Radius

Humerus

Spine of scapula

Acromion

Scapula Teres major

The teres major gets its name from its circular transverse section.

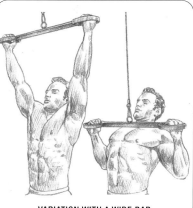

VARIATION WITH A WIDE BAR AND PALMS FACING EACH OTHER

BACK LAT PULL-DOWNS 4

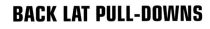

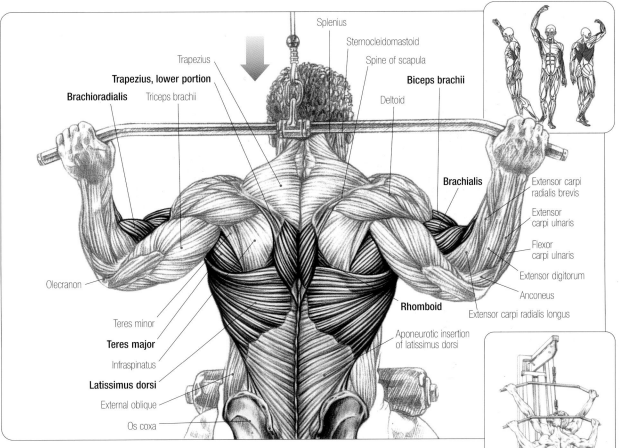

Splenius
Sternocleidomastoid
Spine of scapula
Trapezius
Trapezius, lower portion
Brachioradialis
Triceps brachii
Biceps brachii
Deltoid
Brachialis
Extensor carpi radialis brevis
Extensor carpi ulnaris
Flexor carpi ulnaris
Extensor digitorum
Anconeus
Extensor carpi radialis longus
Rhomboid
Aponeurotic insertion of latissimus dorsi
Olecranon
Teres minor
Teres major
Infraspinatus
Latissimus dorsi
External oblique
Os coxa

ACTION OF TERES MAJOR AND LATISSIMUS DORSI

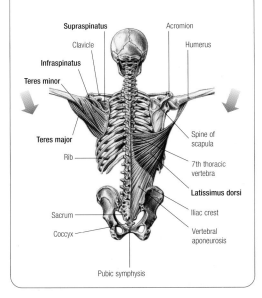

Supraspinatus
Acromion
Clavicle
Humerus
Infraspinatus
Teres minor
Spine of scapula
7th thoracic vertebra
Teres major
Rib
Sacrum
Latissimus dorsi
Iliac crest
Coccyx
Vertebral aponeurosis
Pubic symphysis

Sit facing the machine with the thighs positioned under the pads. Grasp the bar with a wide overhand grip:

- Inhale and pull the bar down to the back of the neck, bringing the elbows alongside the body.
- Exhale at the end of the movement.

This exercise develops the width of the back. It works the latissimus dorsi (mainly the lateral and lower fibers), the teres major, the forearm flexors (biceps brachii, brachialis, and brachioradialis), the rhomboids, and the lower portion of the trapezius. The latter two muscles come into play when the shoulder blades are pulled together. Back lat pull-downs help beginners develop enough strength to move on to chin-ups.

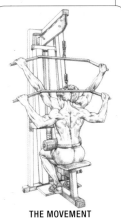

THE MOVEMENT

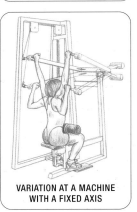

VARIATION AT A MACHINE WITH A FIXED AXIS

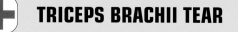

TRICEPS BRACHII TEAR

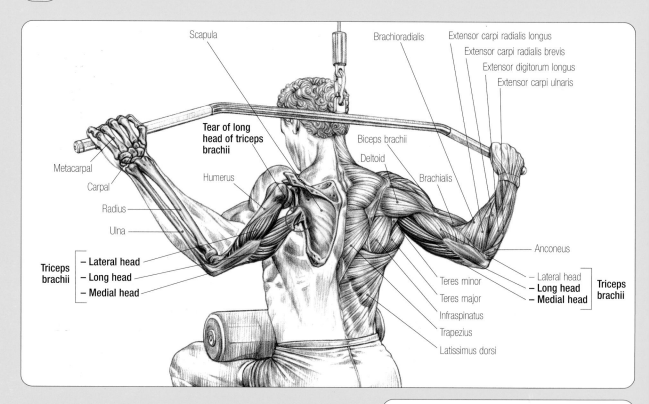

Scapula

Brachioradialis

Extensor carpi radialis longus

Extensor carpi radialis brevis

Extensor digitorum longus

Extensor carpi ulnaris

Tear of long head of triceps brachii

Biceps brachii

Deltoid

Brachialis

Metacarpal

Carpal

Humerus

Radius

Ulna

Triceps brachii
— Lateral head
— Long head
— Medial head

Anconeus

— Lateral head
— Long head
— Medial head

Triceps brachii

Teres minor

Teres major

Infraspinatus

Trapezius

Latissimus dorsi

Although it is not the most-used muscle when working the back, the long head of the triceps brachii is the most frequently injured muscle during back lat pull-downs with heavy weights or during chin-ups with added weight.

The latissimus dorsi is a powerful, fan-shaped muscle that attaches the arm to the rib cage, and whose distal tendon is strongly attached to the humerus.

This is the main climbing muscle.

The long head of the triceps brachii, on the other hand, is a smaller muscle whose main function is to extend the forearm and secondarily to bring the arm toward the rib cage. In this way it complements the action of the latissimus dorsi.

Tearing of the long head of the triceps occurs when the muscle is fatigued, most frequently after an improper warm-up.

It only takes a sudden relaxation of the latissimus dorsi during chin-ups with added weight to immediately shift the tension to the long head of the triceps.

This tendon may partially tear, most often close to its insertion on the scapula. (Fortunately complete tears are infrequent.)

Unlike incapacitating shoulder injuries, which may completely halt upper-body training, a tear in the long head of the triceps is less devastating.

You can still perform back exercises such as seated rows or T-bar rows and movements for the triceps such as forearm extensions at a high pulley with the elbows next to the body despite the injury as long as you begin with lighter weights.

However, a brief rest period is recommended before beginning upper-body training.

Comment: Tearing the long head of the triceps may also occur during bench presses. To prevent this triceps tear, warm up with stretching exercises (see page 31).

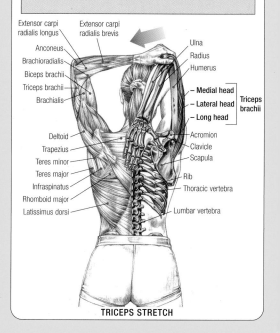

Extensor carpi radialis longus

Extensor carpi radialis brevis

Anconeus

Brachioradialis

Biceps brachii

Triceps brachii

Brachialis

Ulna

Radius

Humerus

— Medial head
— Lateral head
— Long head

Triceps brachii

Deltoid

Trapezius

Teres minor

Teres major

Infraspinatus

Rhomboid major

Latissimus dorsi

Acromion

Clavicle

Scapula

Rib

Thoracic vertebra

Lumbar vertebra

TRICEPS STRETCH

CLOSE-GRIP LAT PULL-DOWNS   5

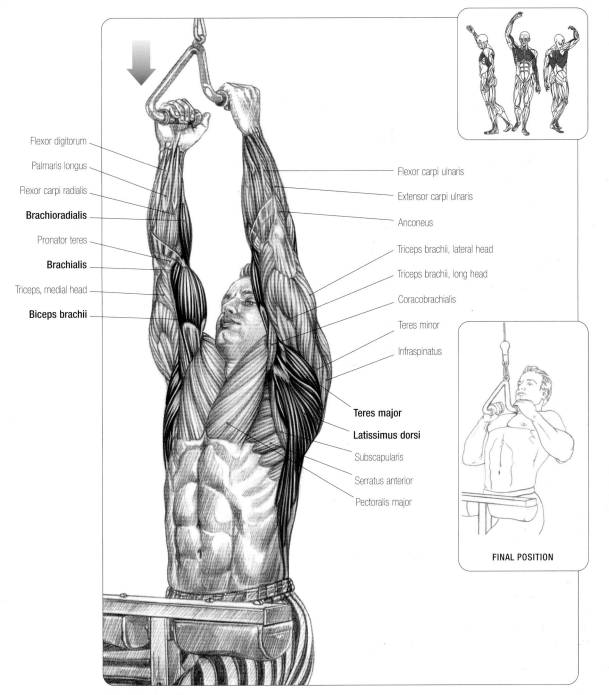

Flexor digitorum

Palmaris longus

Flexor carpi radialis

Brachioradialis

Pronator teres

Brachialis

Triceps, medial head

Biceps brachii

Flexor carpi ulnaris

Extensor carpi ulnaris

Anconeus

Triceps brachii, lateral head

Triceps brachii, long head

Coracobrachialis

Teres minor

Infraspinatus

Teres major

Latissimus dorsi

Subscapularis

Serratus anterior

Pectoralis major

FINAL POSITION

Sit and face the machine with knees positioned under the pads:

• Inhale and bring the handle to the sternum while expanding the chest and leaning slightly back with the torso.

• Exhale at the end of the movement.

This exercise develops the latissimus dorsi and teres major.

When the shoulder blades come together, the trapezius and the posterior deltoid contract.

As with every pulling exercise, the biceps brachii and brachialis contract, and when the palms face each other, the brachioradialis comes into play.

6 SEATED ROWS

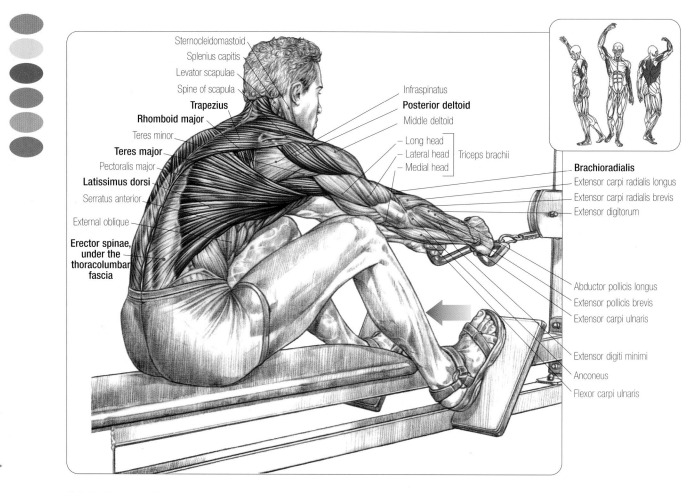

Sternocleidomastoid
Splenius capitis
Levator scapulae
Spine of scapula
Trapezius
Rhomboid major
Teres minor
Teres major
Pectoralis major
Latissimus dorsi
Serratus anterior
External oblique
**Erector spinae,
under the
thoracolumbar
fascia**

Infraspinatus
Posterior deltoid
Middle deltoid
– Long head
– Lateral head Triceps brachii
– Medial head

Brachioradialis
Extensor carpi radialis longus
Extensor carpi radialis brevis
Extensor digitorum

Abductor pollicis longus
Extensor pollicis brevis
Extensor carpi ulnaris

Extensor digiti minimi
Anconeus
Flexor carpi ulnaris

Sit facing the machine, feet resting on the foot pad and the torso bent forward:
- Inhale and bring the handle to the base of the sternum by straightening the back and pulling the elbows back as far as possible.
- Exhale at the end of the movement and return smoothly to the initial position.

This exercise works the bulk of the back. It focuses the effort on the latissimus dorsi, teres major, posterior deltoid, biceps brachii, and brachioradialis, and, at the end of the movement when the shoulder blades come together, the trapezius and rhomboids.

While raising the chest, the spinal muscles (erector spinae) also contribute.

Allowing the weight to pull you on the return helps develop back flexibility.

Attention: To prevent back injury, never round the back when performing seated rows with heavy weights. ⚠

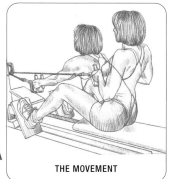

THE MOVEMENT

WIDE GRIP SEATED ROWS | 7

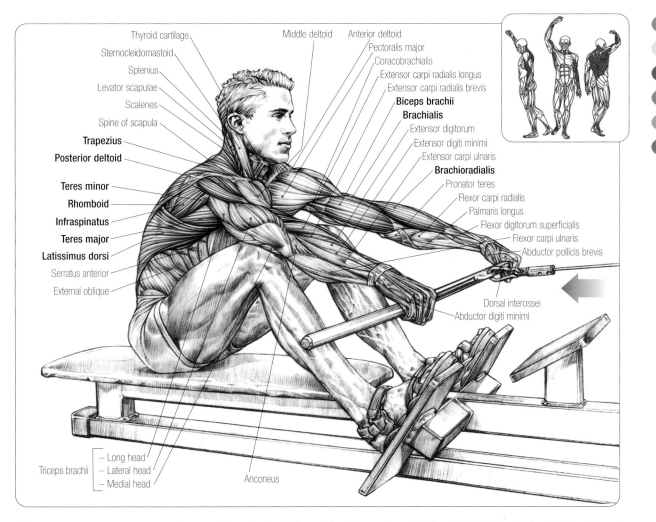

Thyroid cartilage
Sternocleidomastoid
Splenius
Levator scapulae
Scalenes
Spine of scapula
Trapezius
Posterior deltoid
Teres minor
Rhomboid
Infraspinatus
Teres major
Latissimus dorsi
Serratus anterior
External oblique

Triceps brachii
 – Long head
 – Lateral head
 – Medial head

Anconeus

Middle deltoid

Anterior deltoid
Pectoralis major
Coracobrachialis
Extensor carpi radialis longus
Extensor carpi radialis brevis
Biceps brachii
Brachialis
Extensor digitorum
Extensor digiti minimi
Extensor carpi ulnaris
Brachioradialis
Pronator teres
Flexor carpi radialis
Palmaris longus
Flexor digitorum superficialis
Flexor carpi ulnaris
Abductor pollicis brevis
Dorsal interossei
Abductor digiti minimi

Sit facing the machine with your feet on the foot pads and your chest flexed. Grasp the bar with an overhand grip (thumbs to the inside) wider than shoulder-width apart:

- Inhale and pull the bar to your chest, straightening the back and keeping your elbows raised.
- Exhale at the end of the movement and return smoothly to the initial position.

This is an excellent exercise for working the upper back behind the shoulders. The main muscles worked are the latissimus dorsi, teres major, posterior deltoid, infraspinatus, teres minor, arm flexors (biceps brachii, brachialis, brachioradialis), and, with the approximation of the shoulder blades, the rhomboids and the middle part of the trapezius. During the straightening of the chest, the erector spinae are also recruited.

Variation: Hold the bar in an underhand position (thumbs to the outside) to work the inferior part of the trapezius, rhomboids, and biceps brachii.

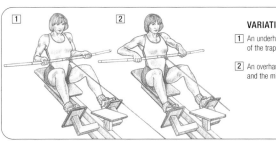

VARIATIONS WITH A WIDE GRIP

1 An underhand grip isolates the inferior portion of the trapezius.

2 An overhand grip isolates the posterior deltoid and the middle portion of the trapezius.

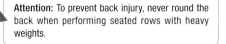

Attention: To prevent back injury, never round the back when performing seated rows with heavy weights.

8 STRAIGHT-ARM LAT PULL-DOWNS

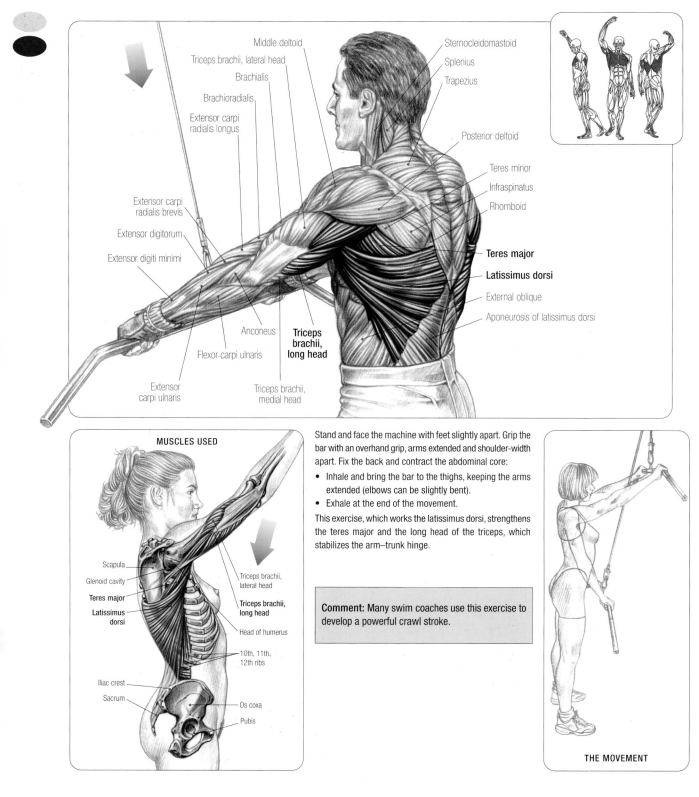

Middle deltoid

Triceps brachii, lateral head

Brachialis

Brachioradialis

Extensor carpi
radialis longus

Sternocleidomastoid

Splenius

Trapezius

Posterior deltoid

Teres minor

Infraspinatus

Rhomboid

Teres major

Latissimus dorsi

External oblique

Aponeurosis of latissimus dorsi

Extensor carpi
radialis brevis

Extensor digitorum

Extensor digiti minimi

Anconeus

Flexor carpi ulnaris

**Triceps
brachii,
long head**

Extensor
carpi ulnaris

Triceps brachii,
medial head

MUSCLES USED

Scapula

Glenoid cavity

Teres major

**Latissimus
dorsi**

Triceps brachii,
lateral head

**Triceps brachii,
long head**

Head of humerus

10th, 11th,
12th ribs

Iliac crest

Sacrum

Os coxa

Pubis

Stand and face the machine with feet slightly apart. Grip the bar with an overhand grip, arms extended and shoulder-width apart. Fix the back and contract the abdominal core:
- Inhale and bring the bar to the thighs, keeping the arms extended (elbows can be slightly bent).
- Exhale at the end of the movement.

This exercise, which works the latissimus dorsi, strengthens the teres major and the long head of the triceps, which stabilizes the arm–trunk hinge.

Comment: Many swim coaches use this exercise to develop a powerful crawl stroke.

THE MOVEMENT

ONE-ARM DUMBBELL ROWS 9

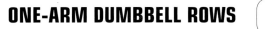

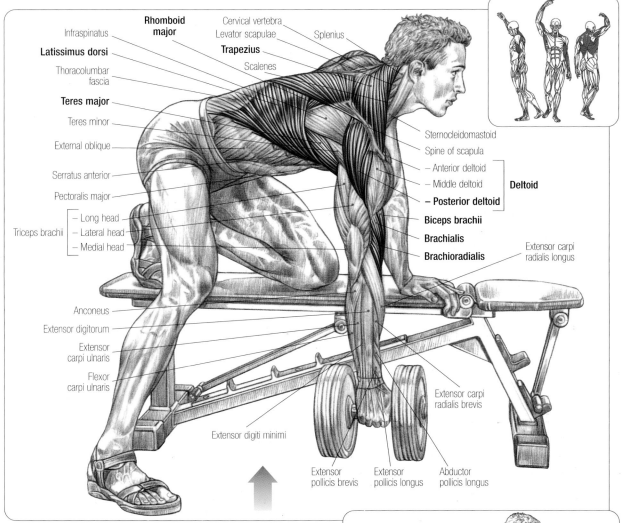

Infraspinatus

Rhomboid major

Cervical vertebra

Levator scapulae

Splenius

Latissimus dorsi

Trapezius

Scalenes

Thoracolumbar fascia

Teres major

Teres minor

External oblique

Serratus anterior

Pectoralis major

Triceps brachii
— Long head
— Lateral head
— Medial head

Sternocleidomastoid

Spine of scapula

— Anterior deltoid

— Middle deltoid

— Posterior deltoid

Deltoid

Biceps brachii

Brachialis

Brachioradialis

Extensor carpi radialis longus

Anconeus

Extensor digitorum

Extensor carpi ulnaris

Flexor carpi ulnaris

Extensor carpi radialis brevis

Extensor digiti minimi

Extensor pollicis brevis

Extensor pollicis longus

Abductor pollicis longus

Grasp a barbell with the palm facing in; use the opposite hand and knee on the bench to support the back:

- Inhale and lift the upper arm and elbow as high as possible next to the body with the elbow bent.
- Exhale at the end of the movement.

To maximize the contraction, rotate the torso slightly toward the working side at the end of the row.

This exercise mainly works the latissimus dorsi, teres major, and posterior deltoid, and, at the end of the contraction, the trapezius and rhomboids. The forearm flexors (biceps brachii, brachialis, and brachioradialis) are also used.

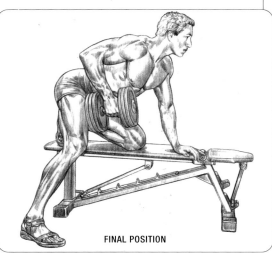

FINAL POSITION

10 DUMBBELL ROWS

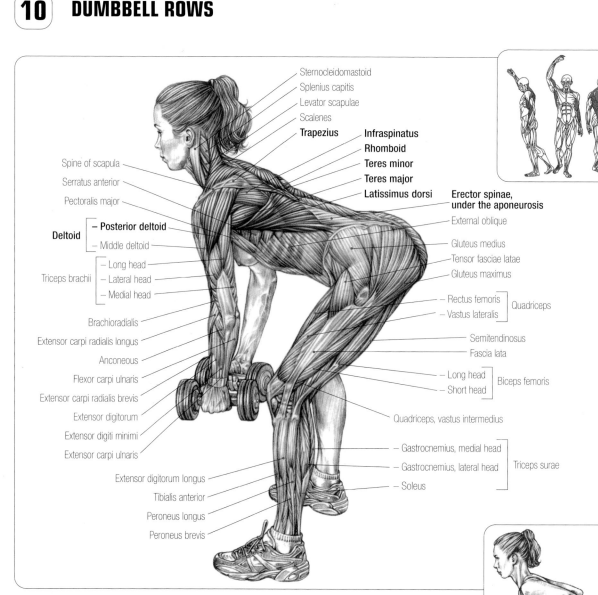

Sternocleidomastoid
Splenius capitis
Levator scapulae
Scalenes
Trapezius
Infraspinatus
Rhomboid
Teres minor
Teres major
Latissimus dorsi
Erector spinae, under the aponeurosis
Spine of scapula
Serratus anterior
Pectoralis major
Deltoid — Posterior deltoid
— Middle deltoid
External oblique
Gluteus medius
Tensor fasciae latae
Gluteus maximus
Triceps brachii — Long head
— Lateral head
— Medial head
— Rectus femoris
— Vastus lateralis
Quadriceps
Brachioradialis
Extensor carpi radialis longus
Anconeous
Flexor carpi ulnaris
Extensor carpi radialis brevis
Extensor digitorum
Extensor digiti minimi
Extensor carpi ulnaris
Semitendinosus
Fascia lata
— Long head
— Short head
Biceps femoris
Quadriceps, vastus intermedius
— Gastrocnemius, medial head
— Gastrocnemius, lateral head
— Soleus
Triceps surae
Extensor digitorum longus
Tibialis anterior
Peroneus longus
Peroneus brevis

Stand with the legs slightly bent and the chest leaning forward at approximately a 45-degree angle. Keep your back very flat and hang your arms by your sides; hold a dumbbell in each hand with an overhand grip, palms facing inward:

- Inhale and isometrically contract the abdominal core. Pull the dumbbells as high as possible, keeping the elbows close to the body. Squeeze the shoulder blades together at the end of the movement.
- Return to the initial position and exhale.

This exercise recruits the latissimus dorsi, teres major, posterior deltoid, forearm flexors (biceps brachii, brachialis, brachioradialis), and, with approximation of the shoulder blades, the rhomboids and trapezius.

The tilted position of the chest works the spinal muscles isometrically.

By varying the angle of the chest, it is possible to focus the work onto specific parts of the back:

1. Keeping the chest up mainly works the superior trapezius.
2. Keeping the chest closer to horizontal works the dorsals, teres major, rhomboids, and middle and inferior trapezius.

! **Attention:** To avoid injury, never round the back during execution of the movement.

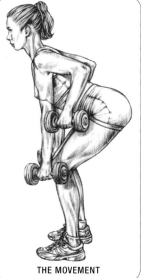

THE MOVEMENT

BARBELL ROWS 11

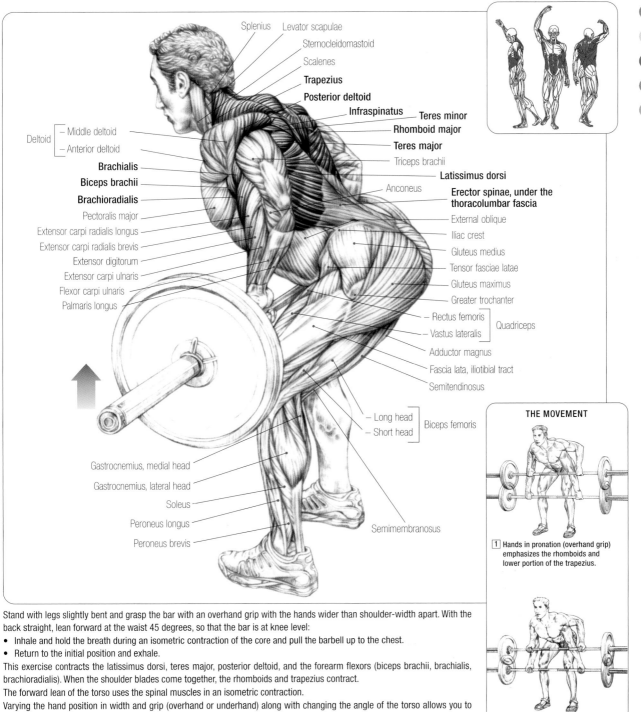

Splenius

Levator scapulae

Sternocleidomastoid

Scalenes

Trapezius

Posterior deltoid

Infraspinatus

Teres minor

Rhomboid major

Teres major

Triceps brachii

Latissimus dorsi

Anconeus

Erector spinae, under the thoracolumbar fascia

External oblique

Iliac crest

Gluteus medius

Tensor fasciae latae

Gluteus maximus

Greater trochanter

– Rectus femoris

– Vastus lateralis

Quadriceps

Adductor magnus

Fascia lata, iliotibial tract

Semitendinosus

– Long head

– Short head

Biceps femoris

Semimembranosus

Deltoid

– Middle deltoid

– Anterior deltoid

Brachialis

Biceps brachii

Brachioradialis

Pectoralis major

Extensor carpi radialis longus

Extensor carpi radialis brevis

Extensor digitorum

Extensor carpi ulnaris

Flexor carpi ulnaris

Palmaris longus

Gastrocnemius, medial head

Gastrocnemius, lateral head

Soleus

Peroneus longus

Peroneus brevis

THE MOVEMENT

1 Hands in pronation (overhand grip) emphasizes the rhomboids and lower portion of the trapezius.

2 Hands in supination (underhand grip) emphasizes the upper portion of the trapezius and the biceps brachii.

Stand with legs slightly bent and grasp the bar with an overhand grip with the hands wider than shoulder-width apart. With the back straight, lean forward at the waist 45 degrees, so that the bar is at knee level:
- Inhale and hold the breath during an isometric contraction of the core and pull the barbell up to the chest.
- Return to the initial position and exhale.

This exercise contracts the latissimus dorsi, teres major, posterior deltoid, and the forearm flexors (biceps brachii, brachialis, brachioradialis). When the shoulder blades come together, the rhomboids and trapezius contract.

The forward lean of the torso uses the spinal muscles in an isometric contraction.

Varying the hand position in width and grip (overhand or underhand) along with changing the angle of the torso allows you to work the back from a variety of angles.

Attention: To prevent injury, never round the back during this exercise. ⚠

12 | T-BAR ROWS

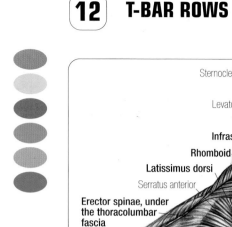

Sternocleidomastoid
Splenius
Levator scapulae
Trapezius
Infraspinatus
Rhomboid
Latissimus dorsi
Serratus anterior

Erector spinae, under the thoracolumbar fascia

Gluteus maximus
Gluteus medius
Iliac crest
Greater trochanter
Tensor fasciae latae
Biceps femoris, long head
Fascia lata, iliotibial tract

Quadriceps
- Rectus femoris
- Vastus lateralis
- Vastus intermedius
- Vastus medialis

Spine of scapula
Posterior deltoid
Acromion
Teres minor
Teres major
Middle deltoid
Pectoralis major
External oblique
Triceps brachii
Brachialis
Brachioradialis
Extensor carpi radialis longus
Anconeus
Extensor digitorum
Extensor carpi radialis brevis
Biceps femoris, long head
Gastrocnemius
Peroneus longus
Extensor digitorum longus
Soleus
Peroneus brevis

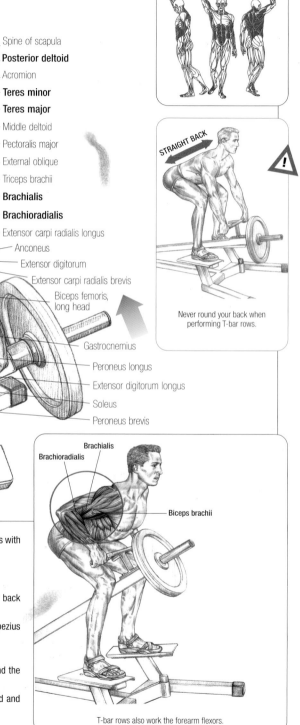

STRAIGHT BACK

Never round your back when performing T-bar rows.

Brachialis
Brachioradialis
Biceps brachii

T-bar rows also work the forearm flexors.

Straddle the bar with the legs slightly bent and lean forward at the waist about 45 degrees with a flat back. Grasp the bar with an overhand grip:

- Inhale and raise the bar to the chest.
- Exhale at the end of the movement.

This exercise is similar to bent rows and allows you to concentrate on working your back because you do not have to focus too much effort on positioning.

This exercise uses mainly the latissimus dorsi, teres major, infraspinatus, rhomboids, trapezius (mainly the middle portion), and the flexors of the forearm.

The forward lean isolates the abdominal and spinal muscles in isometric contraction.

Using a supinated (underhand) grip transfers some of the effort to the biceps brachii and the upper portion of the trapezius at the end of the pull.

Some machines are equipped with parallel handles that allow a grip between pronated and supinated, which contracts the brachioradialis more intensely.

T-BAR ROWS WITH ABDOMINAL SUPPORT 13

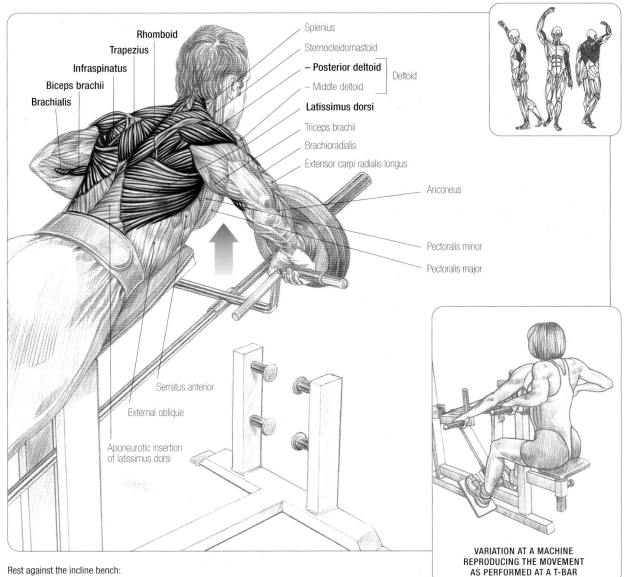

- Splenius
- Sternocleidomastoid
- **– Posterior deltoid**] Deltoid
- – Middle deltoid
- **Latissimus dorsi**
- Triceps brachii
- Brachioradialis
- Extensor carpi radialis longus
- Anconeus
- Pectoralis minor
- Pectoralis major

Rhomboid
Trapezius
Infraspinatus
Biceps brachii
Brachialis

Serratus anterior
External oblique
Aponeurotic insertion of latissimus dorsi

VARIATION AT A MACHINE REPRODUCING THE MOVEMENT AS PERFORMED AT A T-BAR

Rest against the incline bench:

- Inhale and bring the bar to the chest with an overhand grip.
- Exhale at the end of the movement.

This exercise is similar to bent rows and allows you to concentrate on working your back because you do not have to focus too much effort on positioning.

It mainly uses the latissimus dorsi, teres major, posterior deltoid, arm flexors, trapezius, and rhomboids.

Some machines are equipped with an abdominal support, which eliminates the work of the abdominal and spinal muscles. However, when using heavy weights, the rib cage is compressed against the abdominal-support pad, which interferes with breathing and makes the exercise painful to perform.

> **Comment:** A pronated (overhand) hold shifts some of the effort to the biceps brachii and the upper portion of the trapezius at the end of the pull.

14 STIFF-LEGGED DEADLIFTS

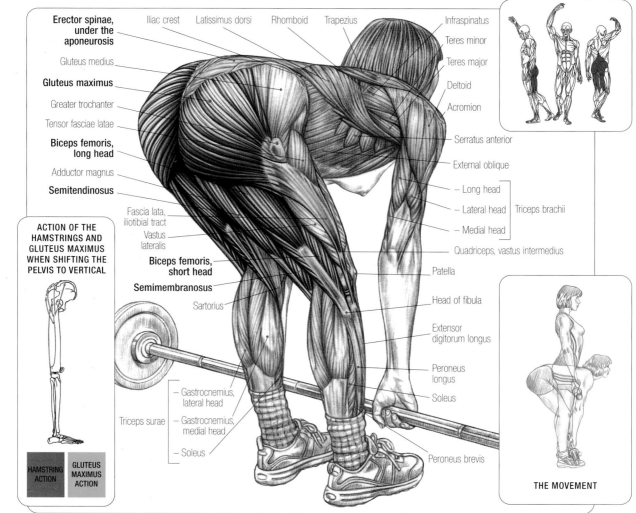

Erector spinae, under the aponeurosis
Iliac crest
Latissimus dorsi
Rhomboid
Trapezius
Infraspinatus
Teres minor
Teres major
Gluteus medius
Deltoid
Gluteus maximus
Acromion
Greater trochanter
Tensor fasciae latae
Serratus anterior
Biceps femoris, long head
External oblique
Adductor magnus
— Long head
Semitendinosus
— Lateral head | Triceps brachii
— Medial head
Fascia lata, iliotibial tract
Quadriceps, vastus intermedius
Vastus lateralis
Biceps femoris, short head
Patella
Semimembranosus
Head of fibula
Sartorius
Extensor digitorum longus
Peroneus longus
Soleus
— Gastrocnemius, lateral head
Triceps surae — Gastrocnemius, medial head
— Soleus
Peroneus brevis

ACTION OF THE HAMSTRINGS AND GLUTEUS MAXIMUS WHEN SHIFTING THE PELVIS TO VERTICAL

| HAMSTRING ACTION | GLUTEUS MAXIMUS ACTION |

THE MOVEMENT

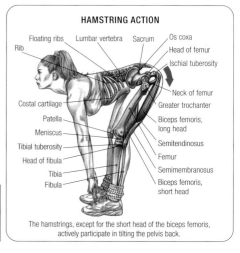

Stand with the feet slightly apart, facing the bar as it rests on the ground:

- Inhale and bend forward at the waist with the chest forward, back arched, and legs as straight as possible.
- Grasp the bar with an overhand grip. Keeping the arms relaxed, stand up straight by rotating the hips. Keep the abdominal muscles tight and a slight arch in the back for support.
- Exhale at the end of the movement.
- Bend forward and return to the initial position, but without returning the bar to the floor.

To avoid injury, keep the back straight.

This exercise contracts the deep spinal muscles on either side of the spinal column that straighten the spine.

Straightening the torso by tilting the pelvis from front to back contracts the gluteus maximus and hamstrings (except the short head of the biceps femoris).

Deadlifting from the ground with extended knees stretches the back of the thighs.

To increase the intensity, stand on a box so that the feet are higher than the bar on the ground.

HAMSTRING ACTION

Floating ribs
Lumbar vertebra
Sacrum
Os coxa
Rib
Head of femur
Ischial tuberosity
Neck of femur
Costal cartilage
Greater trochanter
Patella
Biceps femoris, long head
Meniscus
Semitendinosus
Tibial tuberosity
Femur
Head of fibula
Semimembranosus
Tibia
Biceps femoris, short head
Fibula

The hamstrings, except for the short head of the biceps femoris, actively participate in tilting the pelvis back.

Comment: To stretch the hamstrings, perform the stiff-legged deadlift with very light weights. The greater the weight, the more the gluteal muscles take over from the hamstrings to straighten the pelvis to vertical.

SUMO DEADLIFTS 15

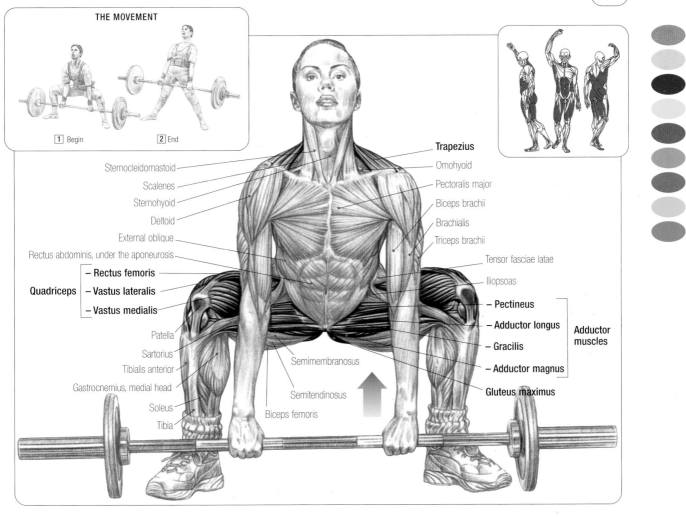

THE MOVEMENT

1 Begin   2 End

Trapezius

Sternocleidomastoid

Scalenes

Sternohyoid

Deltoid

External oblique

Rectus abdominis, under the aponeurosis

Quadriceps
- Rectus femoris
- Vastus lateralis
- Vastus medialis

Patella

Sartorius

Tibialis anterior

Gastrocnemius, medial head

Soleus

Tibia

Semimembranosus

Semitendinosus

Biceps femoris

Omohyoid

Pectoralis major

Biceps brachii

Brachialis

Triceps brachii

Tensor fasciae latae

Iliopsoas

- Pectineus
- Adductor longus
- Gracilis
- Adductor magnus

Adductor muscles

Gluteus maximus

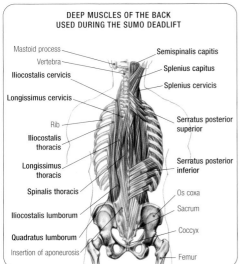

DEEP MUSCLES OF THE BACK USED DURING THE SUMO DEADLIFT

Mastoid process

Vertebra

Iliocostalis cervicis

Longissimus cervicis

Rib

Iliocostalis thoracis

Longissimus thoracis

Spinalis thoracis

Iliocostalis lumborum

Quadratus lumborum

Insertion of aponeurosis

Semispinalis capitis

Splenius capitis

Splenius cervicis

Serratus posterior superior

Serratus posterior inferior

Os coxa

Sacrum

Coccyx

Femur

Stand facing the bar, with legs wider than shoulder-width apart and toes pointing out in line with the knees:

- Inhale and bend the legs until the thighs are horizontal to the ground; grasp the bar with an overhand grip about shoulder-width apart. If you are lifting very heavy weights, use a reverse grip (grasp the bar with one overhand and one underhand grip) to keep the bar from rolling.
- Hold your breath and contract the core, slightly round the back, and extend the legs, bringing the torso vertical and pulling the shoulders back.
- Exhale at the end of the movement.
- Return the bar to the ground while holding your breath. Never round your back.

The difference between this and the classic deadlift is that this exercise works the quadriceps and adductor muscles intensely. Because the pelvis is not as tilted, it works the back less.

Comments: When beginning the movement, slide the bar along the shins. High reps (10 maximum) with light weights strengthen the lumbar region and work the thighs and the gluteal muscles.

When using heavy weights, perform this exercise with great caution to prevent injuries to the hip joints, adductor group of the thighs, and the lumbosacral junction. The sumo deadlift is one of the three powerlifting movements.

16 DEADLIFTS

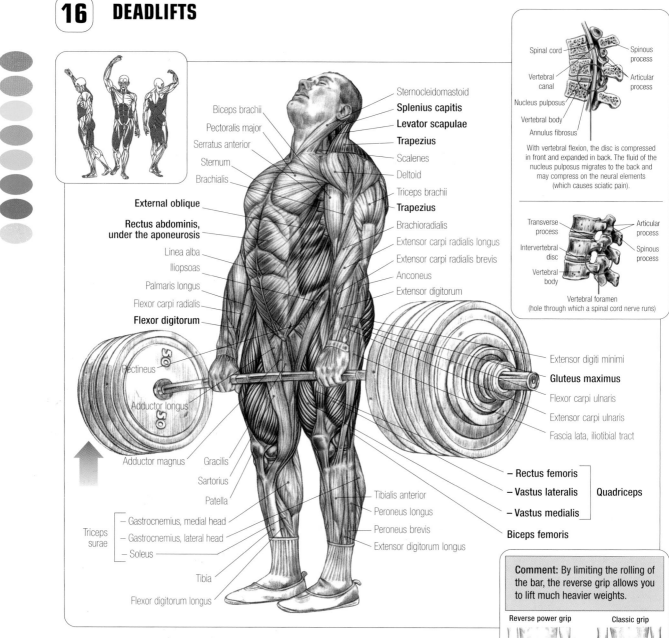

Spinal cord
Spinous process
Vertebral canal
Articular process
Nucleus pulposus
Vertebral body
Annulus fibrosus

With vertebral flexion, the disc is compressed in front and expanded in back. The fluid of the nucleus pulposus migrates to the back and may compress on the neural elements (which causes sciatic pain).

Transverse process
Articular process
Intervertebral disc
Spinous process
Vertebral body

Vertebral foramen
(hole through which a spinal cord nerve runs)

Biceps brachii
Pectoralis major
Serratus anterior
Sternum
Brachialis

External oblique
Rectus abdominis, under the aponeurosis
Linea alba
Iliopsoas
Palmaris longus
Flexor carpi radialis
Flexor digitorum

Pectineus
Adductor longus
Adductor magnus
Gracilis
Sartorius
Patella

Triceps surae
Gastrocnemius, medial head
Gastrocnemius, lateral head
Soleus

Tibia

Flexor digitorum longus

Sternocleidomastoid
Splenius capitis
Levator scapulae
Trapezius
Scalenes
Deltoid
Triceps brachii
Trapezius
Brachioradialis
Extensor carpi radialis longus
Extensor carpi radialis brevis
Anconeus
Extensor digitorum

Extensor digiti minimi
Gluteus maximus
Flexor carpi ulnaris
Extensor carpi ulnaris
Fascia lata, iliotibial tract

– **Rectus femoris**
– **Vastus lateralis**   Quadriceps
– **Vastus medialis**

Biceps femoris

Tibialis anterior
Peroneus longus
Peroneus brevis
Extensor digitorum longus

Comment: By limiting the rolling of the bar, the reverse grip allows you to lift much heavier weights.

Reverse power grip   Classic grip

Stand facing the barbell, legs slightly apart with the abdominal muscles contracted and the back slightly arched. Bend the knees until the thighs are almost parallel to the floor. This position will vary depending on your physical structure and the flexibility of your ankles. (The thighs will be horizontal for someone with short thigh bones and arms. The thighs will be a little above the knees for someone with long thigh bones and arms.) Take an overhand grip on the bar with your hands slightly more than shoulder-width apart. You can also use an over-under grip (one palm faces forward and the other faces back) to prevent the bar from rolling and to work with much heavier weight:

- Inhale, hold the breath, contract the abdominal and low back muscles, and lift the bar by straightening your legs and allowing the bar to slide up the shins.
- When the bar reaches the knees, extend your torso while straightening your legs so you are standing erect with your arms straight down at your sides, exhaling as you complete the movement.
- Hold this straightened position for 2 seconds, then return the weight to the floor, making sure you do not hyperextend or arch your back.

Throughout the exercise, keep your back straight.

This exercise works nearly every muscle in the body and is effective for developing the lumbosacral and trapezius muscles. It also works the gluteal muscles and quadriceps intensely.

The deadlift, along with the bench press and the squat, make up the exercises in powerlifting competitions.

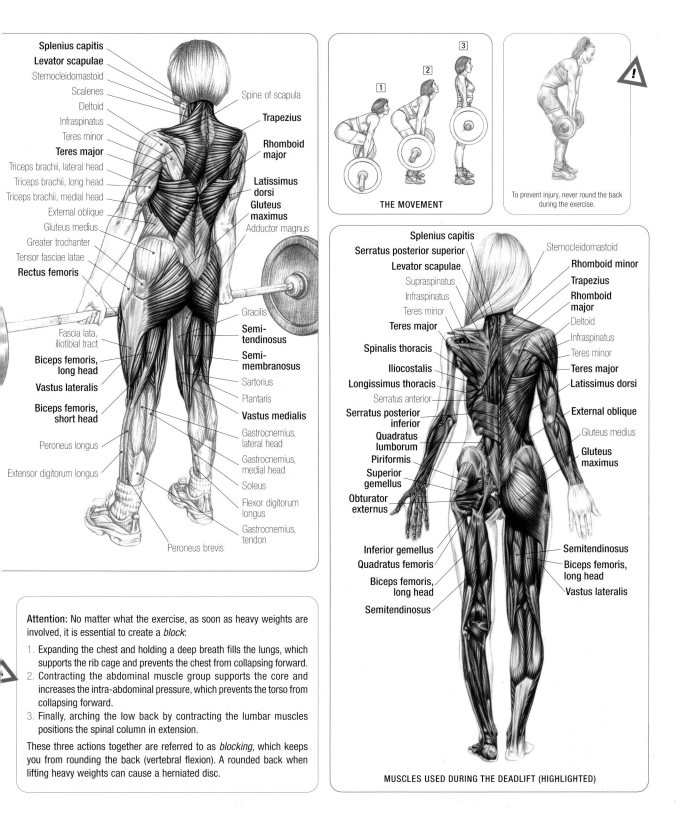

Splenius capitis
Levator scapulae
Sternocleidomastoid
Scalenes
Deltoid
Infraspinatus
Teres minor
Teres major
Triceps brachii, lateral head
Triceps brachii, long head
Triceps brachii, medial head
External oblique
Gluteus medius
Greater trochanter
Tensor fasciae latae
Rectus femoris
Fascia lata, iliotibial tract
Biceps femoris, long head
Vastus lateralis
Biceps femoris, short head
Peroneus longus
Extensor digitorum longus

Spine of scapula
Trapezius
Rhomboid major
Latissimus dorsi
Gluteus maximus
Adductor magnus
Gracilis
Semi-tendinosus
Semi-membranosus
Sartorius
Plantaris
Vastus medialis
Gastrocnemius, lateral head
Gastrocnemius, medial head
Soleus
Flexor digitorum longus
Gastrocnemius, tendon
Peroneus brevis

THE MOVEMENT

To prevent injury, never round the back during the exercise.

Splenius capitis
Serratus posterior superior
Levator scapulae
Supraspinatus
Infraspinatus
Teres minor
Teres major
Spinalis thoracis
Iliocostalis
Longissimus thoracis
Serratus anterior
Serratus posterior inferior
Quadratus lumborum
Piriformis
Superior gemellus
Obturator externus
Inferior gemellus
Quadratus femoris
Biceps femoris, long head
Semitendinosus

Sternocleidomastoid
Rhomboid minor
Trapezius
Rhomboid major
Deltoid
Infraspinatus
Teres minor
Teres major
Latissimus dorsi
External oblique
Gluteus medius
Gluteus maximus
Semitendinosus
Biceps femoris, long head
Vastus lateralis

Attention: No matter what the exercise, as soon as heavy weights are involved, it is essential to create a *block*:

1. Expanding the chest and holding a deep breath fills the lungs, which supports the rib cage and prevents the chest from collapsing forward.
2. Contracting the abdominal muscle group supports the core and increases the intra-abdominal pressure, which prevents the torso from collapsing forward.
3. Finally, arching the low back by contracting the lumbar muscles positions the spinal column in extension.

These three actions together are referred to as *blocking*, which keeps you from rounding the back (vertebral flexion). A rounded back when lifting heavy weights can cause a herniated disc.

MUSCLES USED DURING THE DEADLIFT (HIGHLIGHTED)

✚ BICEPS BRACHII TENDON TEAR

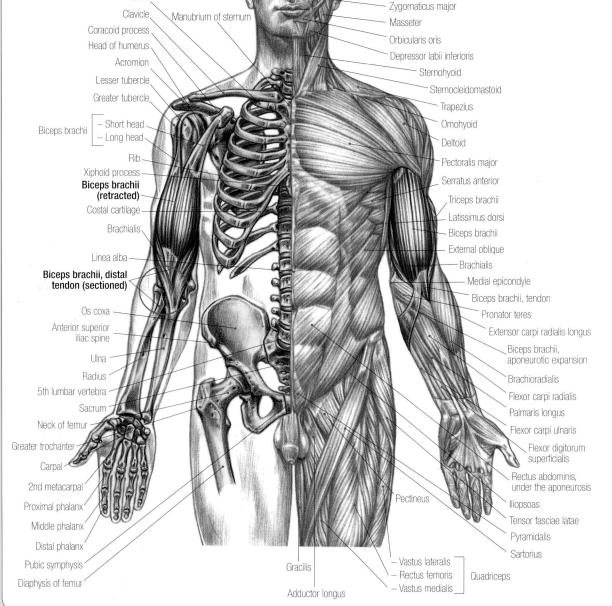

1st rib
Clavicle
Manubrium of sternum
Coracoid process
Head of humerus
Acromion
Lesser tubercle
Greater tubercle
Biceps brachii
— Short head
— Long head
Rib
Xiphoid process
Biceps brachii (retracted)
Costal cartilage
Brachialis
Linea alba
Biceps brachii, distal tendon (sectioned)
Os coxa
Anterior superior iliac spine
Ulna
Radius
5th lumbar vertebra
Sacrum
Neck of femur
Greater trochanter
Carpal
2nd metacarpal
Proximal phalanx
Middle phalanx
Distal phalanx
Pubic symphysis
Diaphysis of femur

Zygomaticus minor
Zygomaticus major
Masseter
Orbicularis oris
Depressor labii inferioris
Sternohyoid
Sternocleidomastoid
Trapezius
Omohyoid
Deltoid
Pectoralis major
Serratus anterior
Triceps brachii
Latissimus dorsi
Biceps brachii
External oblique
Brachialis
Medial epicondyle
Biceps brachii, tendon
Pronator teres
Extensor carpi radialis longus
Biceps brachii, aponeurotic expansion
Brachioradialis
Flexor carpi radialis
Palmaris longus
Flexor carpi ulnaris
Flexor digitorum superficialis
Rectus abdominis, under the aponeurosis
Iliopsoas
Tensor fasciae latae
Pyramidalis
Sartorius

Pectineus
Gracilis
Adductor longus
— Vastus lateralis
— Rectus femoris   Quadriceps
— Vastus medialis

Tearing the long head of the biceps brachii is by far the most common serious sport-related biceps injury.

Generally, it occurs in a muscle, already weakened by tendinitis, after a sudden backward movement of the arm (e.g., during a throw). This movement is relatively common in baseball, tennis, and any sport involving a throwing action, but it also occurs in the snatch in weightlifting. During this motion, tension is suddenly placed on the long head of the biceps brachii, most often where its tendon passes through the bicipital groove of the humerus.

Weightlifting, specifically the deadlift, with heavy weights can cause another characteristic biceps brachii injury.

A common practice when using heavy weights in the deadlift is to use a reverse grip (one overhand grip and one underhand grip) to prevent the bar from rolling in the hands.

This technique, although usually safe, can in rare instances cause the tearing or the pulling away of the inferior tendon of the biceps brachii where the muscle inserts onto the humerus.

During the positive phase of the deadlift, the effort is mainly exerted by the leg, gluteal, back, and abdominal muscles. The arms hang down, completely extended and relaxed.

Unfortunately, the slight shortening caused by contracting either head of the biceps brings the hand into supination (the biceps being the strongest supinator), which with extra heavy weights may cause complete rupture of the tendon at the radius.

This injury occurs at the distal attachment because as the arms hang next to the body, the proximal tension is divided between the short and long heads of the biceps brachii, whereas distally, only one tendinous insertion supports the tension.

Compared to other tendon tears such as the pectoralis major or the adductors of the thigh, in which the pain is unbearable and stops the athlete from continuing, the pain of a biceps tendon tear is relatively mild despite the seriousness of the actual injury. In competitive powerlifting, athletes have continued their lift despite the biceps tendon tear incurred during that lift.

After the accident the diagnosis is obvious: Swelling caused by hemorrhaging appears in the forearm. But what is most striking is the appearance of the biceps brachii, which becomes ball shaped at the upper arm close to the pectoralis major and the deltoid, revealing the brachialis muscle lower down.

Despite the tear, the brachialis, brachioradialis, extensor carpi radialis longus and brevis, and pronator teres muscles can still flex the arm, just not as strongly. Supination of the forearm becomes much more of a problem because the end range of this movement relies only on the supinator muscle.

If this injury is not immediately treated with surgery to reattach the biceps tendon onto the radius, irreversible retraction of the muscle will occur with fibrous change. And although moving the arm will still be possible, there will be permanent loss of strength in flexion and supination. It is possible to prevent this injury by regularly working the biceps, not to develop the muscle, but to strengthen its tendon. For this reason add forearm flexion isolations using a bar in a series of "cheats" by leaning the chest back to give the bar a boost. If practiced regularly, this technique reinforces the distal tendon of the biceps by the tension it places on it. Nevertheless it must be performed carefully without rounding the back to avoid injury.

Pectoralis major
Deltoid
**Biceps brachii
(sectioned and retracted)**
Triceps brachii
Brachialis

**BICEPS BRACHII MUSCLE
RETRACTED WITH TEARING
OF ITS DISTAL TENDON**

NORMAL BICEPS BRACHII MUSCLE

**TYPICAL APPEARANCE OF AN UNTREATED
DISTAL BICEPS TENDON TEAR**

If, after tearing the distal tendon of the biceps brachii, surgery to reattach it to the radius is not performed quickly, permanent retraction and atrophy of the muscle will occur.

Biceps tendon on the arm of the supinated hand can tear during a heavy deadlift.

(17) TRAP BAR DEADLIFTS

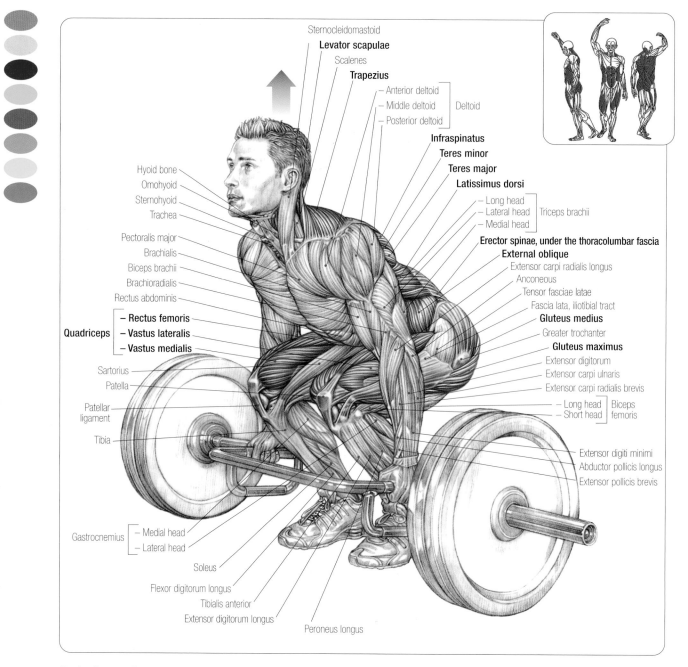

Sternocleidomastoid
Levator scapulae
Scalenes
Trapezius
— Anterior deltoid
— Middle deltoid | Deltoid
— Posterior deltoid
Infraspinatus
Teres minor
Teres major
Latissimus dorsi
— Long head
— Lateral head | Triceps brachii
— Medial head
Erector spinae, under the thoracolumbar fascia
External oblique
Extensor carpi radialis longus
Anconeous
Tensor fasciae latae
Fascia lata, iliotibial tract
Gluteus medius
— Greater trochanter
Gluteus maximus
Extensor digitorum
Extensor carpi ulnaris
Extensor carpi radialis brevis
— Long head | Biceps
— Short head | femoris
Extensor digiti minimi
Abductor pollicis longus
Extensor pollicis brevis

Hyoid bone
Omohyoid
Sternohyoid
Trachea
Pectoralis major
Brachialis
Biceps brachii
Brachioradialis
Rectus abdominis
Quadriceps
— **Rectus femoris**
— **Vastus lateralis**
— **Vastus medialis**
Sartorius
Patella
Patellar ligament
Tibia
Gastrocnemius
— Medial head
— Lateral head
Soleus
Flexor digitorum longus
Tibialis anterior
Extensor digitorum longus
Peroneus longus

Stand well centered in the bar (be careful because poor centering will lead to lateral instability). Legs are slightly apart and back is well fixed and slightly bent:

- Flex the legs in order to bring the thighs close to horizontal; this position can vary depending on the flexibility of the ankles and the individual morphology (for example, for people with short femurs and arms, the thighs will be horizontal; for people with long femurs and arms, the thighs will be more or less higher than horizontal).
- With arms extended, grasp the handles of the bar, carefully centering the grip. (Attention: With heavy weights on a trap bar, a badly adjusted grip will push the bar forward or back.)
- Inhale, contract the abdominal girdle and the lumbar region, and raise the bar by straightening the legs without ever rounding the low back. Exhale at the end of the effort.
- Maintain the extension of the body for 2 seconds, then replace the bar while keeping the abdominal girdle and the lumbar region contracted.

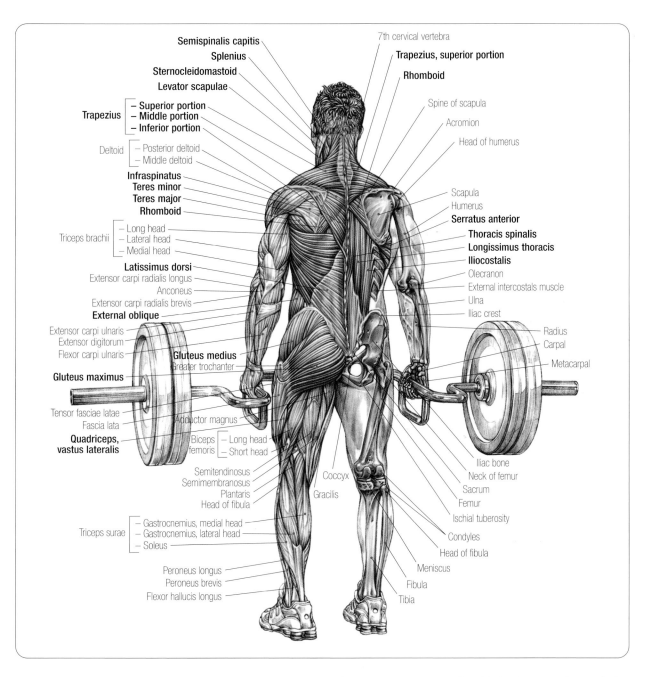

Semispinalis capitis
Splenius
Sternocleidomastoid
Levator scapulae

7th cervical vertebra
Trapezius, superior portion
Rhomboid

Trapezius
– **Superior portion**
– **Middle portion**
– **Inferior portion**

Spine of scapula
Acromion
Head of humerus

Deltoid
– Posterior deltoid
– Middle deltoid

Infraspinatus
Teres minor
Teres major
Rhomboid

Scapula
Humerus
Serratus anterior
Thoracis spinalis
Longissimus thoracis
Iliocostalis

Triceps brachii
– Long head
– Lateral head
– Medial head

Latissimus dorsi
Extensor carpi radialis longus
Anconeus
Extensor carpi radialis brevis
External oblique

Olecranon
External intercostals muscle
Ulna
Iliac crest

Extensor carpi ulnaris
Extensor digitorum
Flexor carpi ulnaris
Gluteus medius
Greater trochanter
Gluteus maximus

Radius
Carpal
Metacarpal

Tensor fasciae latae
Fascia lata
Quadriceps,
vastus lateralis

Adductor magnus
Biceps femoris
– Long head
– Short head

Semitendinosus
Semimembranosus
Plantaris
Head of fibula

Coccyx
Gracilis

Iliac bone
Neck of femur
Sacrum
Femur
Ischial tuberosity

Triceps surae
– Gastrocnemius, medial head
– Gastrocnemius, lateral head
– Soleus

Condyles
Head of fibula
Meniscus

Peroneus longus
Peroneus brevis
Flexor hallucis longus

Fibula
Tibia

As in the classic deadlift (page 104), the deadlift with a trap bar works all the muscles of the body, but the centered position of the bar allows you to decrease the lean of the torso, which will limit the intensity of the work on the lumbar region of the gluteals by throwing some of the effort onto the quadriceps. Thus this movement may be included in a specific program of thigh work and in some cases can replace the squat.

With heavy weights, the superior part of the trapezius is strongly recruited.

Comment: If you have low back pain, this exercise is safer than the classic deadlift.

MUSCLES RECRUITED ACCORDING TO THE DIFFERENT TYPES OF DEADLIFT

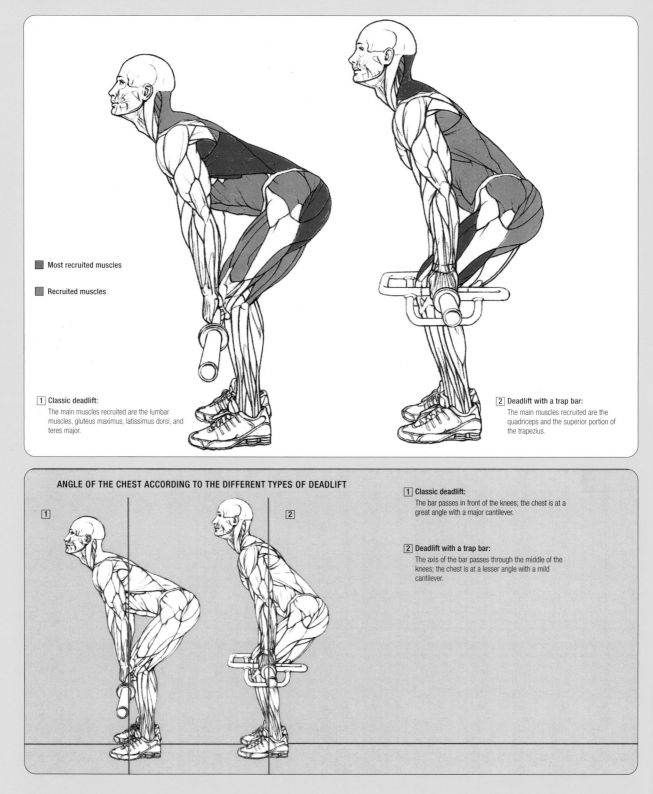

■ Most recruited muscles

■ Recruited muscles

1 **Classic deadlift:**
The main muscles recruited are the lumbar muscles, gluteus maximus, latissimus dorsi, and teres major.

2 **Deadlift with a trap bar:**
The main muscles recruited are the quadriceps and the superior portion of the trapezius.

ANGLE OF THE CHEST ACCORDING TO THE DIFFERENT TYPES OF DEADLIFT

1

2

1 **Classic deadlift:**
The bar passes in front of the knees; the chest is at a great angle with a major cantilever.

2 **Deadlift with a trap bar:**
The axis of the bar passes through the middle of the knees; the chest is at a lesser angle with a mild cantilever.

LOW BACK PAIN

Back pain is the most common problem of the lumbar spine region.

Generally, it is not serious and is most often caused by the shortening of the small, deep vertebral muscles that attach to the transverse processes.

If, during a poorly executed rotation or extension of the spine, one of these muscles is overstretched or is torn, it will automatically shorten along with its neighboring muscles and the superficial erector spinae. The back muscles cramp in pain; however, this cramping limits movement that otherwise might tear or increase the tearing of the small deep muscle.

This general shortening of a portion of the back muscles often disappears when the small deep muscle heals. But sometimes the back pain becomes entrenched, and even after the muscles heal, the local shortening can last several weeks and in some people for years.

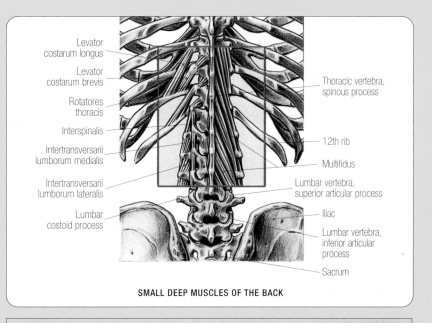

Levator costarum longus
Levator costarum brevis
Rotatores thoracis
Interspinalis
Intertransversarii lumborum medialis
Intertransversarii lumborum lateralis
Lumbar costoid process

Thoracic vertebra, spinous process
12th rib
Multifidus
Lumbar vertebra, superior articular process
Iliac
Lumbar vertebra, inferior articular process
Sacrum

SMALL DEEP MUSCLES OF THE BACK

Comment: Although not serious in and of itself, lumbago, which is a painful contracture of the back muscles, can be part of more serious vertebral injuries such as herniated discs, tears in the paravertebral muscles and ligaments, and fractures.

SHOULD YOU ARCH YOUR BACK?

For people without vertebral problems, arching the back during an exercise is not risky. In fact, with movements such as the squat (page 126) or the deadlift (page 104), where the back tends to round, arching the back can prevent injury. However, for some people arching the back during an exercise can be very dangerous.

- For people suffering from congenital spondylolysis (incomplete fusing of the vertebral arch), putting the lumbar spine in extension can cause the vertebra to slide (spondylolisthesis), which may cause serious nerve compression and lead to sciatica.
- For people who are not fully grown or people experiencing osteoporosis, extending the lumbar spine may lead to spondylolysis because of fractures in the vertebral arch. This fracture in the posterior anchoring system of the vertebra may allow the vertebra to slide forward and seriously compress the neural elements (which leads to sciatica).

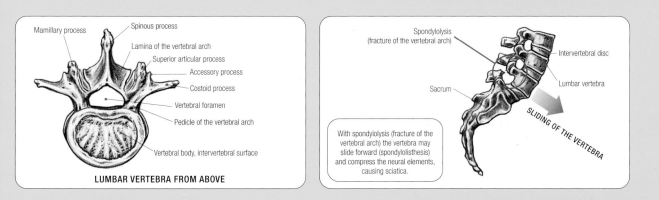

Mamillary process
Spinous process
Lamina of the vertebral arch
Superior articular process
Accessory process
Costoid process
Vertebral foramen
Pedicle of the vertebral arch
Vertebral body, intervertebral surface

LUMBAR VERTEBRA FROM ABOVE

Spondylolysis (fracture of the vertebral arch)
Intervertebral disc
Lumbar vertebra
Sacrum
SLIDING OF THE VERTEBRA

With spondylolysis (fracture of the vertebral arch) the vertebra may slide forward (spondylolisthesis) and compress the neural elements, causing sciatica.

18 BACK EXTENSIONS

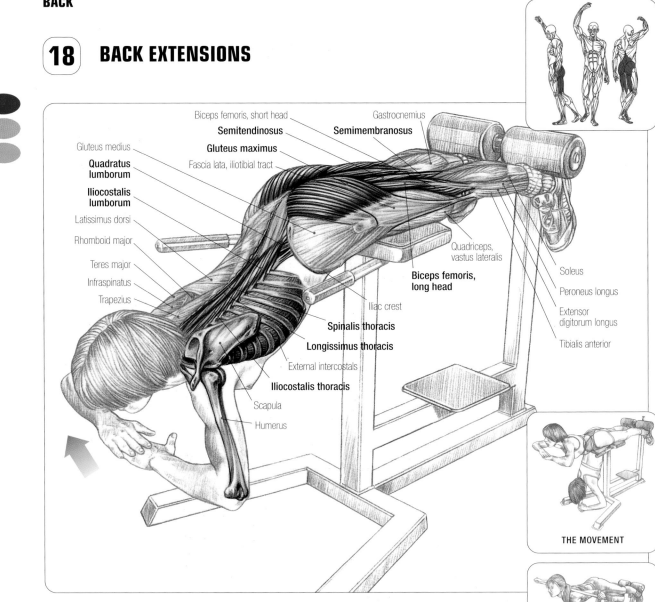

Biceps femoris, short head
Semitendinosus
Semimembranosus
Gastrocnemius

Gluteus medius
Gluteus maximus
Fascia lata, iliotibial tract
Quadratus lumborum
Iliocostalis lumborum
Latissimus dorsi
Rhomboid major
Teres major
Infraspinatus
Trapezius

Quadriceps, vastus lateralis
Biceps femoris, long head
Iliac crest
Spinalis thoracis
Longissimus thoracis
External intercostals
Iliocostalis thoracis
Scapula
Humerus

Soleus
Peroneus longus
Extensor digitorum longus
Tibialis anterior

Lie facedown on a Roman chair and place the ankles under the roller pads. Because the axis of flexion passes through the coxo-femoral joints, the pubic bone should not rest on the support pad:

- With the torso bent forward, extend the back to horizontal.
- Raise the head and continue into hyperextension by arching the lumbar spine. This must be performed carefully to protect your low back.

This exercise mainly develops the group of paraspinal erectors of the spine (iliocostales, longissimus thoracis, spinalis thoracis, splenius, and semispinalis capitis) and quadratus lumborum and, to a lesser degree, the gluteus maximus and the hamstrings, except for the short head of the biceps femoris. Complete flexion of the torso develops the flexibility of the lumbosacral mass. Supporting the pelvis on the bench, so that the axis is displaced to the back of the body, focuses the movement completely at the lumbosacral level but less intensely, given the range of motion and the greater power of the lever arm.

To increase the intensity, sustain the horizontal position of the torso at the end of the extension for a few seconds. Using an incline bench makes this exercise easier for beginners to execute.

Variations

- Performing the torso extension with a bar on the shoulders stabilizes the upper back, which focuses the effort on the lower part of the erector spinae muscles.
- The back extension machine allows you to focus on the lumbosacral mass of the spinal muscles (see page 113, machine back extensions).
- To increase the intensity, perform the exercise while holding a weight to the chest or behind the neck.

THE MOVEMENT

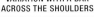

VARIATION WITH A BAR ACROSS THE SHOULDERS

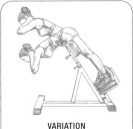

VARIATION EXTENDING AT AN INCLINE BENCH

MACHINE BACK EXTENSIONS 19

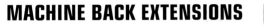

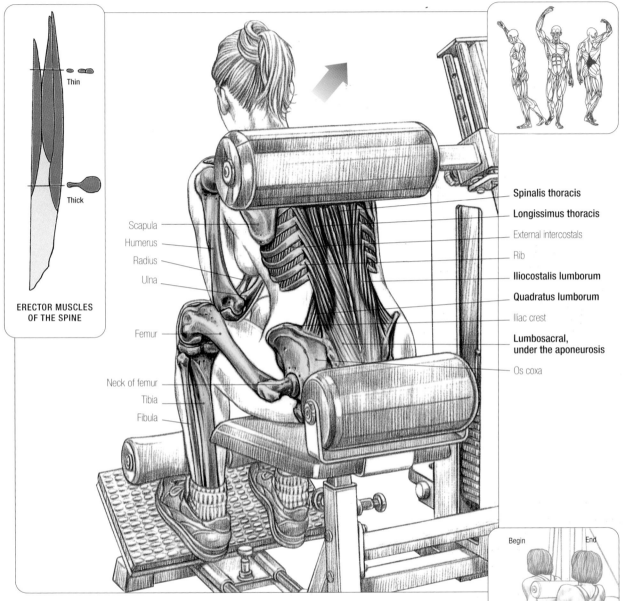

**ERECTOR MUSCLES
OF THE SPINE**

Thin

Thick

Scapula
Humerus
Radius
Ulna

Femur

Neck of femur
Tibia
Fibula

Spinalis thoracis
Longissimus thoracis
External intercostals
Rib
Iliocostalis lumborum
Quadratus lumborum
Iliac crest
Lumbosacral,
under the aponeurosis
Os coxa

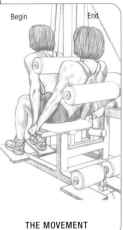

Begin   End

THE MOVEMENT

Sit at the machine, with the torso leaning forward and the pad of the machine at shoulder-blade (scapula) level:

- Inhale and press back, straightening the torso as much as possible.
- Return slowly to the initial position while exhaling and begin again.

This exercise works the erector muscles of the spine, focusing the effort on the low back, specifically the lumbosacral mass of the spinal muscles.

This exercise is excellent for beginners. Done in sets of 10 to 12 repetitions, it develops the strength to progress to more technically demanding exercises for the back.

To perform this exercise with heavier weights, reduce the number of repetitions in the set.

Because the machine regulates the range of motion and the weight, the number of repetitions may vary during the same session.

Example: Two series of 15 repetitions with moderate weights and complete range of performance followed by two series of 7 repetitions with more weights and reduced range.

STRETCHING THE BACK WITH A CHIN-UP BAR

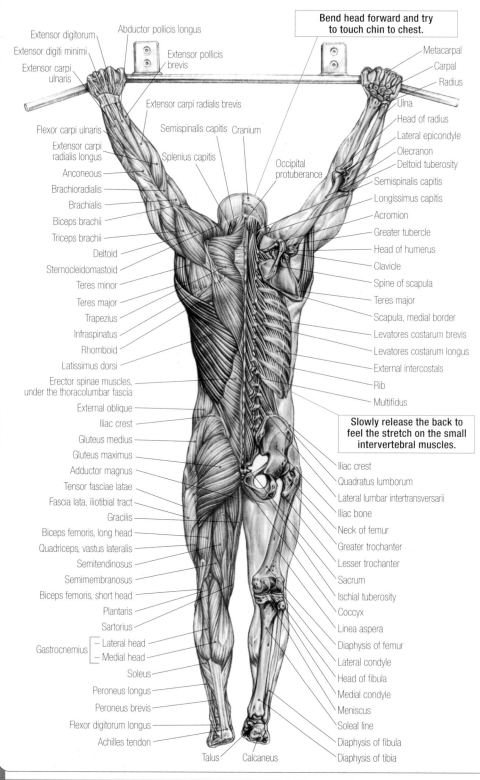

Bend head forward and try to touch chin to chest.

Extensor digitorum
Abductor pollicis longus
Extensor digiti minimi
Extensor pollicis brevis
Extensor carpi ulnaris
Flexor carpi ulnaris
Extensor carpi radialis brevis
Semispinalis capitis
Cranium
Extensor carpi radialis longus
Splenius capitis
Anconeous
Brachioradialis
Occipital protuberance
Brachialis
Biceps brachii
Triceps brachii
Deltoid
Sternocleidomastoid
Teres minor
Teres major
Trapezius
Infraspinatus
Rhomboid
Latissimus dorsi
Erector spinae muscles, under the thoracolumbar fascia
External oblique
Iliac crest
Gluteus medius
Gluteus maximus
Adductor magnus
Tensor fasciae latae
Fascia lata, iliotibial tract
Gracilis
Biceps femoris, long head
Quadriceps, vastus lateralis
Semitendinosus
Semimembranosus
Biceps femoris, short head
Plantaris
Sartorius
Gastrocnemius — Lateral head
— Medial head
Soleus
Peroneus longus
Peroneus brevis
Flexor digitorum longus
Achilles tendon
Talus
Calcaneus

Metacarpal
Carpal
Radius
Ulna
Head of radius
Lateral epicondyle
Olecranon
Deltoid tuberosity
Semispinalis capitis
Longissimus capitis
Acromion
Greater tubercle
Head of humerus
Clavicle
Spine of scapula
Teres major
Scapula, medial border
Levatores costarum brevis
Levatores costarum longus
External intercostals
Rib
Multifidus

Slowly release the back to feel the stretch on the small intervertebral muscles.

Iliac crest
Quadratus lumborum
Lateral lumbar intertransversarii
Iliac bone
Neck of femur
Greater trochanter
Lesser trochanter
Sacrum
Ischial tuberosity
Coccyx
Linea aspera
Diaphysis of femur
Lateral condyle
Head of fibula
Medial condyle
Meniscus
Soleal line
Diaphysis of fibula
Diaphysis of tibia

DIAGRAM OF VERTEBRAE

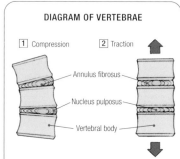

[1] Compression   [2] Traction

Annulus fibrosus
Nucleus pulposus
Vertebral body

[1] When you lift heavy weights, such as during squats or in deadlift exercises, the intervertebral discs can become pinched and the nucleus can migrate to the periphery.

[2] When you hang from a chin-up bar, the small intervertebral ligaments and muscles stretch, the intervertebral disc compression decreases, and the nucleus pulposus can return to its position at the center of the disc.

Hang from a chin-up bar with a wide overhand grip (thumbs facing each other):

- Inhale and exhale slowly, concentrating on the relaxation of your body, which allows the back muscles to relax and the pressure inside the discs to equilibrate as well as relax the small paravertebral muscles (interconnecting the vertebrae), which are often painfully contracted.

- When you are relaxed, lean your head forward, trying to touch your sternum with your chin. This will stretch the upper and middle back.

To accentuate the stretch, swing gently or ask a partner to grasp your hips on each side and slowly pull down.

This stretch is fundamental. When practiced regularly at the end of squat and deadlift sessions (or any other heavyweight exercises that would have compressed the spine), it helps over time to limit the deterioration of the intervertebral discs and reduces the risk of disc herniation (see page 134).

Variation: If you grip strongly with the hands, the latissimus dorsi and teres major muscles are stretched more intensely.

Comment: During this exercise, you often hear cracking of the spine followed by a pleasant feeling of freedom and relaxation of the vertebral column.

These cracking sounds are caused by the release of the paravertebral muscles acting like a bellows that, when opened, decompresses the small intervertebral and costovertebral articulations.

UPRIGHT ROWS 20

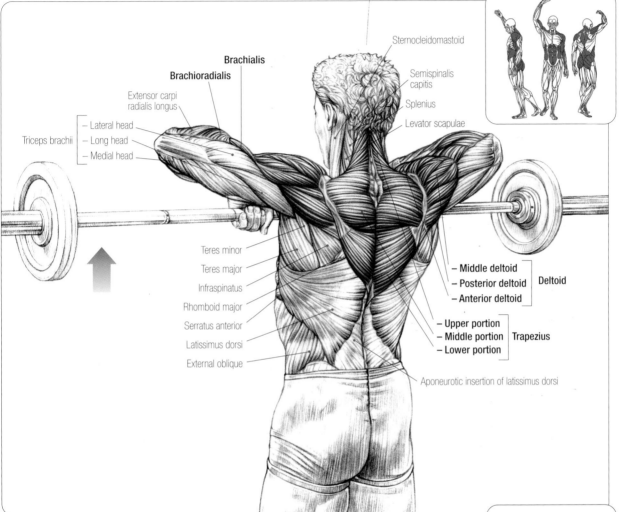

Sternocleidomastoid

Brachialis

Brachioradialis

Semispinalis capitis

Extensor carpi radialis longus

Splenius

Levator scapulae

Triceps brachii
– Lateral head
– Long head
– Medial head

Teres minor

Teres major

Infraspinatus

Rhomboid major

Serratus anterior

Latissimus dorsi

External oblique

– Middle deltoid
– Posterior deltoid
– Anterior deltoid

Deltoid

– Upper portion
– Middle portion
– Lower portion

Trapezius

Aponeurotic insertion of latissimus dorsi

Stand with the legs slightly apart, keeping the back straight and grasping the barbell with an overhand grip. The grip should be hand width or slightly wider:

- Inhale and pull the barbell up along the front of the body to the chin, raising the elbows as high as possible.
- Exhale and lower the barbell with a controlled movement.

This exercise mainly uses the superior portion of the trapezius as well as the deltoids, levator scapulae, biceps brachii, brachialis, forearm muscles, abdominal muscles, gluteal muscles, and lumbosacral group.

A wider grip uses the deltoid more than the trapezius.

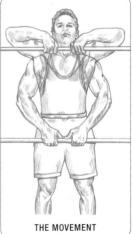

THE MOVEMENT

21 BARBELL SHRUGS

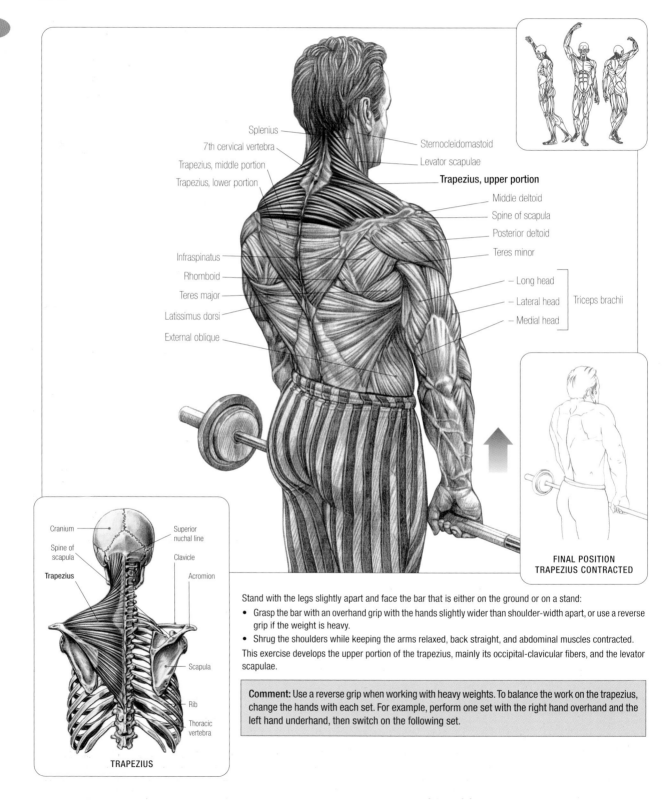

Splenius

7th cervical vertebra

Trapezius, middle portion

Trapezius, lower portion

Sternocleidomastoid

Levator scapulae

Trapezius, upper portion

Middle deltoid

Spine of scapula

Posterior deltoid

Teres minor

Infraspinatus

Rhomboid

Teres major

Latissimus dorsi

External oblique

– Long head

– Lateral head

– Medial head

Triceps brachii

**FINAL POSITION
TRAPEZIUS CONTRACTED**

Cranium

Spine of scapula

Trapezius

Superior nuchal line

Clavicle

Acromion

Scapula

Rib

Thoracic vertebra

TRAPEZIUS

Stand with the legs slightly apart and face the bar that is either on the ground or on a stand:
- Grasp the bar with an overhand grip with the hands slightly wider than shoulder-width apart, or use a reverse grip if the weight is heavy.
- Shrug the shoulders while keeping the arms relaxed, back straight, and abdominal muscles contracted.

This exercise develops the upper portion of the trapezius, mainly its occipital-clavicular fibers, and the levator scapulae.

Comment: Use a reverse grip when working with heavy weights. To balance the work on the trapezius, change the hands with each set. For example, perform one set with the right hand overhand and the left hand underhand, then switch on the following set.

DUMBBELL SHRUGS **22**

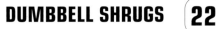

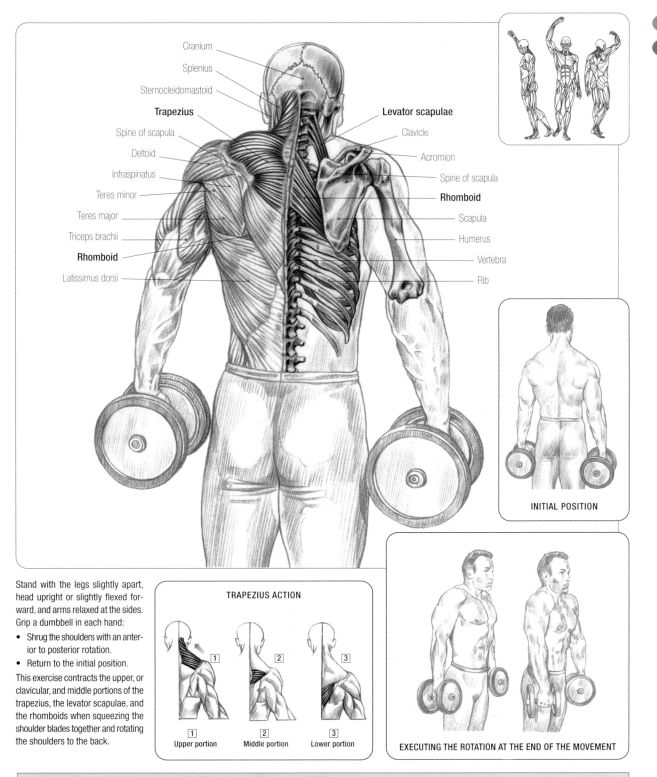

Cranium
Splenius
Sternocleidomastoid
Trapezius
Spine of scapula
Deltoid
Infraspinatus
Teres minor
Teres major
Triceps brachii
Rhomboid
Latissimus dorsi

Levator scapulae
Clavicle
Acromion
Spine of scapula
Rhomboid
Scapula
Humerus
Vertebra
Rib

INITIAL POSITION

Stand with the legs slightly apart, head upright or slightly flexed forward, and arms relaxed at the sides. Grip a dumbbell in each hand:

- Shrug the shoulders with an anterior to posterior rotation.
- Return to the initial position.

This exercise contracts the upper, or clavicular, and middle portions of the trapezius, the levator scapulae, and the rhomboids when squeezing the shoulder blades together and rotating the shoulders to the back.

TRAPEZIUS ACTION

1 Upper portion
2 Middle portion
3 Lower portion

EXECUTING THE ROTATION AT THE END OF THE MOVEMENT

Comment: It is impossible to rotate the shoulders when using heavy weights.

23 TRAP BAR SHRUGS

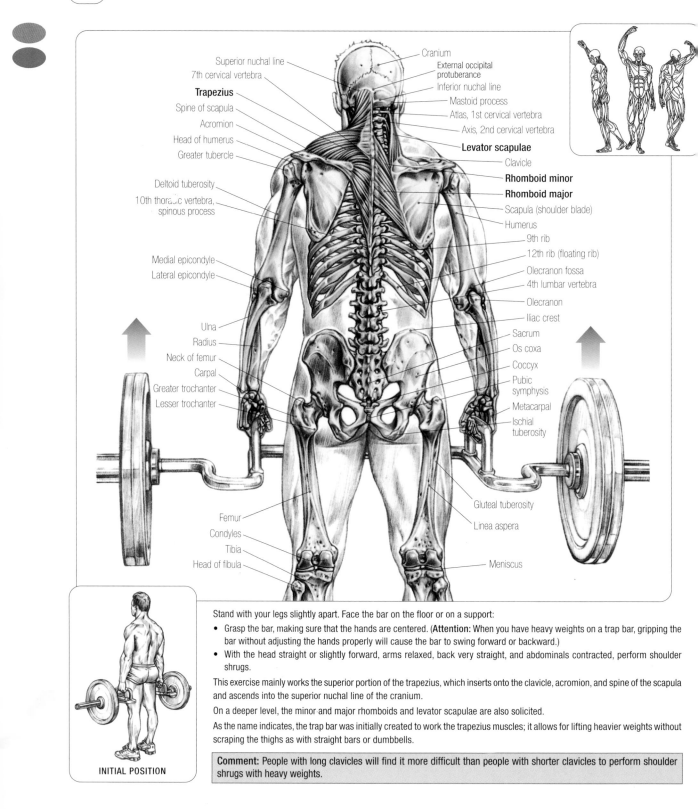

Superior nuchal line
7th cervical vertebra
Trapezius
Spine of scapula
Acromion
Head of humerus
Greater tubercle
Deltoid tuberosity
10th thoracic vertebra, spinous process
Medial epicondyle
Lateral epicondyle
Ulna
Radius
Neck of femur
Carpal
Greater trochanter
Lesser trochanter
Femur
Condyles
Tibia
Head of fibula

Cranium
External occipital protuberance
Inferior nuchal line
Mastoid process
Atlas, 1st cervical vertebra
Axis, 2nd cervical vertebra
Levator scapulae
Clavicle
Rhomboid minor
Rhomboid major
Scapula (shoulder blade)
Humerus
9th rib
12th rib (floating rib)
Olecranon fossa
4th lumbar vertebra
Olecranon
Iliac crest
Sacrum
Os coxa
Coccyx
Pubic symphysis
Metacarpal
Ischial tuberosity
Gluteal tuberosity
Linea aspera
Meniscus

INITIAL POSITION

Stand with your legs slightly apart. Face the bar on the floor or on a support:

- Grasp the bar, making sure that the hands are centered. (**Attention:** When you have heavy weights on a trap bar, gripping the bar without adjusting the hands properly will cause the bar to swing forward or backward.)
- With the head straight or slightly forward, arms relaxed, back very straight, and abdominals contracted, perform shoulder shrugs.

This exercise mainly works the superior portion of the trapezius, which inserts onto the clavicle, acromion, and spine of the scapula and ascends into the superior nuchal line of the cranium.

On a deeper level, the minor and major rhomboids and levator scapulae are also solicited.

As the name indicates, the trap bar was initially created to work the trapezius muscles; it allows for lifting heavier weights without scraping the thighs as with straight bars or dumbbells.

Comment: People with long clavicles will find it more difficult than people with shorter clavicles to perform shoulder shrugs with heavy weights.

MACHINE SHRUGS 24

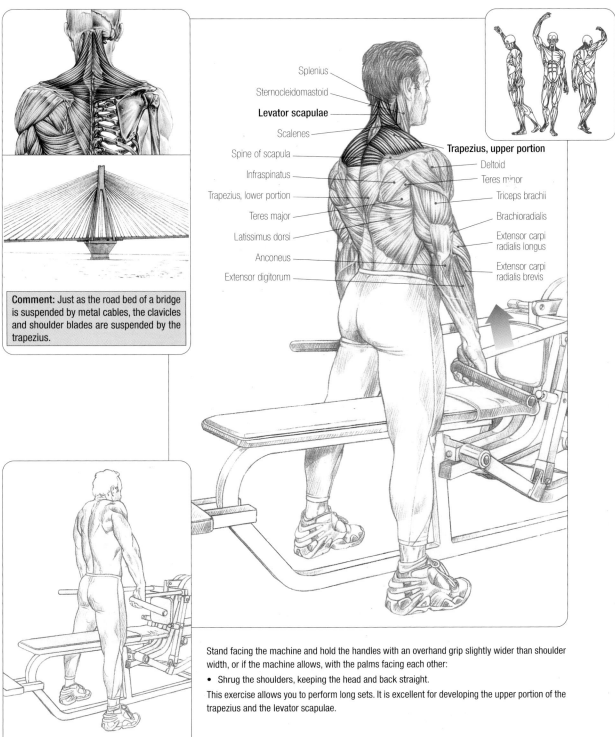

Splenius
Sternocleidomastoid
Levator scapulae
Scalenes
Spine of scapula
Infraspinatus
Trapezius, lower portion
Teres major
Latissimus dorsi
Anconeus
Extensor digitorum

Trapezius, upper portion
Deltoid
Teres minor
Triceps brachii
Brachioradialis
Extensor carpi radialis longus
Extensor carpi radialis brevis

Comment: Just as the road bed of a bridge is suspended by metal cables, the clavicles and shoulder blades are suspended by the trapezius.

**FINAL POSITION
TRAPEZIUS CONTRACTED**

Stand facing the machine and hold the handles with an overhand grip slightly wider than shoulder width, or if the machine allows, with the palms facing each other:

- Shrug the shoulders, keeping the head and back straight.

This exercise allows you to perform long sets. It is excellent for developing the upper portion of the trapezius and the levator scapulae.

STRETCHING THE DELTOIDS, TRAPEZIUS, AND NECK

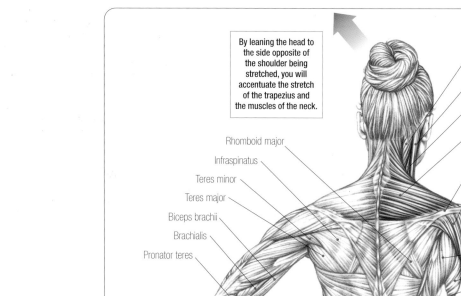

By leaning the head to the side opposite of the shoulder being stretched, you will accentuate the stretch of the trapezius and the muscles of the neck.

Splenius capitis

Sternocleidomastoid

Levator scapulae

Trapezius

Spine of scapula

— Posterior deltoid ⎤ Deltoid
— Middle deltoid ⎦

Rhomboid major

Infraspinatus

Teres minor

Teres major

Biceps brachii

Brachialis

Pronator teres

— Long head ⎤
— Lateral head ⎥ Triceps brachii
— Medial head ⎦

Latissimus dorsi

Anconeus

Flexor carpi radialis

Palmaris longus

Flexor carpi ulnaris

Flexor digitorum superficialis

Biceps brachii, aponeurotic expansion

Pull the hand slowly.

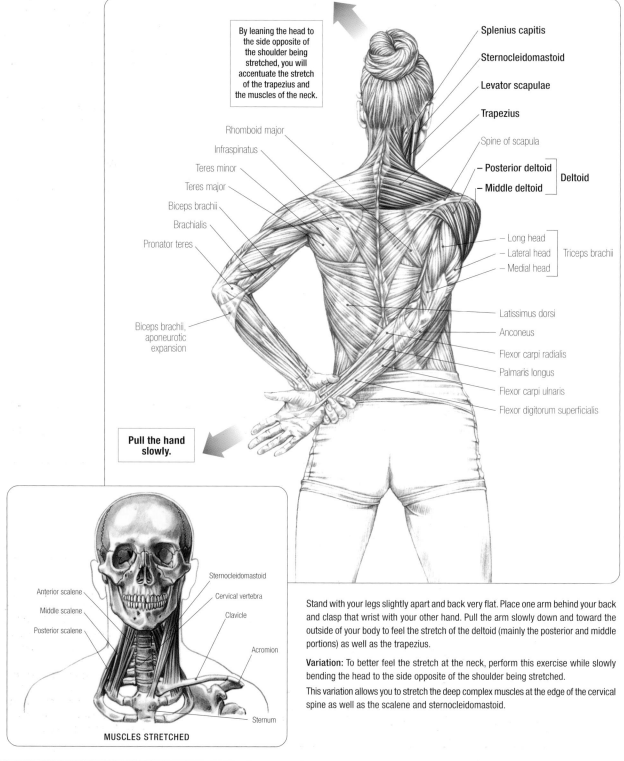

Anterior scalene

Middle scalene

Posterior scalene

Sternocleidomastoid

Cervical vertebra

Clavicle

Acromion

Sternum

MUSCLES STRETCHED

Stand with your legs slightly apart and back very flat. Place one arm behind your back and clasp that wrist with your other hand. Pull the arm slowly down and toward the outside of your body to feel the stretch of the deltoid (mainly the posterior and middle portions) as well as the trapezius.

Variation: To better feel the stretch at the neck, perform this exercise while slowly bending the head to the side opposite of the shoulder being stretched.

This variation allows you to stretch the deep complex muscles at the edge of the cervical spine as well as the scalene and sternocleidomastoid.

STRETCHING THE TRAPEZIUS AND NECK

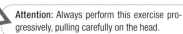

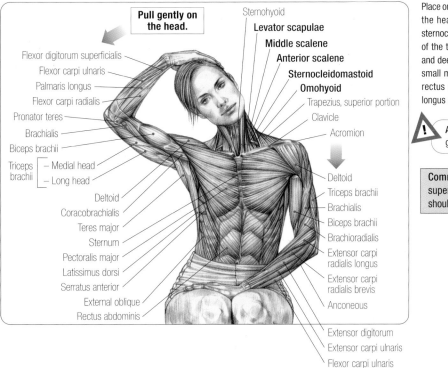

Pull gently on the head.

Flexor digitorum superficialis
Flexor carpi ulnaris
Palmaris longus
Flexor carpi radialis
Pronator teres
Brachialis
Biceps brachii
Triceps brachii — Medial head
— Long head
Deltoid
Coracobrachialis
Teres major
Sternum
Pectoralis major
Latissimus dorsi
Serratus anterior
External oblique
Rectus abdominis

Sternohyoid
Levator scapulae
Middle scalene
Anterior scalene
Sternocleidomastoid
Omohyoid
Trapezius, superior portion
Clavicle
Acromion
Deltoid
Triceps brachii
Brachialis
Biceps brachii
Brachioradialis
Extensor carpi radialis longus
Extensor carpi radialis brevis
Anconeous
Extensor digitorum
Extensor carpi ulnaris
Flexor carpi ulnaris

Place one hand over your head and pull gently, bending the head to the side. This exercise stretches the sternocleidomastoid, scalene group, superior portion of the trapezius, splenius capitis, splenius cervices, and deeper in the semispinalis capitis as well as the small muscles of the spine such as the longus colli, rectus capitis anterior, rectus capitis lateralis, and longus capitis.

⚠️ **Attention:** Always perform this exercise progressively, pulling carefully on the head.

Comment: To better feel the stretch on the superior portion of the trapezius, lower the shoulder at the same time.

ABOUT THE NECK

In quadrupeds as well as the anthropomorphic ape, such as the gorilla, the muscles of the neck are particularly powerful and developed to maintain the head and prevent it from dropping forward.

But in humans, who have moved to complete bipedal uprightness with the head perched at the top of the spine, the muscles of the neck no longer serve to powerfully hold the head up but more to subtly balance the head on the spine.

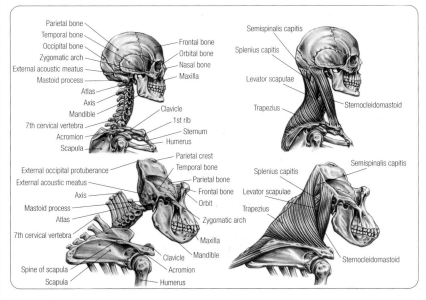

Parietal bone
Temporal bone
Occipital bone
Zygomatic arch
External acoustic meatus
Mastoid process
Atlas
Axis
Mandible
7th cervical vertebra
Acromion
Scapula
Frontal bone
Orbital bone
Nasal bone
Maxilla
Clavicle
1st rib
Sternum
Humerus

Semispinalis capitis
Splenius capitis
Levator scapulae
Trapezius
Sternocleidomastoid

External occipital protuberance
External acoustic meatus
Axis
Mastoid process
Atlas
7th cervical vertebra
Spine of scapula
Scapula
Parietal crest
Temporal bone
Parietal bone
Frontal bone
Orbit
Zygomatic arch
Maxilla
Clavicle
Mandible
Acromion
Humerus

Splenius capitis
Levator scapulae
Trapezius
Semispinalis capitis
Sternocleidomastoid

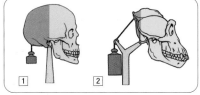

1 In human evolution, the smaller face and the development of the bipedal stance and encephalon has caused the occipital foramen to move toward the center of the cranial base. The head positioned at the top of the spine requires the muscles of the neck to play only a subtle stabilizing role.

2 In the gorilla, a partial quadruped with a bigger face along with the posterior position of the occipital foramen, the muscles of the neck are particularly well developed and powerful to prevent the head from falling forward.

5
LEGS

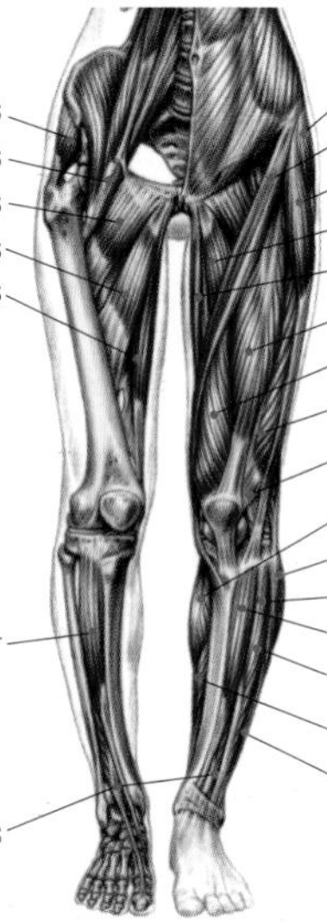

Gluteus minimus
Iliopsoas
Pectineus
Adductor longus
Adductor magnus

Gluteus medius
Sartorius
Tensor fasciae latae
Adductor longus
Gracilis
– Rectus femoris
– Vastus medialis
– Vastus lateralis
– Vastus intermedius
– Medial head
– Lateral head
Peroneus longus
Tibialis anterior
Extensor digitorum longus
Soleus
Peroneus brevis

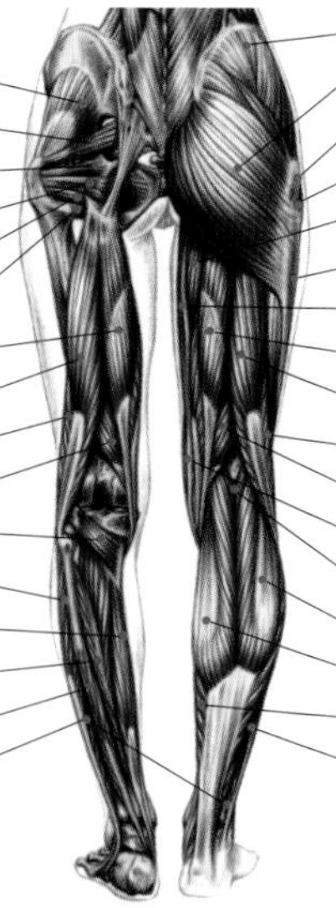

Quadriceps

Gastrocnemius

Tibialis anterior

Extensor hallucis longus

Gluteus minimus
Piriformis
Superior gemellus
Obturator internus
Inferior gemellus
Quadratus femoris
Semimembranosus
Biceps femoris
– Long head
– Short head
Semimembranosus
Popliteus
Peroneus longus
Flexor digitorum longus
Tibialis posterior
Flexor hallucis longus
Peroneus brevis

Gluteus medius
Gluteus maximus
Greater trochanter
Tensor fasciae latae
Adductor magnus
Fascia lata, iliotibial tract
Gracilis
Semitendinosus
– Long head
– Short head
Semimembranosus
Sartorius
Plantaris
– Lateral head
– Medial head
Soleus
Peroneus longus

Biceps fe

Gastroc

DUMBBELL SQUATS $\boxed{1}$

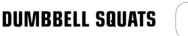

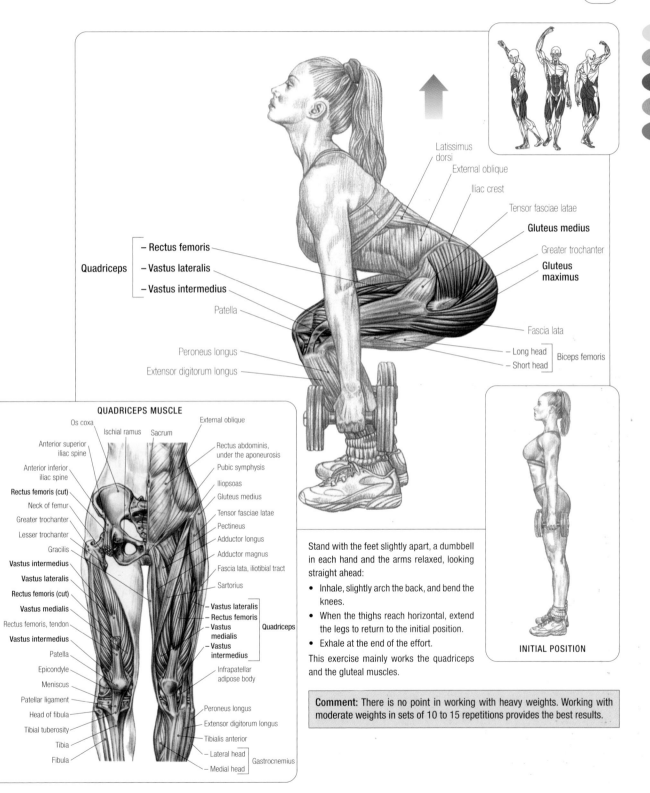

Latissimus dorsi

External oblique

Iliac crest

Tensor fasciae latae

Gluteus medius

Greater trochanter

Gluteus maximus

Fascia lata

– Long head
– Short head
Biceps femoris

Quadriceps
– **Rectus femoris**
– **Vastus lateralis**
– **Vastus intermedius**

Patella

Peroneus longus

Extensor digitorum longus

QUADRICEPS MUSCLE

Os coxa
Ischial ramus
Sacrum
External oblique

Anterior superior iliac spine

Anterior inferior iliac spine

Rectus abdominis, under the aponeurosis

Pubic symphysis

Iliopsoas

Gluteus medius

Tensor fasciae latae

Pectineus

Adductor longus

Adductor magnus

Fascia lata, iliotibial tract

Sartorius

Rectus femoris (cut)
Neck of femur
Greater trochanter
Lesser trochanter
Gracilis
Vastus intermedius
Vastus lateralis
Rectus femoris (cut)
Vastus medialis
Rectus femoris, tendon
Vastus intermedius
Patella
Epicondyle
Meniscus
Patellar ligament
Head of fibula
Tibial tuberosity
Tibia
Fibula

– **Vastus lateralis**
– **Rectus femoris**
– **Vastus medialis**
– **Vastus intermedius**
Quadriceps

Infrapatellar adipose body

Peroneus longus

Extensor digitorum longus

Tibialis anterior

– Lateral head
– Medial head
Gastrocnemius

Stand with the feet slightly apart, a dumbbell in each hand and the arms relaxed, looking straight ahead:

- Inhale, slightly arch the back, and bend the knees.
- When the thighs reach horizontal, extend the legs to return to the initial position.
- Exhale at the end of the effort.

This exercise mainly works the quadriceps and the gluteal muscles.

Comment: There is no point in working with heavy weights. Working with moderate weights in sets of 10 to 15 repetitions provides the best results.

INITIAL POSITION

2 SQUATS WITH A DUMBBELL HELD BETWEEN THE LEGS

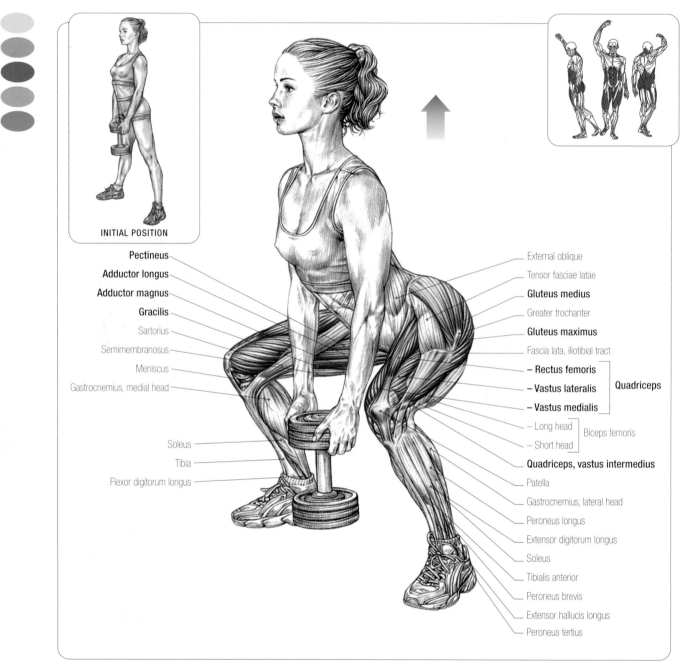

INITIAL POSITION

Pectineus
Adductor longus
Adductor magnus
Gracilis
Sartorius
Semimembranosus
Meniscus
Gastrocnemius, medial head

Soleus
Tibia
Flexor digitorum longus

External oblique
Tensor fasciae latae
Gluteus medius
Greater trochanter
Gluteus maximus
Fascia lata, iliotibial tract
– Rectus femoris
– Vastus lateralis   Quadriceps
– Vastus medialis
– Long head   Biceps femoris
– Short head
Quadriceps, vastus intermedius
Patella
Gastrocnemius, lateral head
Peroneus longus
Extensor digitorum longus
Soleus
Tibialis anterior
Peroneus brevis
Extensor hallucis longus
Peroneus tertius

Stand with your legs apart and toes pointing out. Hold a dumbbell in your hands:
- Look straight ahead, arch your back slightly, inhale, and bend your knees.
- When the thighs reach horizontal, extend your legs to return to the initial position.
- Exhale at the end of the movement.

This exercise works the quadriceps as well as the gluteal muscles.

Comment: The wide-leg position works the adductors.

FRONT SQUATS ③

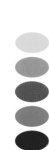

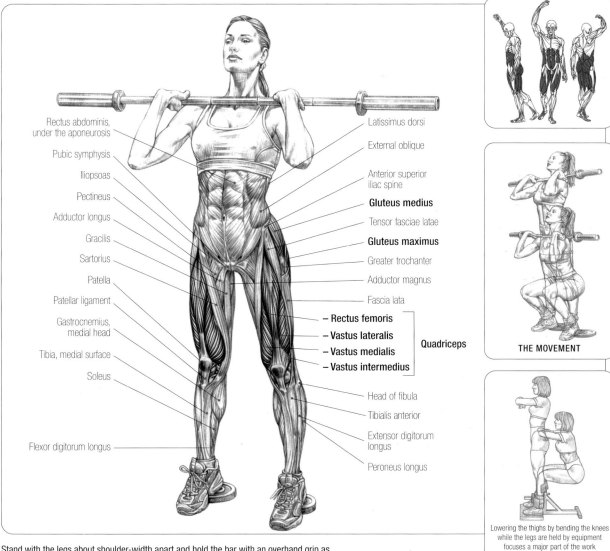

Rectus abdominis, under the aponeurosis
Pubic symphysis
Iliopsoas
Pectineus
Adductor longus
Gracilis
Sartorius
Patella
Patellar ligament
Gastrocnemius, medial head
Tibia, medial surface
Soleus
Flexor digitorum longus

Latissimus dorsi
External oblique
Anterior superior iliac spine
Gluteus medius
Tensor fasciae latae
Gluteus maximus
Greater trochanter
Adductor magnus
Fascia lata
– Rectus femoris
– Vastus lateralis
– Vastus medialis
– Vastus intermedius
Head of fibula
Tibialis anterior
Extensor digitorum longus
Peroneus longus

Quadriceps

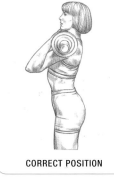

THE MOVEMENT

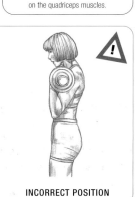

Lowering the thighs by bending the knees while the legs are held by equipment focuses a major part of the work on the quadriceps muscles.

Stand with the legs about shoulder-width apart and hold the bar with an overhand grip as it rests on the upper pectoral muscles and the anterior deltoid:

- Inhale deeply to maintain intrathoracic pressure, which prevents the torso from collapsing forward, slightly arch the low back, contract the abdominal core, and bend the knees to lower the thighs horizontal to the floor.
- Return to the initial position and exhale at the end of the movement.

Stick out the chest and raise the elbows as high as possible to prevent the barbell from sliding forward.

Even though the barbell is in front, keep the back upright and don't lean the torso forward. To make the exercise easier, place blocks under the heels.

This type of squat focuses a greater part of the effort onto the quadriceps and is performed with lighter weights than the classic squat. This exercise also contracts the gluteal muscles, hamstrings, abdominal core, and the erector spinae. This is a movement frequently used in weight training because it corresponds perfectly with the work the thighs do at the end of a snatch.

CORRECT POSITION   **INCORRECT POSITION**

4 SQUATS

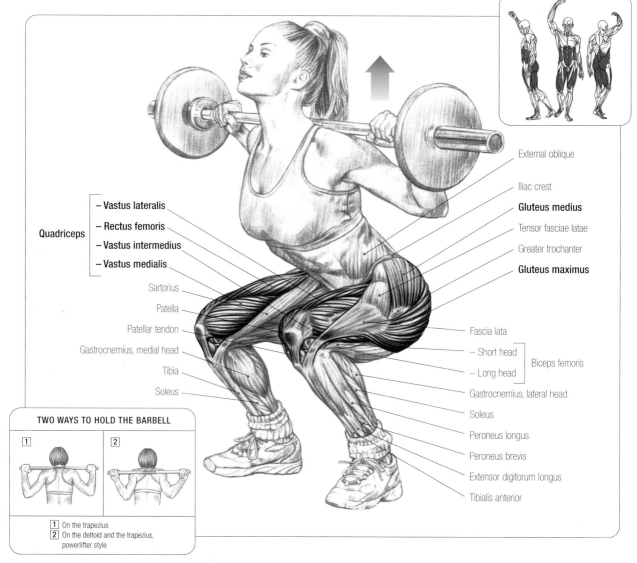

Quadriceps
- Vastus lateralis
- Rectus femoris
- Vastus intermedius
- Vastus medialis

Sartorius

Patella

Patellar tendon

Gastrocnemius, medial head

Tibia

Soleus

External oblique

Iliac crest

Gluteus medius

Tensor fasciae latae

Greater trochanter

Gluteus maximus

Fascia lata

- Short head
- Long head } Biceps femoris

Gastrocnemius, lateral head

Soleus

Peroneus longus

Peroneus brevis

Extensor digitorum longus

Tibialis anterior

TWO WAYS TO HOLD THE BARBELL

① ②

① On the trapezius
② On the deltoid and the trapezius, powerlifter style

The squat is the number one bodybuilding movement: It uses nearly the entire muscular system, and it also works the cardiovascular system. It helps develop thoracic expansion, and therefore, respiratory capacity:

- With the barbell resting on a stand, slide under the bar and place it on the trapezius a bit higher than the posterior deltoid. Grasp the bar firmly with the hands at a comfortable width and the elbows back.

- Inhale deeply (to maintain the intrathoracic pressure, which will prevent the torso from collapsing forward), slightly arch the back by rotating the pelvis forward, contract the abdominal core, look straight ahead, and remove the barbell from the stand.

- Step back one or two steps and stop with both feet parallel to each other (or toes pointing slightly outward) and about shoulder-width apart. Bend forward from the hips (the axis of flexion should pass through the coxofemoral joints) and avoid rounding the back in order to prevent injury.

- When the thighs are horizontal to the floor, straighten the legs and lift the torso to return to the initial position.

- Exhale at the end of the movement.

The squat mainly works the quadriceps, gluteal muscles, adductor group, erector spinae, abdominal muscles, and the hamstrings.

Comment: The squat is one of the best exercises for developing the shape of the buttocks.

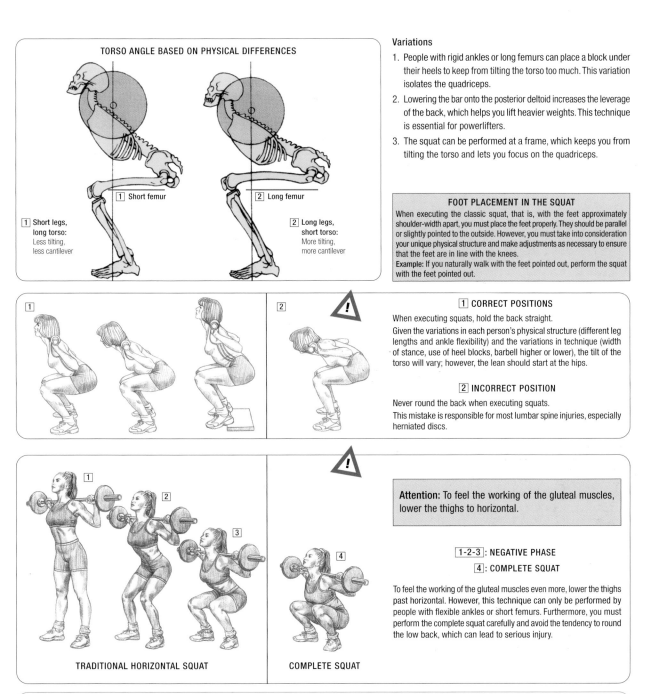

TORSO ANGLE BASED ON PHYSICAL DIFFERENCES

1 Short femur   2 Long femur

1 Short legs,
long torso:
Less tilting,
less cantilever

2 Long legs,
short torso:
More tilting,
more cantilever

Variations

1. People with rigid ankles or long femurs can place a block under their heels to keep from tilting the torso too much. This variation isolates the quadriceps.

2. Lowering the bar onto the posterior deltoid increases the leverage of the back, which helps you lift heavier weights. This technique is essential for powerlifters.

3. The squat can be performed at a frame, which keeps you from tilting the torso and lets you focus on the quadriceps.

FOOT PLACEMENT IN THE SQUAT

When executing the classic squat, that is, with the feet approximately shoulder-width apart, you must place the feet properly. They should be parallel or slightly pointed to the outside. However, you must take into consideration your unique physical structure and make adjustments as necessary to ensure that the feet are in line with the knees.

Example: If you naturally walk with the feet pointed out, perform the squat with the feet pointed out.

1 CORRECT POSITIONS

When executing squats, hold the back straight.

Given the variations in each person's physical structure (different leg lengths and ankle flexibility) and the variations in technique (width of stance, use of heel blocks, barbell higher or lower), the tilt of the torso will vary; however, the lean should start at the hips.

2 INCORRECT POSITION

Never round the back when executing squats.

This mistake is responsible for most lumbar spine injuries, especially herniated discs.

Attention: To feel the working of the gluteal muscles, lower the thighs to horizontal.

1-2-3 : NEGATIVE PHASE

4 : COMPLETE SQUAT

To feel the working of the gluteal muscles even more, lower the thighs past horizontal. However, this technique can only be performed by people with flexible ankles or short femurs. Furthermore, you must perform the complete squat carefully and avoid the tendency to round the low back, which can lead to serious injury.

TRADITIONAL HORIZONTAL SQUAT

COMPLETE SQUAT

Attention: No matter what the exercise, as soon as heavy weights are involved, it is essential to create a *block*.

1. Expanding the chest and holding a deep breath fills the lungs, which supports the rib cage and prevents the chest from collapsing forward.

2. Contracting the abdominal muscle group supports the core and increases the intra-abdominal pressure, which prevents the torso from collapsing forward.

3. Finally, arching the low back by contracting the lumbar muscles positions the spinal column in extension.

These three actions together are referred to as *blocking*, which keeps you from rounding the back (vertebral flexion). A rounded back when lifting heavy weights can cause a herniated disc.

SQUAT-SPECIFIC STRETCH

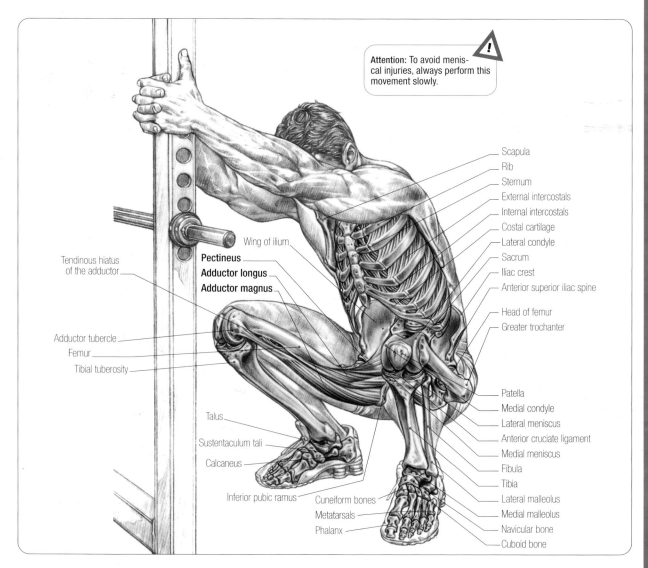

Attention: To avoid meniscal injuries, always perform this
movement slowly.

Scapula
Rib
Sternum
External intercostals
Internal intercostals
Costal cartilage
Lateral condyle
Sacrum
Iliac crest
Anterior superior iliac spine
Head of femur
Greater trochanter
Patella
Medial condyle
Lateral meniscus
Anterior cruciate ligament
Medial meniscus
Fibula
Tibia
Lateral malleolus
Medial malleolus
Navicular bone
Cuboid bone

Wing of ilium
Pectineus
Adductor longus
Adductor magnus

Tendinous hiatus
of the adductor

Adductor tubercle
Femur
Tibial tuberosity

Talus
Sustentaculum tali
Calcaneus

Inferior pubic ramus
Cuneiform bones
Metatarsals
Phalanx

To avoid tearing muscles when practicing the squat, do some stretching exercises at the beginning of the workout while warming up and between the first series.

One stretching exercise most often performed by powerlifters involves crouching deeply while holding onto a stable support such as the post of a weight training machine.

This move, corresponding perfectly to the flexion of a squat, allows the adductors to be stretched favorably, especially the adductor magnus; this muscle is frequently injured during excessive tilting of the torso with heavy weights.

The quadriceps (except for the rectus femoris), gluteus maximus, and the deep external rotator muscles of the hip stabilize and also slow down the anterior tilting in the crouch position.

Comment: To really feel the stretch on the inside of the leg, you can shift your body weight from one leg to the other.

POWER SQUATS

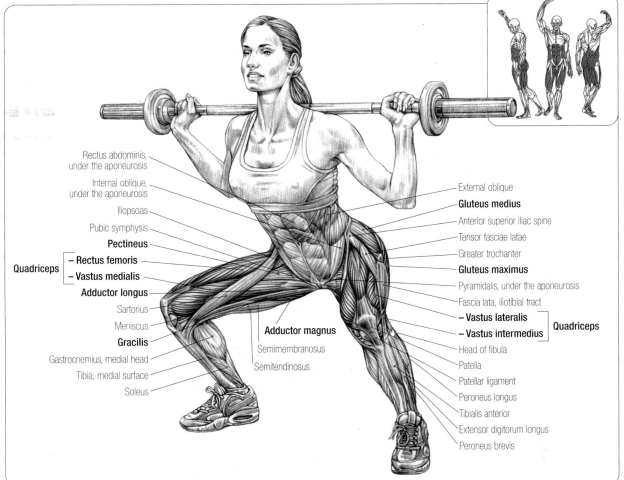

Rectus abdominis, under the aponeurosis
Internal oblique, under the aponeurosis
Iliopsoas
Pubic symphysis
Pectineus
Quadriceps [**– Rectus femoris**
– Vastus medialis
Adductor longus
Sartorius
Meniscus
Gracilis
Gastrocnemius, medial head
Tibia, medial surface
Soleus

Adductor magnus
Semimembranosus
Semitendinosus

External oblique
Gluteus medius
Anterior superior iliac spine
Tensor fasciae latae
Greater trochanter
Gluteus maximus
Pyramidalis, under the aponeurosis
Fascia lata, iliotibial tract
– Vastus lateralis] **Quadriceps**
– Vastus intermedius
Head of fibula
Patella
Patellar ligament
Peroneus longus
Tibialis anterior
Extensor digitorum longus
Peroneus brevis

This movement is performed the same as the classic squat, except that the legs are farther apart and the toes point out, which works the inner thigh intensely.

The working muscles are as follows:

- Quadriceps
- Adductor muscle group (adductor magnus, adductor longus, adductor brevis, adductor pectineus, and gracilis)
- Gluteal muscles
- Hamstrings
- Abdominal muscles
- Lumbosacral muscle group

Comment: In the squat with legs farther apart, the torso is more upright at the bottom of the squat than in the classic squat. Some powerlifters choose the wide-leg technique in order to limit the stress on the back. However, certain powerlifters using heavy weights prefer the classic squat for relieving pressure on the low back because the torso can rest on the thighs at the bottom of the movement.

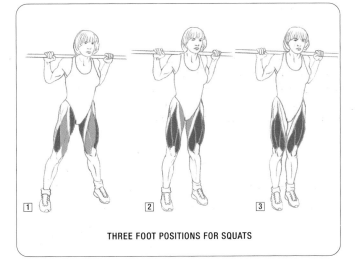

THREE FOOT POSITIONS FOR SQUATS

ADAPTING TRAINING TO YOUR MORPHOLOGY

Short-Limbed and Long-Limbed People

In weightlifting, it is important to consider your individual morphological type in your choice of form for exercises, particularly the squat and deadlift. Both these exercises work the muscles quite differently in short-limbed and long-limbed people.

A short-limbed person is someone with a proportionately longer torso and shorter limbs, whereas a long-limbed person has a relatively shorter torso and longer extremities. This has nothing to do with waistline, muscular development, or fat (a person can be short and long limbed or tall, thin, and short limbed).

Short-limbed people will be more adept at performing a squat. In fact, because of the shortness of the femur, the torso will tilt only a little, limiting the stress on the low back and the hamstring muscles, allowing the movement to be performed in relative security, and focusing almost completely on the quadriceps. It is therefore not surprising that almost all squat champions are in this morphological category. Extreme examples are the dwarves monopolizing the podiums in the small categories in powerlifting.

Long-limbed people will have more difficulty performing the squat. In fact, because of the length of the femurs, the torso will lean forward dramatically. This will place a dangerous amount of tension on the hamstring muscles as well as the adductor magnus and the gracilis. Long-limbed people constantly need to struggle to avoid training in an anterior imbalance.

People with long limbs will also have to concentrate on the position of the back to avoid rounding it, a fault that can lead to severe vertebral injuries—that is, disc herniation.

This type of long-limbed squat intensely works the gluteus maximus muscles (which come into play when straightening the pelvis and thus the chest) as well as the erector spinae muscles, which struggle against the rounding of the back.

The squat is excellent for developing powerful gluteals and good lumbar muscles in long-limbed people, but they will need to concentrate a great deal on their positioning.

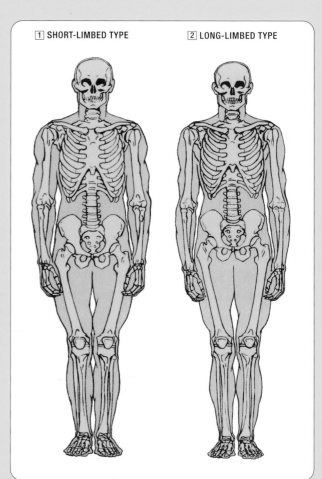

1 SHORT-LIMBED TYPE   2 LONG-LIMBED TYPE

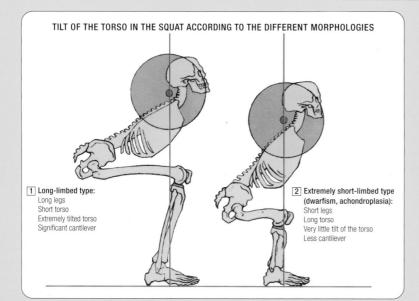

TILT OF THE TORSO IN THE SQUAT ACCORDING TO THE DIFFERENT MORPHOLOGIES

1 Long-limbed type:
Long legs
Short torso
Extremely tilted torso
Significant cantilever

2 Extremely short-limbed type (dwarfism, achondroplasia):
Short legs
Long torso
Very little tilt of the torso
Less cantilever

Furthermore, the squat exercise becomes dangerous as soon as heavier weights are added. Long-limbed people who wish to target the work onto the quadriceps should work with machines, especially the hack squat (page 136).

Short-limbed people dominate squat competitions, but they don't do as well in deadlift competitions. Because of their shorter extremities, they are forced to flex the legs while grasping the bar on the floor. They must bring the femurs practically horizontal. Initiating the movement in this position requires an enormous amount of energy.

Long-limbed people initiate the deadlift with legs partially bent, a position in which the quadriceps can push the most. Despite a greater forward tilt of the back and more intense work on the gluteals and the erector spinae muscles, their morphology allows them to lift significantly heavier weights than short-limbed people can. This is why long-limbed people are essentially the champions of the deadlift.

Flexibility of the Ankles

Flexibility of the ankles has a big influence on the execution of the squat.

Whether it is due to a musculotendinous restriction (such as in retraction of the calves) or bone restriction, if dorsiflexion (raising the front part of the foot) is limited, the squat technique will be profoundly altered.

In fact, the lack of flexibility at the ankles will limit the forward tilt of the tibias and therefore the anterior movement of the knees. This forces the squat to be performed with the gluteals very far back and the back very tilted forward, which works the gluteals and erector spinae intensely.

An excessive tilt of the torso caused by limited ankle flexibility puts a dangerous amount of tension on the posterior muscles of the thigh as well as the adductors magnus and gracilis, increasing the risk of muscle tears.

Furthermore, the lowering of the femurs below horizontal forces the lower back to round, increasing the danger of vertebral injuries.

This squat demands enormous concentration in order to maintain the correct position. Because of its risks, the use of heavier weights is limited.

Notice that stiff ankles also limit the flexion of the legs even though the thighs arrive at horizontal.

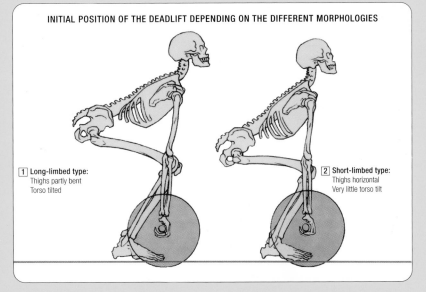

INITIAL POSITION OF THE DEADLIFT DEPENDING ON THE DIFFERENT MORPHOLOGIES

1 Long-limbed type: Thighs partly bent Torso tilted

2 Short-limbed type: Thighs horizontal Very little torso tilt

Finally, the greater cantilever than in the classic squat forces the quadriceps to provide a greater force to extend the legs.

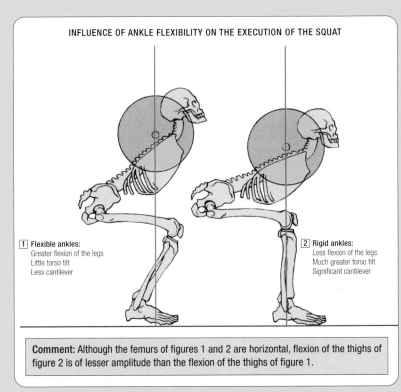

INFLUENCE OF ANKLE FLEXIBILITY ON THE EXECUTION OF THE SQUAT

1 Flexible ankles: Greater flexion of the legs Little torso tilt Less cantilever

2 Rigid ankles: Less flexion of the legs Much greater torso tilt Significant cantilever

Comment: Although the femurs of figures 1 and 2 are horizontal, flexion of the thighs of figure 2 is of lesser amplitude than the flexion of the thighs of figure 1.

Improving Your Squat Position

To limit the stress on the low back and hamstring muscles, it is possible, as the powerlifters do, to lower the bar to the level of the posterior deltoids. This technique allows you to reduce the cantilever and increase the power of the lift from the back, which allows you to take on more weight.

Using a block under your heels or weightlifting or powerlifting shoes with rigid raised heels reduces the cantilever by limiting the backward movement of the gluteals as the knees move forward, allowing for greater amplitude of flexion of the knees. This technique enables you to feel the work of the quadriceps muscles while limiting the tilt of the torso and the work of the gluteus maximus muscles and the erector spinae.

The combination of bar placement and raised heels allows you to take on significantly heavier weight. It is recommended for people with long limbs or rigid ankles.

Squat With the Bar in Front to Target the Quadriceps

By limiting the tilt of the torso, the squat with the bar in front reduces the work of the low back and limits the stress on the hamstring muscles and adductor magnus.

However, by increasing the cantilever, the anterior position of the bar forces the quadriceps to work harder to extend the thigh over the lower leg.

Thus, this is the premier squat for the thighs. However, it always works with much lower weight than the classic squat. For greater stability, always execute it with raised heels.

Unfortunately, this squat is difficult for people with long limbs. A more inclined torso makes it more difficult to hold the bar, which you might drop by falling forward.

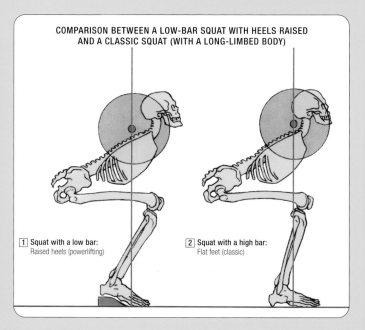

COMPARISON BETWEEN A LOW-BAR SQUAT WITH HEELS RAISED AND A CLASSIC SQUAT (WITH A LONG-LIMBED BODY)

1 Squat with a low bar:
Raised heels (powerlifting)

2 Squat with a high bar:
Flat feet (classic)

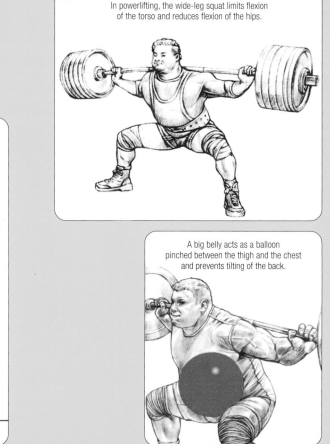

In powerlifting, the wide-leg squat limits flexion of the torso and reduces flexion of the hips.

A big belly acts as a balloon pinched between the thigh and the chest and prevents tilting of the back.

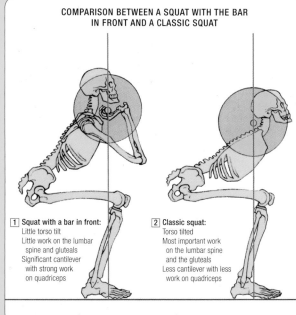

COMPARISON BETWEEN A SQUAT WITH THE BAR IN FRONT AND A CLASSIC SQUAT

1 Squat with a bar in front:
Little torso tilt
Little work on the lumbar spine and gluteals
Significant cantilever with strong work on quadriceps

2 Classic squat:
Torso tilted
Most important work on the lumbar spine and the gluteals
Less cantilever with less work on quadriceps

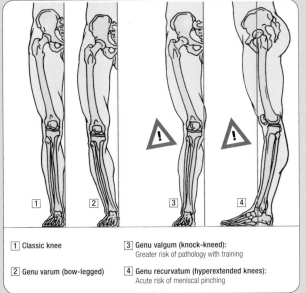

1 Classic knee

2 Genu varum (bow-legged)

3 Genu valgum (knock-kneed):
Greater risk of pathology with training

4 Genu recurvatum (hyperextended knees):
Acute risk of meniscal pinching

Spreading the Legs to Raise the Torso

With the squat, in order to limit excessive and dangerous tilting of the torso, you can position the legs wider apart by turning the toes out. Certain powerlifters take this technique to the extreme by placing the legs in almost a full split (which also allows them to limit their leg flexion).

The squat with widespread legs requires good flexibility of the adductor muscles of the leg and an adequate structure of the coxofemoral articulation. Therefore, not everyone can perform this type of squat.

The Advantage of a Big Belly

A big belly presses against the thighs and helps limit flexion of the hips and rounding of the back. It also protects the small of the back and limits the risk of disc herniation. This physical characteristic is common among many powerlifters and heavyweight lifters.

The Different Kinds of Knees

In weightlifting, it is important to take into account individual variations of morphology, especially in the knees.

Although bow-leggedness (genu varum) does not present more risk than normal legs, knock-kneed legs (genu valgum) or hyperextended knees (genu recurvatum) may even be a contraindication to weightlifting with heavy weights.

Genu valgum is generally found in these people:

1. Those who were overweight during their youth. During that time, the bones of the legs are not yet fully developed and still malleable, so they became deformed and develop the X shape.

2. Women, who tend to have wider hips due to their reproductive function. This can increase the angle of the femurs.

If the genu valgum is too great, the articulation is overused. The medial collateral ligament is overstretched and the lateral meniscus along with the articular surfaces covered with cartilage of the lateral condyle of the femur and the lateral external tuberosity of the tibia are subjected to excessive friction, which can lead to overuse pathologies.

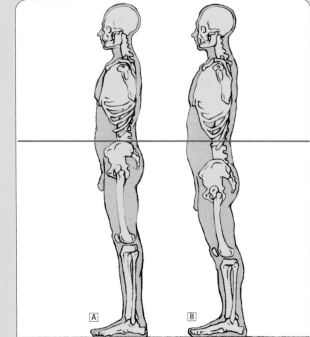

TYPE A: Long legs, short torso
TYPE B: Short legs, long torso

Comment: It is important to take into account the relationship between the length of the torso and the length of the leg.

Type A: People whose legs are proportionately longer than the torso will find it more difficult to perform a squat correctly without leaning too far forward with the chest.

However, limiting the cantilever helps a person with a short torso execute the good morning, the classic deadlift, and the stiff-legged deadlift.

Type B: People whose torsos are proportionately longer than the legs will find it easier to perform the squat safely without excessively leaning forward. It is therefore not surprising that the greatest powerlifting champions specializing in the squat have this type of morphology.

Genu recurvatum is mainly found in people who are very supple (referred to as hypermobile), especially women, in whom this frequent ligamentous and muscular hyperlaxity is directly related to the reproductive function.

Rarely pathological, the recurvatum knee can involve complications such as a pinched meniscus, which occurs when the knee moves rapidly into hyperextension and the menisci do not have the time to slide, or during exercises with heavy weights, which force hyperextension of the thigh.

For this reason, people who have pathological recurvatum should never completely lock the knees at the end of extension during the squat or leg press.

DISC HERNIATION

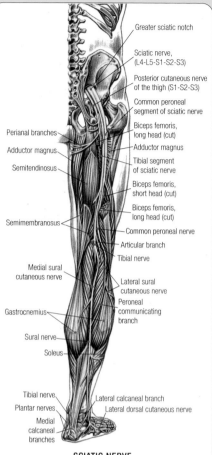

Greater sciatic notch

Sciatic nerve,
(L4-L5-S1-S2-S3)

Posterior cutaneous nerve
of the thigh (S1-S2-S3)

Common peroneal
segment of sciatic nerve

Perineal branches

Biceps femoris,
long head (cut)

Adductor magnus

Adductor magnus

Semitendinosus

Tibial segment
of sciatic nerve

Biceps femoris,
short head (cut)

Biceps femoris,
long head (cut)

Semimembranosus

Common peroneal nerve

Articular branch

Tibial nerve

Medial sural
cutaneous nerve

Lateral sural
cutaneous nerve

Peroneal
communicating
branch

Gastrocnemius

Sural nerve

Soleus

Tibial nerve,
Plantar nerves

Lateral calcaneal branch

Lateral dorsal cutaneous nerve

Medial
calcaneal
branches

**SCIATIC NERVE
AND POSTERIOR CUTANEOUS NERVE OF THIGH**

Disc herniation is a relatively frequent injury in weightlifting, most often caused by incorrect back position during the squat, deadlift, or bent row.

When executing these exercises, the main thing to avoid is rounding the back (vertebral flexion), which expands the back of the disc and pinches the front of it.

If the intervertebral disc is cracked or aging, the gelatinous liquid of the nucleus pulposus migrates backward and can compress on the spinal cord or the roots of the spinal nerves. Symptoms depend on the type of lesion, the amount of nucleus pulposus pushed out, and the surface that is compressed. The nucleus pulposus can bulge or, worse, explode through the annulus fibrosus, which surrounds it, and sometimes tear the posterior ligament that connects the vertebrae to each other. Compression of the neural elements caused by the tearing of the annulus fibrosus is particularly painful and incapacitating.

In weight training, herniations usually occur at the lumbar level and most frequently between the third and fourth or between the fourth and fifth lumbar vertebrae. The pain is dull and deep, sometimes accompanied by swelling and tingling. The pain is located in the middle of the back or more often to one side, radiating to the gluteal muscles, pelvis, and pubis and down the leg following the path of the sciatic nerve (hence the name sciatica to define this type of pain). Generally, disc herniations are spontaneously reabsorbed, and the pain eventually disappears. But in some cases, the bulge in the disc does not disappear and continues to press painfully against the nerves, or a detached piece of intervertebral cartilage compresses the neural elements.

In both these cases, a surgeon can remove the part that is pressing against the nerves.

To prevent disc herniation, use proper form when performing risky exercises such as the squat, deadlift, good morning, and bent row.

Attention: No matter what the exercise, as soon as heavy weights are involved, it is essential to create a *block*.
1. Expanding the chest and holding a deep breath fills the lungs, which supports the rib cage and prevents the chest from collapsing forward.
2. Contracting the abdominal muscle group supports the core and increases the intra-abdominal pressure, which prevents the torso from collapsing forward.
3. Finally, arching the low back by contracting the lumbar muscles positions the spinal column in extension.

These three actions together are referred to as *blocking*, which keeps you from rounding the back (vertebral flexion). A rounded back when lifting heavy weights can cause a herniated disc.

Comment: After a heavy workout, stretch the back by hanging from a chinning bar and focusing on relaxing the body. This allows the muscles to relax and rebalance the pressures inside the intervertebral discs.

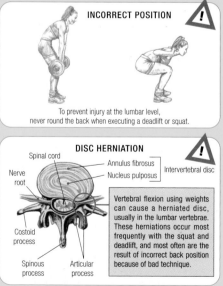

INCORRECT POSITION

To prevent injury at the lumbar level,
never round the back when executing a deadlift or squat.

DISC HERNIATION

Spinal cord

Annulus fibrosus

Nerve
root

Nucleus pulposus

Intervertebral disc

Costoid
process

Spinous
process

Articular
process

Vertebral flexion using weights can cause a herniated disc, usually in the lumbar vertebrae. These herniations occur most frequently with the squat and deadlift, and most often are the result of incorrect back position because of bad technique.

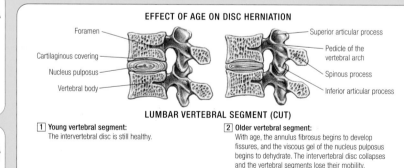

EFFECT OF AGE ON DISC HERNIATION

Foramen

Superior articular process

Cartilaginous covering

Pedicle of the
vertebral arch

Nucleus pulposus

Spinous process

Vertebral body

Inferior articular process

LUMBAR VERTEBRAL SEGMENT (CUT)

1 **Young vertebral segment:**
The intervertebral disc is still healthy.

2 **Older vertebral segment:**
With age, the annulus fibrosus begins to develop fissures, and the viscous gel of the nucleus pulposus begins to dehydrate. The intervertebral disc collapses and the vertebral segments lose their mobility.

From the age of 30, the intervertebral discs degenerate, and the annulus fibrosus can crack as the nucleus pulposus begins to dehydrate. The discs of older athletes are more rigid and less elastic, and the mobility of the spine is limited. On the other hand, as the viscous gel of the nucleus pulposus gradually dehydrates, it becomes less likely that it will be displaced and compress against the nerve.

In comparison, disc herniation in a young person involves the movement of a greater amount of the gelatinous fluid of the nucleus pulposus, causing more compression, pain, and incapacity of the neural elements. Disc herniation therefore occurs more frequently with young athletes.

INCLINE LEG PRESSES 6

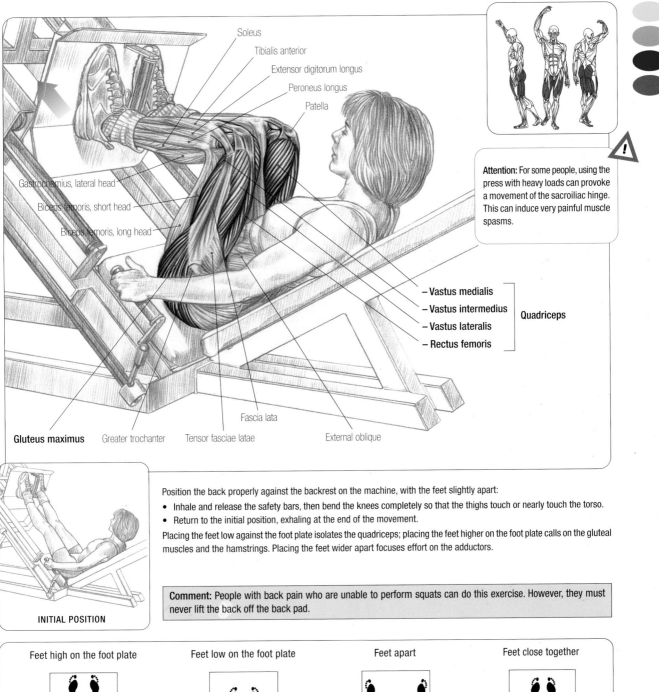

Soleus
Tibialis anterior
Extensor digitorum longus
Peroneus longus
Patella

Gastrocnemius, lateral head
Biceps femoris, short head
Biceps femoris, long head

– **Vastus medialis**
– **Vastus intermedius**
– **Vastus lateralis**
– **Rectus femoris**

Quadriceps

Gluteus maximus   Greater trochanter   Tensor fasciae latae   External oblique

Fascia lata

Attention: For some people, using the press with heavy loads can provoke a movement of the sacroiliac hinge. This can induce very painful muscle spasms.

INITIAL POSITION

Position the back properly against the backrest on the machine, with the feet slightly apart:
- Inhale and release the safety bars, then bend the knees completely so that the thighs touch or nearly touch the torso.
- Return to the initial position, exhaling at the end of the movement.

Placing the feet low against the foot plate isolates the quadriceps; placing the feet higher on the foot plate calls on the gluteal muscles and the hamstrings. Placing the feet wider apart focuses effort on the adductors.

Comment: People with back pain who are unable to perform squats can do this exercise. However, they must never lift the back off the back pad.

Feet high on the foot plate	Feet low on the foot plate	Feet apart	Feet close together

Strong use of the gluteal muscles and the hamstrings	**Strong use of the quadriceps**	**Strong use of the adductors**	**Strong use of the quadriceps**

7 HACK SQUATS

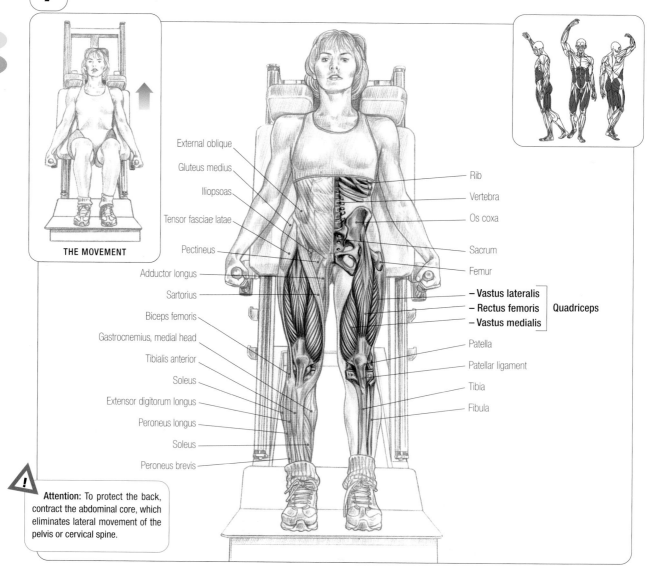

THE MOVEMENT

External oblique
Gluteus medius
Iliopsoas
Tensor fasciae latae
Pectineus
Adductor longus
Sartorius
Biceps femoris
Gastrocnemius, medial head
Tibialis anterior
Soleus
Extensor digitorum longus
Peroneus longus
Soleus
Peroneus brevis

Rib
Vertebra
Os coxa
Sacrum
Femur
– Vastus lateralis
– Rectus femoris   Quadriceps
– Vastus medialis
Patella
Patellar ligament
Tibia
Fibula

Attention: To protect the back, contract the abdominal core, which eliminates lateral movement of the pelvis or cervical spine.

Stand with the legs straight and feet slightly apart, back against the back pad, and shoulders positioned under the shoulder pads. (Hack refers to a "yoke." The pads are reminiscent of the collar placed around the neck of draft animals.):

• Inhale and release the safety catch.
• Bend the knees, then return to the initial position.
• Exhale at the end of the exercise.

This movement focuses the effort on the quadriceps. The more the feet are forward, the more the gluteal muscles will be used.

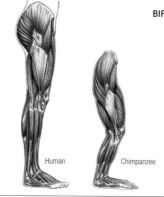

Human   Chimpanzee

BIPEDAL ADAPTATION

In the chimpanzee, our closest relative, the well-developed torso is paired with an underdeveloped gluteus maximus, which makes raising the trunk and standing erect difficult and causes an awkward two-footed gait.

The human is the only primate who has completely adapted to walking upright on two legs. Besides the well-developed gluteus maximus, the entire human structure has adapted to walking on two legs. For example, the torso is relatively small, which makes holding it erect easier, and, unlike the gorilla or chimpanzee, humans can lock the knee joint when it is extended, which makes standing much less tiring.

BOX SQUATS 8

THE MOVEMENT

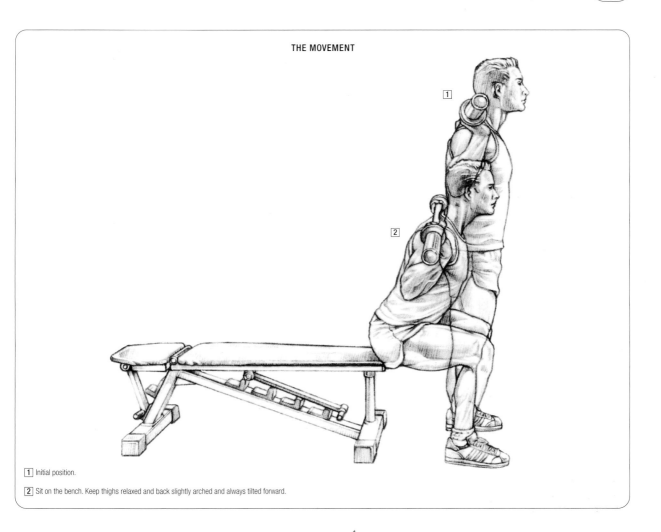

1 Initial position.

2 Sit on the bench. Keep thighs relaxed and back slightly arched and always tilted forward.

The box squat is mainly used by powerlifters with the goal of strengthening the intensity of the squat.

This technique involves performing a squat by sitting on a bench for one or two seconds before standing. In a classic squat, the tension accumulated in the muscles during the negative (lowering) phase, as in stretching an elastic, is released during the positive (standing up) phase. Sitting down on a bench during the box squat relaxes the muscles of the thighs so that they cannot use the accumulated energy from the descent for the ascent.

For this reason, with the same amount of weight, the effort of the quadriceps is more intense in the classic box squat. Thus, it is a very good movement for focusing the work onto the thighs.

This movement can be included in a program for long-legged athletes who have difficulty feeling the quadriceps work during a squat. Furthermore, initiating a squat from a sitting position helps develop the automatic pushing reflex in the classic squat, making the positive standing phase quicker and more powerful.

! **Attention:** Although the box squat is an excellent movement, you must perform the box squat very carefully, always controlling the lowering in order to sit gently onto the bench. If the lowering phase is too rapid and the gluteals slam down on the bench, the shock and the excessive pressure on the vertebral articulations can cause serious trauma.

Comment: Special benches are adjustable in height and adaptable to individual morphologies. Their cushioned seats minimize the shock of the lowering phase and limit the risk of vertebral injury by compression.

To perform the movement properly, always keep the back slightly tilted. If the back is too straight when you're standing up from the bench, it will be impossible to perform the exercise.

9 LEG EXTENSIONS

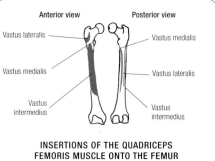

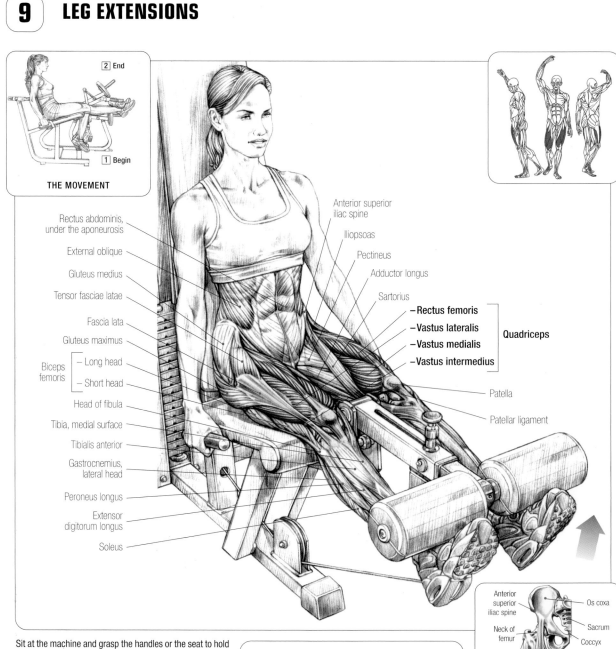

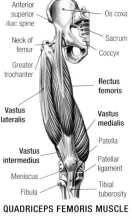

THE MOVEMENT

Rectus abdominis, under the aponeurosis

External oblique

Gluteus medius

Tensor fasciae latae

Fascia lata

Gluteus maximus

Biceps femoris
— Long head
— Short head

Head of fibula

Tibia, medial surface

Tibialis anterior

Gastrocnemius, lateral head

Peroneus longus

Extensor digitorum longus

Soleus

Anterior superior iliac spine

Iliopsoas

Pectineus

Adductor longus

Sartorius

— Rectus femoris
— Vastus lateralis
— Vastus medialis
— Vastus intermedius
} Quadriceps

Patella

Patellar ligament

Anterior superior iliac spine

Neck of femur

Greater trochanter

Vastus lateralis

Vastus intermedius

Meniscus

Fibula

Os coxa

Sacrum

Coccyx

Rectus femoris

Vastus medialis

Patella

Patellar ligament

Tibial tuberosity

QUADRICEPS FEMORIS MUSCLE

Sit at the machine and grasp the handles or the seat to hold the torso immobile. Bend the knees and place the ankles under the ankle pads.

- Inhale and raise the legs to horizontal.
- Exhale at the end of the exercise.

This is the best exercise for isolating the quadriceps. The greater the angle of the backrest, the farther toward the back the pelvis rotates. This exercise stretches the rectus femoris (the midline biarticular portion of the quadriceps), which makes the work on it more intense while extending the legs.

This movement is recommended for beginners so that they can develop enough strength to move on to more technically demanding exercises.

Anterior view   Posterior view

Vastus lateralis

Vastus medialis

Vastus intermedius

Vastus medialis

Vastus lateralis

Vastus intermedius

INSERTIONS OF THE QUADRICEPS FEMORIS MUSCLE ONTO THE FEMUR

STRETCHING THE QUADRICEPS

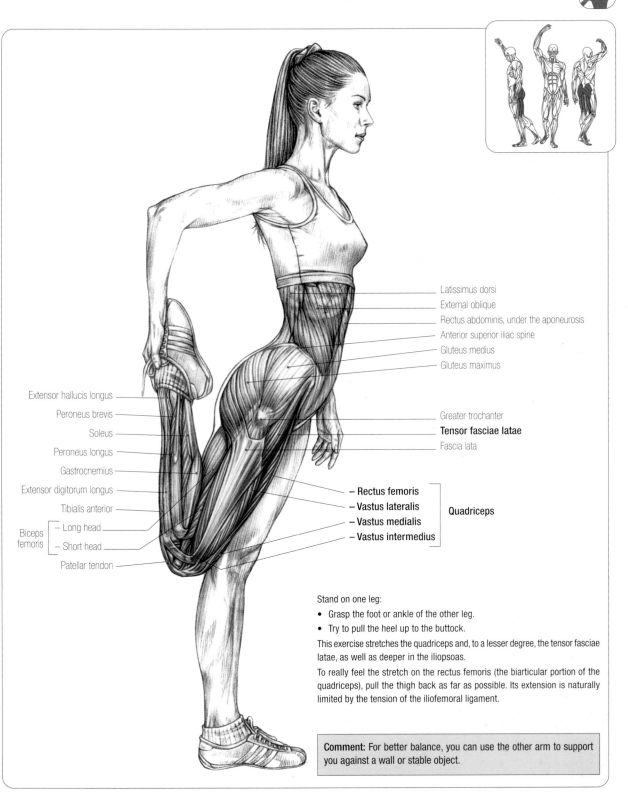

Latissimus dorsi
External oblique
Rectus abdominis, under the aponeurosis
Anterior superior iliac spine
Gluteus medius
Gluteus maximus

Extensor hallucis longus
Peroneus brevis
Soleus
Peroneus longus
Gastrocnemius
Extensor digitorum longus
Tibialis anterior

Biceps femoris — Long head
— Short head

Patellar tendon

Greater trochanter
Tensor fasciae latae
Fascia lata

— **Rectus femoris**
— **Vastus lateralis**
— **Vastus medialis**
— **Vastus intermedius**

Quadriceps

Stand on one leg:

- Grasp the foot or ankle of the other leg.
- Try to pull the heel up to the buttock.

This exercise stretches the quadriceps and, to a lesser degree, the tensor fasciae latae, as well as deeper in the iliopsoas.

To really feel the stretch on the rectus femoris (the biarticular portion of the quadriceps), pull the thigh back as far as possible. Its extension is naturally limited by the tension of the iliofemoral ligament.

Comment: For better balance, you can use the other arm to support you against a wall or stable object.

10 LYING LEG CURLS

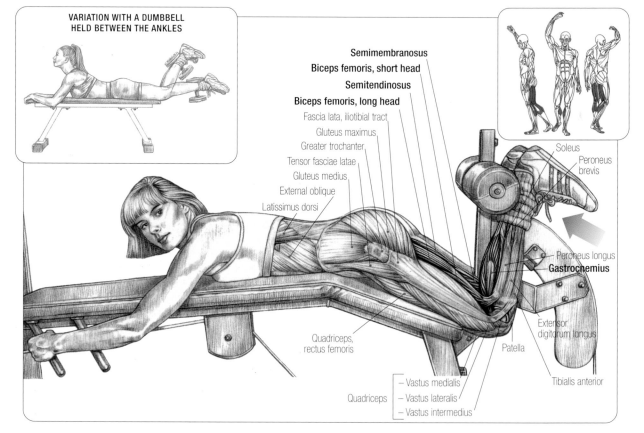

VARIATION WITH A DUMBBELL
HELD BETWEEN THE ANKLES

Semimembranosus
Biceps femoris, short head
Semitendinosus
Biceps femoris, long head
Fascia lata, iliotibial tract
Gluteus maximus
Greater trochanter
Tensor fasciae latae
Gluteus medius
External oblique
Latissimus dorsi

Soleus
Peroneus brevis

Peroneus longus
Gastrocnemius

Extensor digitorum longus

Quadriceps, rectus femoris

Patella

Tibialis anterior

Quadriceps
– Vastus medialis
– Vastus lateralis
– Vastus intermedius

Lie facedown on the machine. Grasp the handles, extend both legs, and position the ankles under the ankle pads:

- Inhale and bend both legs at the same time, trying to touch the gluteal muscles with the heels.
- Exhale at the end of the effort.
- Return to the initial position with a controlled movement.

This exercise works the hamstring group and gastrocnemius and deeper, the popliteus muscle. In theory, during flexion, it is possible to target the semitendinosus and semimembranosus by internally rotating the feet, or to target the long and short heads of the biceps femoris by externally rotating the feet. But in practice, this proves to be difficult, and only emphasis on the hamstrings and the gastrocnemius can be easily achieved:

- Point the toes (plantar flexion) to feel the effort in the hamstrings.
- Flex the feet (dorisflexion) to feel the effort in the gastrocnemius.

Variation: This exercise may be performed by alternating the legs.

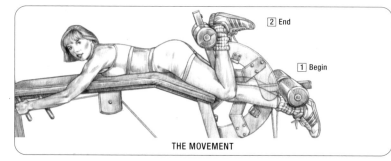

2 End

1 Begin

THE MOVEMENT

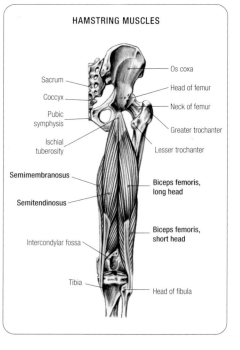

HAMSTRING MUSCLES

Os coxa
Head of femur
Neck of femur
Greater trochanter
Lesser trochanter

Sacrum
Coccyx
Pubic symphysis
Ischial tuberosity

Semimembranosus
Semitendinosus

Biceps femoris, long head

Biceps femoris, short head

Intercondylar fossa

Tibia

Head of fibula

STANDING LEG CURLS 11

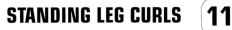

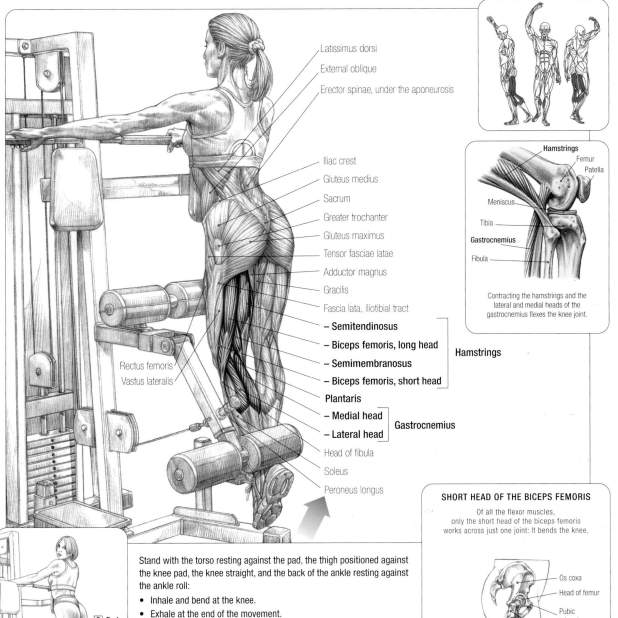

Latissimus dorsi

External oblique

Erector spinae, under the aponeurosis

Iliac crest

Gluteus medius

Sacrum

Greater trochanter

Gluteus maximus

Tensor fasciae latae

Adductor magnus

Gracilis

Fascia lata, iliotibial tract

– Semitendinosus

– Biceps femoris, long head

– Semimembranosus

– Biceps femoris, short head   **Hamstrings**

Plantaris

– Medial head

– Lateral head   **Gastrocnemius**

Head of fibula

Soleus

Peroneus longus

Rectus femoris

Vastus lateralis

Hamstrings
Femur
Patella

Meniscus

Tibia

Gastrocnemius

Fibula

Contracting the hamstrings and the lateral and medial heads of the gastrocnemius flexes the knee joint.

THE MOVEMENT

2 End

1 Begin

Stand with the torso resting against the pad, the thigh positioned against the knee pad, the knee straight, and the back of the ankle resting against the ankle roll:

- Inhale and bend at the knee.
- Exhale at the end of the movement.

This exercise uses the hamstring group (semitendinosus and semimembranosus and the long and short heads of the biceps femoris) and, to a lesser extent, the gastrocnemius. To engage the gastrocnemius more, simply bend at the ankle when bending at the knee. To decrease its participation, which is often the goal, simply point the toes.

SHORT HEAD OF THE BICEPS FEMORIS

Of all the flexor muscles, only the short head of the biceps femoris works across just one joint: It bends the knee.

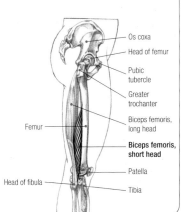

Os coxa

Head of femur

Pubic tubercle

Greater trochanter

Biceps femoris, long head

Femur

Biceps femoris, short head

Patella

Head of fibula

Tibia

12 SEATED LEG CURLS

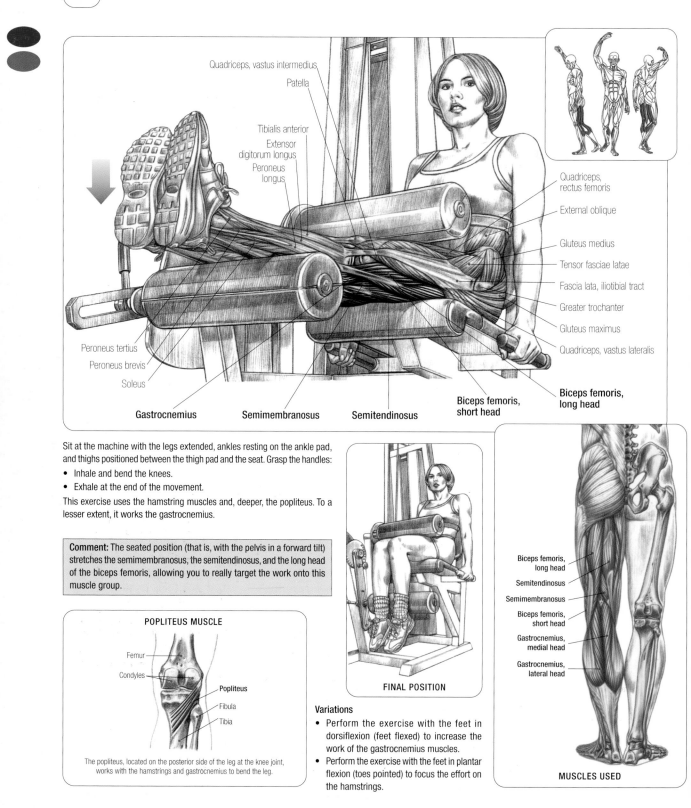

Quadriceps, vastus intermedius

Patella

Tibialis anterior

Extensor digitorum longus

Peroneus longus

Peroneus tertius

Peroneus brevis

Soleus

Gastrocnemius

Semimembranosus

Semitendinosus

Biceps femoris, short head

Biceps femoris, long head

Quadriceps, vastus lateralis

Gluteus maximus

Greater trochanter

Fascia lata, iliotibial tract

Tensor fasciae latae

Gluteus medius

External oblique

Quadriceps, rectus femoris

Sit at the machine with the legs extended, ankles resting on the ankle pad, and thighs positioned between the thigh pad and the seat. Grasp the handles:

• Inhale and bend the knees.
• Exhale at the end of the movement.

This exercise uses the hamstring muscles and, deeper, the popliteus. To a lesser extent, it works the gastrocnemius.

Comment: The seated position (that is, with the pelvis in a forward tilt) stretches the semimembranosus, the semitendinosus, and the long head of the biceps femoris, allowing you to really target the work onto this muscle group.

POPLITEUS MUSCLE

Femur

Condyles

Popliteus

Fibula

Tibia

The popliteus, located on the posterior side of the leg at the knee joint, works with the hamstrings and gastrocnemius to bend the leg.

FINAL POSITION

Variations

• Perform the exercise with the feet in dorsiflexion (feet flexed) to increase the work of the gastrocnemius muscles.
• Perform the exercise with the feet in plantar flexion (toes pointed) to focus the effort on the hamstrings.

Biceps femoris, long head

Semitendinosus

Semimembranosus

Biceps femoris, short head

Gastrocnemius, medial head

Gastrocnemius, lateral head

MUSCLES USED

✚ HAMSTRING MUSCLE TEARS

ACTION OF THE HAMSTRING MUSCLES DURING THE SQUAT

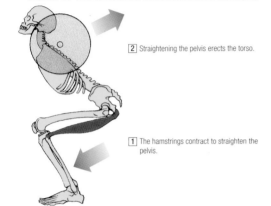

2 Straightening the pelvis erects the torso.

1 The hamstrings contract to straighten the pelvis.

While performing the squat, the hamstring muscles contract to straighten the pelvis, which at the same time prevents the torso from tilting too far forward (as long as the pelvis is aligned with the torso by contracting the abdominal and lumbar muscles).

In bodybuilding, hamstring tears occur frequently. This injury occurs most often during the squat when the torso is too far forward. The hamstring muscle group, with the exception of the short head of biceps femoris, is in an extremely stretched position and contracts forcefully to straighten the pelvis. This can lead to tearing, most often at the high or middle portion of the muscle group.

Hamstring tears can also occur when working at a leg curl machine using heavy weights. This most often occurs at the beginning of the movement when the legs are extended and the muscles are stretched.

Although in general, the tears in hamstring muscle fibers are not extensive and not serious (it is rare to see a significant tear in the muscle or its tendinous insertion), they are always painful and prone to complications.

In fact, fibrous scarring frequently occurs after a tear in this muscle group, which creates friction that is especially painful and incapacitating during sport activity. Furthermore, this inelastic scar tissue is liable to tear during intense effort.

Preventing Hamstring Tearing

To prevent muscle tears, perform either a specific stretching workout or incorporate hamstring stretches during a lifting workout between sets of squats and deadlifts and exercises for the back of the thigh.

Certain weightlifting exercises, such as good mornings or stiff-legged deadlifts, can be considered the best hamstring protectors because of their combined action of muscle strengthening and stretching.

After Hamstring Tearing

To prevent the formation of fibrous scar tissue in the hamstrings, it is essential to reeducate the muscles as soon as possible. A week after a tear, you must perform gentle stretches for the back of the thighs. The goal is to stretch the injured muscles and especially to soften the scar so that it doesn't tear when you resume training.

HAMSTRING MUSCLES

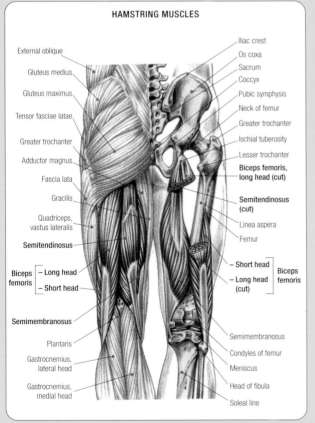

External oblique
Gluteus medius
Gluteus maximus
Tensor fasciae latae
Greater trochanter
Adductor magnus
Fascia lata
Gracilis
Quadriceps, vastus lateralis
Semitendinosus
Biceps femoris — Long head / — Short head
Semimembranosus
Plantaris
Gastrocnemius, lateral head
Gastrocnemius, medial head

Iliac crest
Os coxa
Sacrum
Coccyx
Pubic symphysis
Neck of femur
Greater trochanter
Ischial tuberosity
Lesser trochanter
Biceps femoris, long head (cut)
Semitendinosus (cut)
Linea aspera
Femur
— Short head / — Long head (cut) **Biceps femoris**
Semimembranosus
Condyles of femur
Meniscus
Head of fibula
Soleal line

RETRACTION OF THE HAMSTRINGS

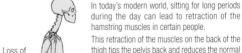

Loss of lumbar curve
Pelvis in posterior tilt
Hamstring muscles

Retraction of the hamstrings causes the pelvis to tip back (posterior rotation), which reduces the lumbar curve and sets the stage for vertebral injuries.

In today's modern world, sitting for long periods during the day can lead to retraction of the hamstring muscles in certain people.

This retraction of the muscles on the back of the thigh tips the pelvis back and reduces the normal curvature of the spine.

This causes the person to adopt poor posture with the pelvis tucked under and the back rounded, which over time can lead to vertebral injuries. To limit this relatively frequently occurring retraction of the hamstrings, stretching movements such as an easy good morning with straight legs and the stiff-legged deadlift are recommended. Hamstring stretches after a hamstring workout are also recommended.

Comment: A massage therapist can also treat fibrous scars by using massage or mechanical techniques aimed at softening the lesion.

13 GOOD MORNINGS

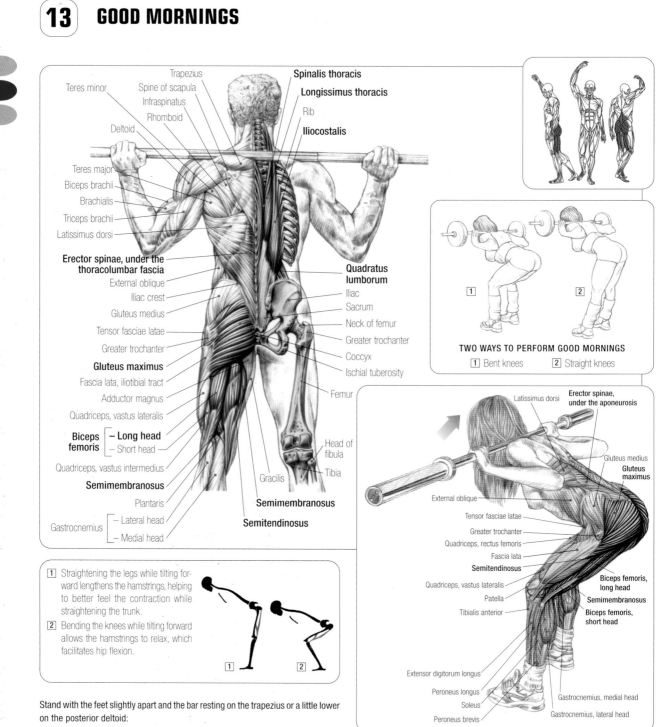

TWO WAYS TO PERFORM GOOD MORNINGS

1 Bent knees   2 Straight knees

Labels (left figure, from top): Trapezius, Teres minor, Spine of scapula, Infraspinatus, Rhomboid, Deltoid, Teres major, Biceps brachii, Brachialis, Triceps brachii, Latissimus dorsi, **Erector spinae, under the thoracolumbar fascia**, External oblique, Iliac crest, Gluteus medius, Tensor fasciae latae, Greater trochanter, **Gluteus maximus**, Fascia lata, iliotibial tract, Adductor magnus, Quadriceps, vastus lateralis, **Biceps femoris** — Long head — Short head, Quadriceps, vastus intermedius, **Semimembranosus**, Plantaris, **Gastrocnemius** — Lateral head — Medial head

Labels (center top): **Spinalis thoracis**, **Longissimus thoracis**, Rib, **Iliocostalis**, **Quadratus lumborum**, Iliac, Sacrum, Neck of femur, Greater trochanter, Coccyx, Ischial tuberosity, Femur, Head of fibula, Tibia, Gracilis, **Semimembranosus**, **Semitendinosus**

Labels (right figure): Latissimus dorsi, **Erector spinae, under the aponeurosis**, Gluteus medius, **Gluteus maximus**, External oblique, Tensor fasciae latae, Greater trochanter, Quadriceps, rectus femoris, Fascia lata, **Semitendinosus**, Quadriceps, vastus lateralis, Patella, Tibialis anterior, **Biceps femoris, long head**, **Semimembranosus**, **Biceps femoris, short head**, Extensor digitorum longus, Peroneus longus, Soleus, Peroneus brevis, Gastrocnemius, medial head, Gastrocnemius, lateral head

1 Straightening the legs while tilting forward lengthens the hamstrings, helping to better feel the contraction while straightening the trunk.

2 Bending the knees while tilting forward allows the hamstrings to relax, which facilitates hip flexion.

Stand with the feet slightly apart and the bar resting on the trapezius or a little lower on the posterior deltoid:

- Inhale and bend the torso forward, keeping the back straight. The axis of rotation should pass through the coxofemoral joints.
- Return to the initial position and exhale.

To make the exercise easier, bend slightly at the knees.

This movement, which works the gluteus maximus and the spinal group, is especially noteworthy for the action on the hamstrings (except the short head of the biceps femoris, which only flexes the knee). Besides knee flexion, the main function of the hamstrings is to tip the pelvis back (posterior rotation) and straighten the torso when the pelvis is locked to the torso through isometric contraction of the abdominal core and the lumbosacral muscle group.

To better feel the work of the hamstrings, don't work with heavy weights. In the negative phase, the good morning is excellent for stretching the back of the thighs. Worked regularly, it helps prevent injury when executing a heavy squat.

STRETCHING THE HAMSTRINGS

Stand on one leg, slightly bending at the knee; the other leg is extended with the foot in dorsiflexion:

- Place the hands on the thighs and slightly arch the back. Slowly bend the torso forward, concentrating on the feeling of stretching at the back of the thigh. The tilt occurs at the pelvis.
- Maintain this position for 20 seconds. Return slowly to the initial position and change sides.

This exercise mainly stretches the hamstring muscle group and adductor magnus as well as the gastrocnemius, soleus, and, to a lesser degree, gluteus maximus.

Variation: Stand on one leg with the other leg extended and resting on a bench with the foot in dorsiflexion:

- Place the hands on the thigh of the leg that is extended. Slightly arch the back and slowly tilt the torso forward, focusing on the feeling of stretching at the back of the thigh. The tilt occurs at the pelvis.
- Maintain the position for 20 seconds. Return slowly to the initial position and change sides.

To better focus on the stretching of the hamstrings, relax the calf muscles by putting the front foot into plantar flexion.

Attention: In weightlifting, the main function of stretching movements is to equalize the muscle fiber tension inside the muscle and limit the risk of injury.

With heavy weights, if the muscle fiber tension is not homogeneous, the tightest fibers risk tearing.

For this reason, at the beginning of the training session during the first warm-up series, perform a few stretching exercises specific to the muscle groups that will be worked.

Always perform the stretching movements gently and in moderation to protect the articulations and to avoid excessive stretching of the ligaments. Excessive and aggressive stretching risks destabilizing the articulation and generating pathological inflammation.

Comment: To avoid injury in the squat and the deadlift, practice this stretch at the beginning of a session by incorporating it among the first series.

External oblique
Latissimus dorsi
Erector spinae, under the aponeurosis
Iliac crest

Keep the back slightly arched.

Tensor fasciae latae
Gluteus medius
Greater trochanter

The tilt of the torso occur at the level of the hip joint.

Quadriceps
– Rectus femoris
– Vastus lateralis
– Vastus medialis
– Vastus intermedius

Gluteus maximus
Fascia lata
Adductor magnus
Semitendinosus

– Long head
– Short head Biceps femoris

Semimembranosus
Gastrocnemius
Peroneus longus
Soleus

Patella
Patellar ligament
Head of fibula
Extensor digitorum longus
Tibialis anterior
Peroneus tertius
Extensor hallucis longus
Peroneus brevis

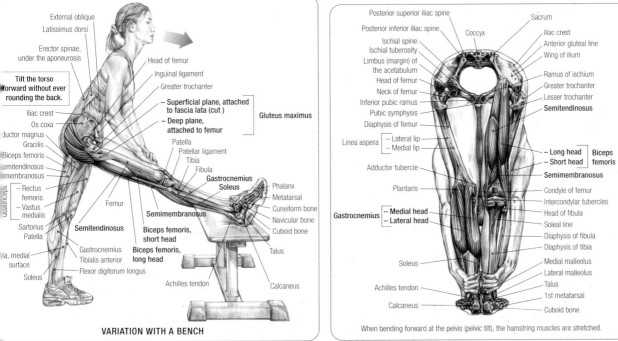

External oblique
Latissimus dorsi
Erector spinae, under the aponeurosis

Tilt the torso forward without ever rounding the back.

Iliac crest
Os coxa
Adductor magnus
Gracilis
Biceps femoris
Semitendinosus
Semimembranosus
– Rectus femoris
– Vastus medialis
Sartorius
Patella
Tibia, medial surface
Soleus

Head of femur
Inguinal ligament
Greater trochanter

– Superficial plane, attached to fascia lata (cut)
– Deep plane, attached to femur   Gluteus maximus

Patella
Patellar ligament
Tibia
Fibula
Gastrocnemius
Soleus
Phalanx
Metatarsal
Cuneiform bone
Navicular bone
Cuboid bone
Talus
Calcaneus

Femur
Semimembranosus
Biceps femoris, short head
Biceps femoris, long head
Semitendinosus
Gastrocnemius
Tibialis anterior
Flexor digitorum longus
Achilles tendon

VARIATION WITH A BENCH

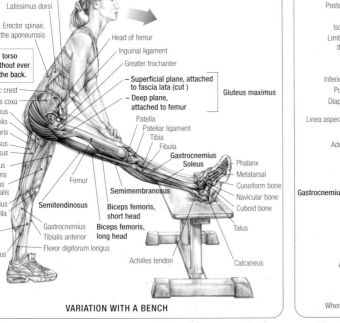

Posterior superior iliac spine
Posterior inferior iliac spine
Ischial spine
Ischial tuberosity
Limbus (margin) of the acetabulum
Head of femur
Neck of femur
Inferior pubic ramus
Pubic symphysis
Diaphysis of femur
Linea aspera – Lateral lip
– Medial lip
Adductor tubercle
Plantaris
Gastrocnemius – Medial head
– Lateral head
Soleus
Achilles tendon
Calcaneus

Coccyx
Sacrum
Iliac crest
Anterior gluteal line
Wing of ilium
Ramus of ischium
Greater trochanter
Lesser trochanter
Semitendinosus
– Long head Biceps
– Short head femoris
Semimembranosus
Condyle of femur
Intercondylar tubercles
Head of fibula
Soleal line
Diaphysis of fibula
Diaphysis of tibia
Medial malleolus
Lateral malleolus
Talus
1st metatarsal
Cuboid bone

When bending forward at the pelvis (pelvic tilt), the hamstring muscles are stretched.

14 CABLE ADDUCTIONS

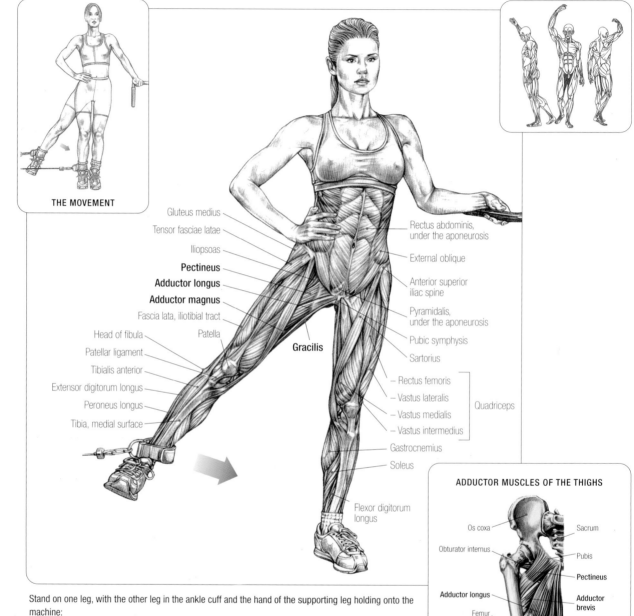

THE MOVEMENT

Gluteus medius

Tensor fasciae latae

Iliopsoas

Pectineus

Adductor longus

Adductor magnus

Fascia lata, iliotibial tract

Head of fibula

Patellar ligament

Tibialis anterior

Extensor digitorum longus

Peroneus longus

Tibia, medial surface

Patella

Gracilis

Rectus abdominis, under the aponeurosis

External oblique

Anterior superior iliac spine

Pyramidalis, under the aponeurosis

Pubic symphysis

Sartorius

– Rectus femoris

– Vastus lateralis

– Vastus medialis   Quadriceps

– Vastus intermedius

Gastrocnemius

Soleus

Flexor digitorum longus

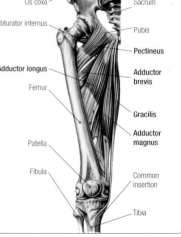

ADDUCTOR MUSCLES OF THE THIGHS

Os coxa

Obturator internus

Adductor longus

Femur

Patella

Fibula

Sacrum

Pubis

Pectineus

Adductor brevis

Gracilis

Adductor magnus

Common insertion

Tibia

Stand on one leg, with the other leg in the ankle cuff and the hand of the supporting leg holding onto the machine:

• Pull the cable across the support leg.

This exercise works the adductor group (pectineus; adductors brevis, longus, and magnus; and gracilis). To develop definition of the inside of the thighs, perform sets of high repetitions.

MACHINE ADDUCTIONS 15

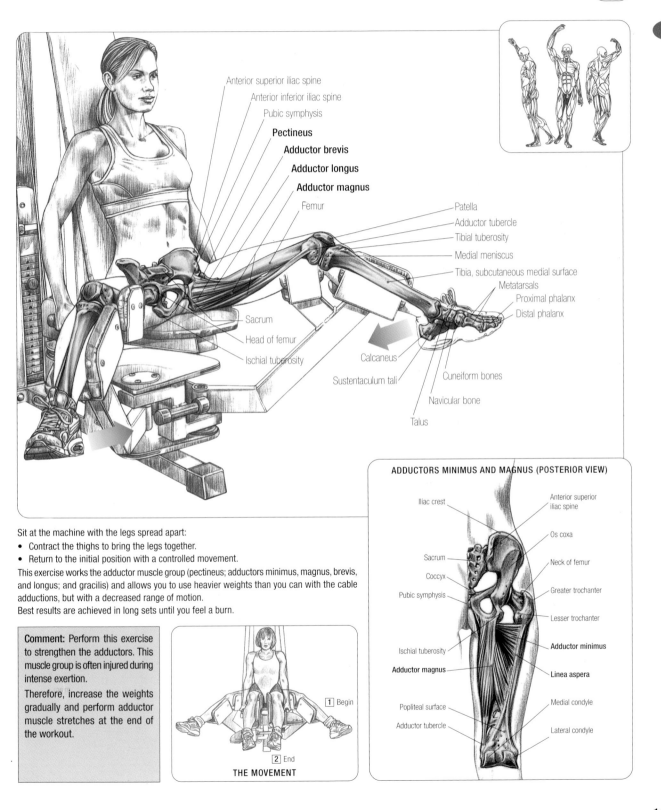

Anterior superior iliac spine
Anterior inferior iliac spine
Pubic symphysis
Pectineus
Adductor brevis
Adductor longus
Adductor magnus
Femur
Patella
Adductor tubercle
Tibial tuberosity
Medial meniscus
Tibia, subcutaneous medial surface
Metatarsals
Proximal phalanx
Distal phalanx
Sacrum
Head of femur
Ischial tuberosity
Calcaneus
Sustentaculum tali
Cuneiform bones
Navicular bone
Talus

ADDUCTORS MINIMUS AND MAGNUS (POSTERIOR VIEW)

Iliac crest
Anterior superior iliac spine
Os coxa
Sacrum
Neck of femur
Coccyx
Pubic symphysis
Greater trochanter
Lesser trochanter
Ischial tuberosity
Adductor minimus
Adductor magnus
Linea aspera
Popliteal surface
Medial condyle
Adductor tubercle
Lateral condyle

Sit at the machine with the legs spread apart:
- Contract the thighs to bring the legs together.
- Return to the initial position with a controlled movement.

This exercise works the adductor muscle group (pectineus; adductors minimus, magnus, brevis, and longus; and gracilis) and allows you to use heavier weights than you can with the cable adductions, but with a decreased range of motion.

Best results are achieved in long sets until you feel a burn.

Comment: Perform this exercise to strengthen the adductors. This muscle group is often injured during intense exertion.

Therefore, increase the weights gradually and perform adductor muscle stretches at the end of the workout.

1 Begin

2 End
THE MOVEMENT

16 FLEXION AND EXTENSION OF THE FEET

Trapezius

Deltoid

Teres minor

Infraspinatus

Teres major

Triceps

Latissimus dorsi

External oblique

Gluteus medius

5th lumbar vertebra

Iliac crest

Sacrum

Coccyx

Pubic symphysis

Iliac spine

Neck of femur

Ischial tuberosity

Greater trochanter

Lesser trochanter

Diaphysis of femur

Linea asperas

Medial condyle

Lateral condyle

Gluteus maximus

Greater trochanter

Adductor magnus

Semitendinosus

Gracilis

Quadriceps, vastus lateralis

– Long head
– Short head | Biceps femoris

Semimembranosus

Adductor tubercle

Gastrocnemius — Lateral head
— Medial head

Line of the soleus muscle

Femur

Plantaris

Head of fibula

Soleus

Gastrocnemius (cut)

The space between the tibia and fibula is filled with an interosseous membrane. This creates a sufficiently large, flat surface for attaching the muscles of the calf.

Fibula

Tibia

Tibialis posterior

Flexor hallucis longus

Flexor digitorum longus

Calcaneal tuberosity

Talus

Sustenaculum tali

Quadratus plantae

Flexor digitorum longus, tendon

Flexor hallucis longus, tendon

Soleus

Peroneus longus

Peroneus brevis

Achilles tendon

Medial malleolus

Lateral malleolus

Calcaneus

Navicular bone

Cuboid bone

Cuneiform bones

Metatarsals

Abductor hallucis

Flexor digitorum brevis

Abductor digiti minimi

Stand on a step with one hand holding a wall or railing for stability:

• Slowly dorsiflex your feet (lower your heels) to get a good stretch in the calves.

• Then plantar flex (rise up on your toes) while keeping the knees extended or slightly bent.

Perform this exercise slowly in a long series until you feel a burn.

The combined action of muscle contraction and stretching makes this movement ideal as a warm-up at the beginning of a training session for the calves with the purpose of avoiding injury, or at the end of the session in order to really feel the muscle contraction.

This exercise mainly works the triceps surae (made up of the two gastrocnemius and the soleus) as well as the flexor hallucis longus, tibialis posterior, and flexor digitorum longus (these last three muscles are located deeper).

Comment: This movement is also excellent for stretching the muscles of the plantar surface of the foot, such as the flexor digitorum brevis and the quadratus plantae, and for making the plantar aponeurosis more supple.

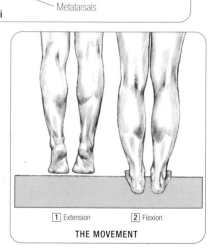

1 Extension   2 Flexion

THE MOVEMENT

STANDING CALF RAISES 17

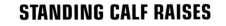

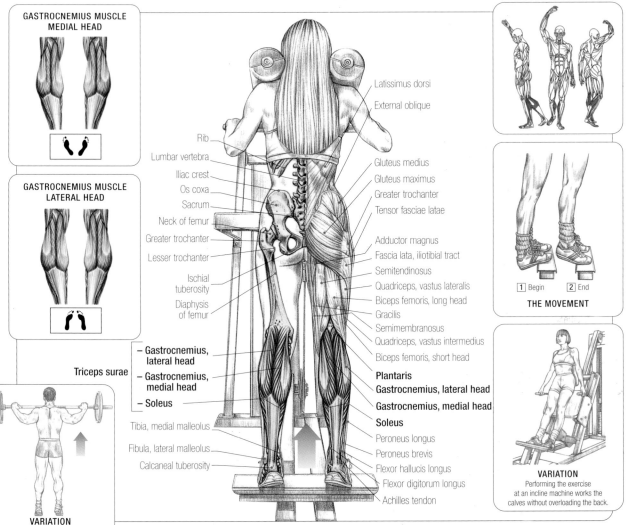

GASTROCNEMIUS MUSCLE MEDIAL HEAD

GASTROCNEMIUS MUSCLE LATERAL HEAD

Triceps surae

VARIATION
STANDING BARBELL CALF RAISES

Latissimus dorsi
External oblique
Rib
Lumbar vertebra
Iliac crest
Os coxa
Sacrum
Neck of femur
Greater trochanter
Lesser trochanter
Ischial tuberosity
Diaphysis of femur
Gluteus medius
Gluteus maximus
Greater trochanter
Tensor fasciae latae
Adductor magnus
Fascia lata, iliotibial tract
Semitendinosus
Quadriceps, vastus lateralis
Biceps femoris, long head
Gracilis
Semimembranosus
Quadriceps, vastus intermedius
Biceps femoris, short head

– Gastrocnemius, lateral head
– Gastrocnemius, medial head
– Soleus

Plantaris
Gastrocnemius, lateral head
Gastrocnemius, medial head
Soleus
Peroneus longus
Peroneus brevis
Flexor hallucis longus
Flexor digitorum longus
Achilles tendon

Tibia, medial malleolus
Fibula, lateral malleolus
Calcaneal tuberosity

THE MOVEMENT
1 Begin   2 End

VARIATION
Performing the exercise at an incline machine works the calves without overloading the back.

Stand at the machine with a straight back, shoulders under the pads, and the balls of the feet on the foot plate, with the calves relaxed and the heels hanging down:

• Rise up by extending (plantar flex) the feet, keeping the knees straight.

This exercise uses the triceps surae (made up of the soleus and the lateral and medial heads of the gastrocnemius). Move the feet through the complete range of flexion with each repetition in order to stretch the muscles properly. In theory, it is possible to isolate the medial gastrocnemius by pointing the toes out and to isolate the lateral gastrocnemius by pointing the toes in. But in practice, this is difficult to achieve. Only separating the work of the soleus and gastrocnemius is easy to achieve. This is done by flexing the knees to relax the gastrocnemius and to put more effort on the soleus.

Variations: Perform the exercise at a frame with a wedge under the feet or with a free bar without the wedge for more balance; however, this reduces the amplitude of movement.

Comment: The triceps surae is an extremely powerful, tough muscle group that alone raises the entire weight of the body thousands of times in a day when we walk. Don't hesitate to work it with heavy weights.

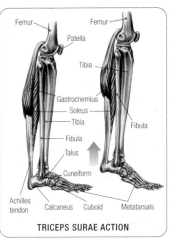

Femur
Femur
Patella
Tibia
Gastrocnemius
Soleus
Tibia
Fibula
Fibula
Talus
Cuneiform
Achilles tendon
Calcaneus
Cuboid
Metatarsals

TRICEPS SURAE ACTION

18 ONE-LEG TOE RAISES

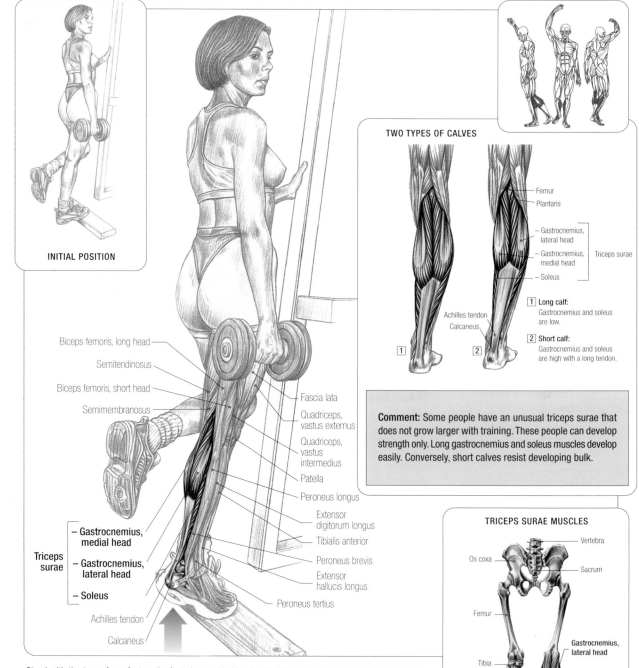

INITIAL POSITION

TWO TYPES OF CALVES

Femur
Plantaris
Gastrocnemius, lateral head
Gastrocnemius, medial head
Triceps surae
Soleus
Achilles tendon
Calcaneus

1 Long calf: Gastrocnemius and soleus are low.

2 Short calf: Gastrocnemius and soleus are high with a long tendon.

Comment: Some people have an unusual triceps surae that does not grow larger with training. These people can develop strength only. Long gastrocnemius and soleus muscles develop easily. Conversely, short calves resist developing bulk.

Biceps femoris, long head
Semitendinosus
Biceps femoris, short head
Semimembranosus
Fascia lata
Quadriceps, vastus externus
Quadriceps, vastus intermedius
Patella
Peroneus longus
Extensor digitorum longus
Tibialis anterior
Peroneus brevis
Extensor hallucis longus
Peroneus tertius

Triceps surae
– Gastrocnemius, medial head
– Gastrocnemius, lateral head
– Soleus
Achilles tendon
Calcaneus

TRICEPS SURAE MUSCLES

Vertebra
Os coxa
Sacrum
Femur
Gastrocnemius, lateral head
Tibia
Fibula
Gastrocnemius, medial head
Soleus
Achilles tendon
Calcaneus

Stand with the toes of one foot on the foot plate and hold a dumbbell in one hand and use the other hand for support and balance:

• Rise up on the toes (plantar flexion), keeping the knee joint straight or slightly flexed.
• Return to the initial position.

This exercise contracts the triceps surae. Completely flex the foot with each repetition in order to stretch the triceps surae properly. Optimal results are obtained through long sets until you feel a burn.

DONKEY CALF RAISES 19

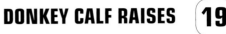

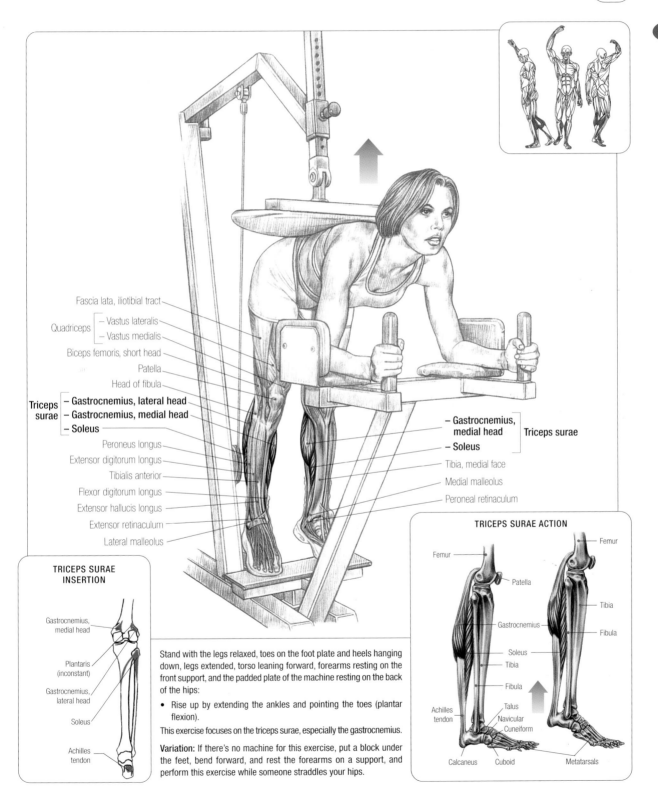

Fascia lata, iliotibial tract

Quadriceps — Vastus lateralis
— Vastus medialis

Biceps femoris, short head

Patella

Head of fibula

Triceps surae
— Gastrocnemius, lateral head
— Gastrocnemius, medial head
— Soleus

Peroneus longus

Extensor digitorum longus

Tibialis anterior

Flexor digitorum longus

Extensor hallucis longus

Extensor retinaculum

Lateral malleolus

— Gastrocnemius, medial head
— Soleus
Triceps surae

Tibia, medial face

Medial malleolus

Peroneal retinaculum

TRICEPS SURAE INSERTION

Gastrocnemius, medial head

Plantaris (inconstant)

Gastrocnemius, lateral head

Soleus

Achilles tendon

TRICEPS SURAE ACTION

Femur

Patella

Gastrocnemius

Tibia

Fibula

Achilles tendon

Femur

Tibia

Gastrocnemius

Fibula

Soleus

Tibia

Fibula

Talus
Navicular
Cuneiform

Calcaneus   Cuboid   Metatarsals

Stand with the legs relaxed, toes on the foot plate and heels hanging down, legs extended, torso leaning forward, forearms resting on the front support, and the padded plate of the machine resting on the back of the hips:

- Rise up by extending the ankles and pointing the toes (plantar flexion).

This exercise focuses on the triceps surae, especially the gastrocnemius.

Variation: If there's no machine for this exercise, put a block under the feet, bend forward, and rest the forearms on a support, and perform this exercise while someone straddles your hips.

20 SEATED MACHINE CALF RAISES

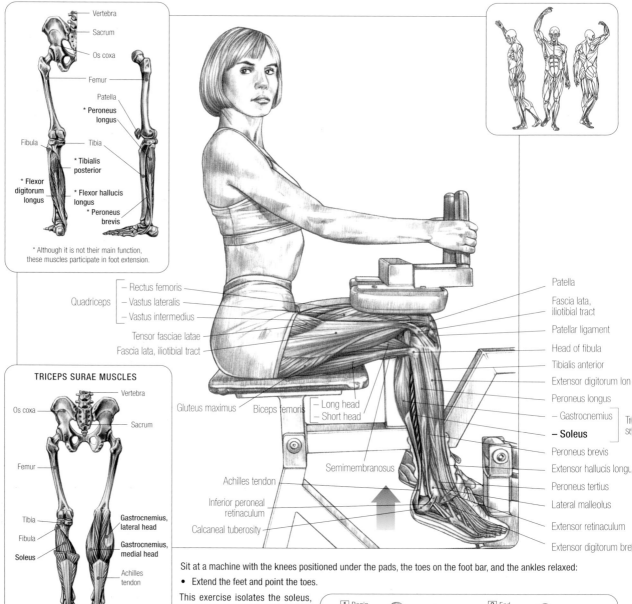

Vertebra

Sacrum

Os coxa

Femur

Patella

* Peroneus longus

Fibula

Tibia

* Tibialis posterior

* Flexor digitorum longus

* Flexor hallucis longus

* Peroneus brevis

*Although it is not their main function, these muscles participate in foot extension.

Quadriceps — Rectus femoris — Vastus lateralis — Vastus intermedius

Tensor fasciae latae

Fascia lata, iliotibial tract

Patella

Fascia lata, iliotibial tract

Patellar ligament

Head of fibula

Tibialis anterior

Extensor digitorum lon

Peroneus longus

– Gastrocnemius

– Soleus

Peroneus brevis

Extensor hallucis longu

Peroneus tertius

Lateral malleolus

Extensor retinaculum

Extensor digitorum bre

Gluteus maximus   Biceps femoris — Long head — Short head

Semimembranosus

Achilles tendon

Inferior peroneal retinaculum

Calcaneal tuberosity

TRICEPS SURAE MUSCLES

Vertebra

Os coxa

Sacrum

Femur

Tibia

Fibula

Soleus

Gastrocnemius, lateral head

Gastrocnemius, medial head

Achilles tendon

Calcaneus

Sit at a machine with the knees positioned under the pads, the toes on the foot bar, and the ankles relaxed:

• Extend the feet and point the toes.

This exercise isolates the soleus, whose name is derived from its resemblance to the flat fish, the sole.

(This muscle inserts at the top at the tibia and fibula under the knee joint and attaches at the bottom to the calcaneus by the Achilles tendon. Its purpose is to extend the feet at the ankles.)

Bending at the knees relaxes the gastrocnemius, which attaches at the top above the knee joint and at the bottom onto the Achilles tendon, and reduces its contribution to ankle extension.

Variation: You can also perform this exercise by sitting on a bench with a wedge under the feet and a barbell resting on the thighs. Wrap the bar for comfort.

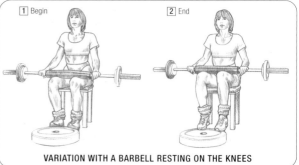

1 Begin   2 End

VARIATION WITH A BARBELL RESTING ON THE KNEES

SEATED BARBELL CALF RAISES 21

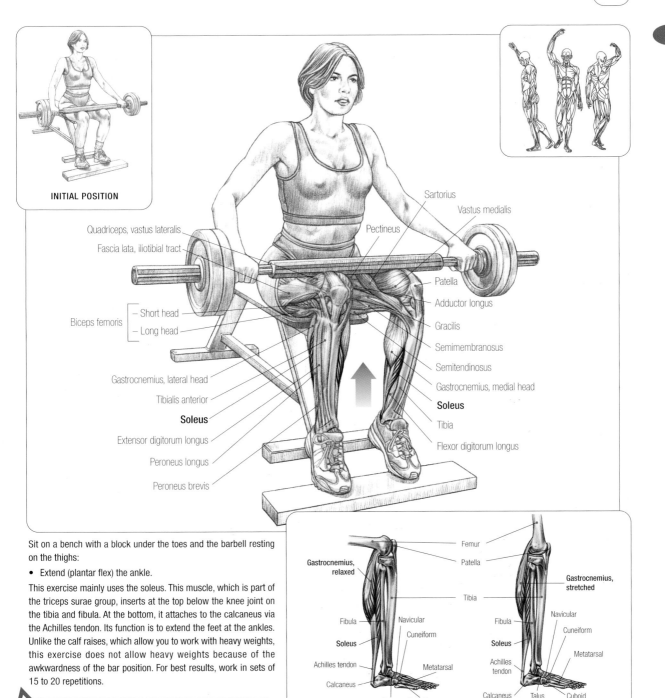

INITIAL POSITION

Sartorius
Vastus medialis
Pectineus
Quadriceps, vastus lateralis
Fascia lata, iliotibial tract
Patella
Adductor longus
Biceps femoris
— Short head
— Long head
Gracilis
Semimembranosus
Semitendinosus
Gastrocnemius, lateral head
Gastrocnemius, medial head
Tibialis anterior
Soleus
Soleus
Tibia
Extensor digitorum longus
Flexor digitorum longus
Peroneus longus
Peroneus brevis

Sit on a bench with a block under the toes and the barbell resting on the thighs:

• Extend (plantar flex) the ankle.

This exercise mainly uses the soleus. This muscle, which is part of the triceps surae group, inserts at the top below the knee joint on the tibia and fibula. At the bottom, it attaches to the calcaneus via the Achilles tendon. Its function is to extend the feet at the ankles. Unlike the calf raises, which allow you to work with heavy weights, this exercise does not allow heavy weights because of the awkwardness of the bar position. For best results, work in sets of 15 to 20 repetitions.

⚠ **Attention:** Cushion the bar on the thighs with a rubber pad or a folded towel to reduce pain.

Variation: You can also perform this exercise without additional weights while sitting on a chair or bench. In this case, work in very long sets until you feel a burn.

Gastrocnemius, relaxed
Femur
Patella
Gastrocnemius, stretched
Tibia
Fibula
Navicular
Cuneiform
Fibula
Navicular
Cuneiform
Soleus
Soleus
Metatarsal
Achilles tendon
Metatarsal
Achilles tendon
Calcaneus
Calcaneus
Talus
Cuboid
Talus
Cuboid

1

When the knees are bent, the gastrocnemius muscle, which attaches above the knee, is relaxed. In this position, it weakly assists ankle extension because most of the work is done by the soleus.

2

Conversely, when the knee is straight, the gastrocnemius is stretched. In this position, it actively participates in ankle extension and completes the action of the soleus.

STRETCHING THE CALF

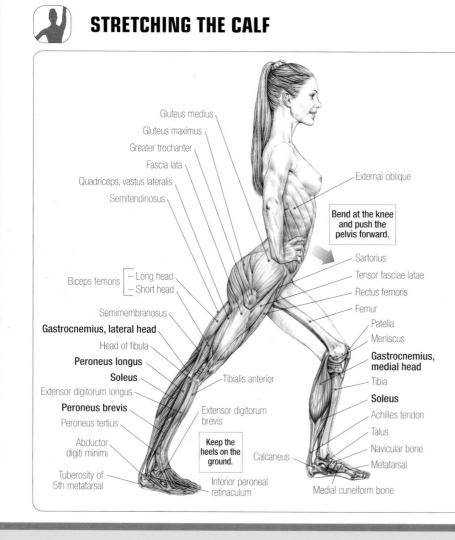

Gluteus medius

Gluteus maximus

Greater trochanter

Fascia lata

Quadriceps, vastus lateralis

Semitendinosus

External oblique

Bend at the knee and push the pelvis forward.

Biceps femoris [— Long head
— Short head

Sartorius

Tensor fasciae latae

Rectus femoris

Femur

Patella

Meniscus

Semimembranosus

Gastrocnemius, lateral head

Head of fibula

Peroneus longus

Soleus

Extensor digitorum longus

Peroneus brevis

Peroneus tertius

Abductor digiti minimi

Tuberosity of 5th metatarsal

Tibialis anterior

Extensor digitorum brevis

Keep the heels on the ground.

Inferior peroneal retinaculum

Gastrocnemius, medial head

Tibia

Soleus

Achilles tendon

Talus

Navicular bone

Metatarsal

Medial cuneiform bone

Calcaneus

Stand with your hands on your hips, with one leg forward in a lunge stance, the other leg extended behind, and your feet in line with the knees:

- Bend the forward knee by advancing with your pelvis, being careful to always keep the back leg extended with the heel on the ground.
- Hold this position until you feel the stretch on the posterior leg.

This exercise mainly solicits the triceps surae, which is made up of the gastrocnemius and the soleus; the flexor digitorum muscles; and the tibialis posterior located deeper beneath the triceps surae. To a lesser degree it solicits the peroneus longus and brevis.

SHORT CALF, LONG CALF

There are great individual differences in the shape of calves. A large part of these morphological variations developed during the first human migrations as evolutionary adaptation to climate. Thus Black Africans commonly have legs that are proportionately longer, a dropped plantar arch (flat feet), and a relatively long calcaneus. This osseous configuration of the leg and foot creates an excellent lever at the ankle with a minimum of triceps surae muscle (the muscle of the calf is short, slender, and high with a long tendon), which produces powerful extension of the foot while walking. On the other hand, Nordic people frequently have legs that are proportionately shorter with a very prominent plantar arch and a short, close calcaneus. This osseous conformation of the leg and foot with a shorter lever requires a voluminous and not very economical triceps surae that reaches far down for extension while walking. This type of long, bulky calf is in fact adapted for cold climates. It conserves the heat of the body, offering a minimal exterior surface and limiting the thermal exchanges and incapacitating, if not fatal, chilling during periods of intense cold. Although often considered more attractive, the long and bulky calf is less well adapted for running and more vulnerable to muscle tearing. Thus, this type of calf needs a more careful warm-up and requires stretching movements before and after intense training sessions.

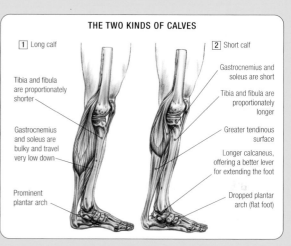

THE TWO KINDS OF CALVES

1 Long calf

Tibia and fibula are proportionately shorter

Gastrocnemius and soleus are bulky and travel very low down

Prominent plantar arch

2 Short calf

Gastrocnemius and soleus are short

Tibia and fibula are proportionately longer

Greater tendinous surface

Longer calcaneus, offering a better lever for extending the foot

Dropped plantar arch (flat foot)

6 BUTTOCKS

Gluteal Muscles, a Human Characteristic

Although some of the larger primates occasionally walk, humans are the only primates and one of the few mammals that have completely adapted to two-legged locomotion. One of the structural features directly related to this way of getting around is the significant development of the gluteus maximus muscle, which has become the biggest and most powerful muscle in the human body.

The development of the gluteal muscles is truly a human characteristic. In comparison, the gluteal muscles in quadrupeds are proportionately underdeveloped, and the hindquarters of the horse, which some consider as typical for animals, are in fact made up of the hamstrings (the back of the thigh in humans).

In humans, the gluteus maximus, which extends the hip, does not play an important role in walking. Instead, the hamstrings play the major role in straightening the pelvis (hip extension) with each stride. Just put your hand on the buttocks while walking, and you can feel that they do not contract much.

However, as soon as the effort becomes significant, such as when walking uphill, walking quickly, or running, the gluteal action is called into play to extend the hip and erect the torso.

These biomechanical points help explain why in exercises for the gluteal muscles and the hamstrings, such as good mornings (see page 144) and stiff-legged deadlifts (see page 102), either the gluteal muscles or the hamstrings are isolated depending on the amount of weight involved.

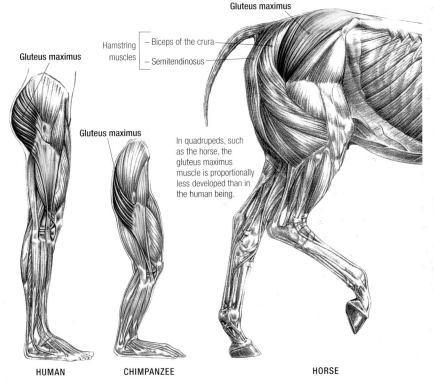

Gluteus maximus

Gluteus maximus

Hamstring muscles — Biceps of the crura
— Semitendinosus

Gluteus maximus

Gluteus maximus

In quadrupeds, such as the horse, the gluteus maximus muscle is proportionally less developed than in the human being.

HUMAN　　　CHIMPANZEE　　　HORSE

1 BARBELL LUNGES

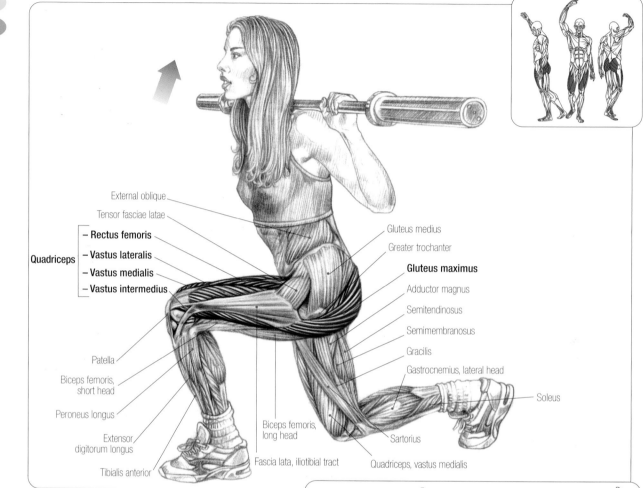

External oblique
Tensor fasciae latae
Rectus femoris
Quadriceps
Vastus lateralis
Vastus medialis
Vastus intermedius

Patella
Biceps femoris, short head
Peroneus longus
Extensor digitorum longus
Tibialis anterior

Gluteus medius
Greater trochanter
Gluteus maximus
Adductor magnus
Semitendinosus
Semimembranosus
Gracilis
Gastrocnemius, lateral head
Soleus

Biceps femoris, long head
Fascia lata, iliotibial tract
Sartorius
Quadriceps, vastus medialis

Stand with the legs slightly apart and the bar behind the neck resting on the trapezius muscles:

- Inhale and take a big step forward, keeping the trunk as straight as possible.
- Lunge until the front thigh is horizontal to the floor or slightly less.
- Exhale and return to the initial position.

This exercise, which works the gluteus maximus intensely, can be performed two different ways: either by taking a small step (which isolates the quadriceps) or taking a big step (which isolates the hamstrings and gluteus maximus and stretches the rectus femoris and iliopsoas of the back leg).

Comment: Because the front leg must support almost all the weight in the lunge position and the exercise demands a good sense of balance, begin with very light weights.

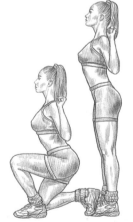
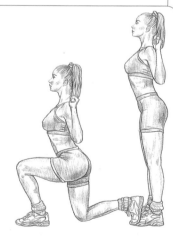

1 Execution with a small step predominantly works the quadriceps.

2 Execution with a big step predominantly works the gluteus maximus.

DUMBBELL LUNGES 2

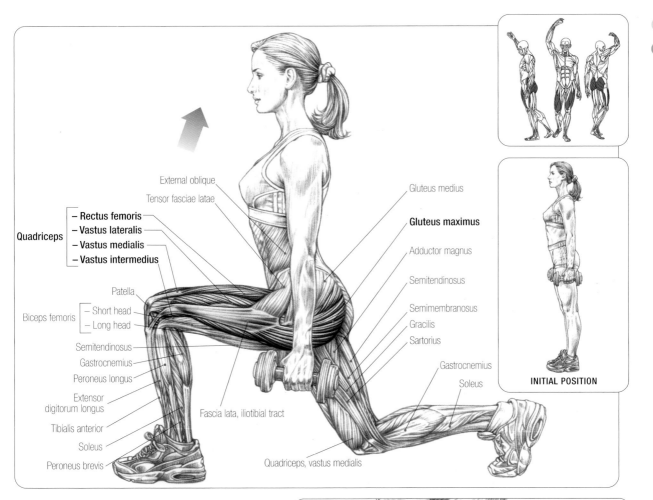

Quadriceps
- – **Rectus femoris**
- – **Vastus lateralis**
- – **Vastus medialis**
- – **Vastus intermedius**

External oblique

Tensor fasciae latae

Patella

Biceps femoris
- – Short head
- – Long head

Semitendinosus

Gastrocnemius

Peroneus longus

Extensor digitorum longus

Tibialis anterior

Soleus

Peroneus brevis

Fascia lata, iliotibial tract

Quadriceps, vastus medialis

Gluteus medius

Gluteus maximus

Adductor magnus

Semitendinosus

Semimembranosus

Gracilis

Sartorius

Gastrocnemius

Soleus

INITIAL POSITION

Stand with the legs slightly apart and hold a dumbbell in each hand:
- Inhale and take a big step forward, keeping the torso as straight as possible.
- When the forward thigh reaches horizontal or slightly below, use tonic extension to return to the initial position.
- Exhale at the end of the movement.

This exercise mainly works the gluteus maximus and quadriceps.

The bigger the step, the more the gluteus maximus of the forward leg is used and the iliopsoas and rectus femoris of the back leg are stretched.

A smaller step isolates the quadriceps of the forward leg.

You can perform a complete set on one side and then the other or work the legs alternately during the same set.

Comment: Because all of the weight is supported by the front leg in the lunge position and the exercise requires a good sense of balance, work with light weights to protect the knee.

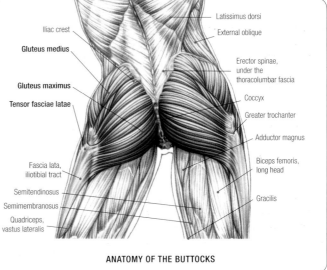

Iliac crest

Gluteus medius

Gluteus maximus

Tensor fasciae latae

Fascia lata, iliotibial tract

Semitendinosus

Semimembranosus

Quadriceps, vastus lateralis

Latissimus dorsi

External oblique

Erector spinae, under the thoracolumbar fascia

Coccyx

Greater trochanter

Adductor magnus

Biceps femoris, long head

Gracilis

ANATOMY OF THE BUTTOCKS

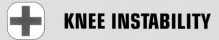

KNEE INSTABILITY

When the knee is extended, the medial and lateral collateral ligaments are stretched and prevent rotation of the joint. When you are standing, the knee locks in extension, and there is no need for muscle tension to stabilize the joint.

When the knee is bent, the medial and lateral collateral ligaments are relaxed. In this position, muscle tension provides the stability.

When the knee flexes and rotates, the meniscus travels forward. Then, if extension is not controlled, the meniscus may not return to its normal position fast enough and becomes pinched between the condyles, which can tear the meniscus. If a piece of the meniscus is severed when it is pinched, surgery may be necessary to remove it.

With asymmetrical exercises such as the lunge (see pages 156 and 157), control the speed and the form of the movement to protect the knee.

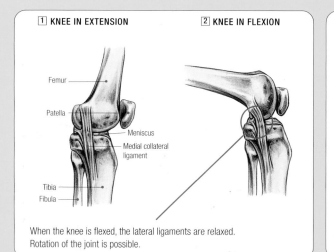

When the knee is flexed, the lateral ligaments are relaxed. Rotation of the joint is possible.

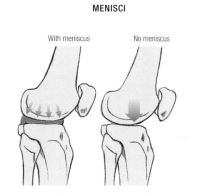

One of the main functions of the meniscus is to disperse pressure in the knee joint by increasing the supporting surface area for the femur on the tibia, avoiding premature wear on the articular surfaces.

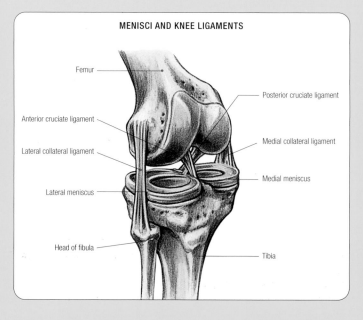

CABLE BACK KICKS 3

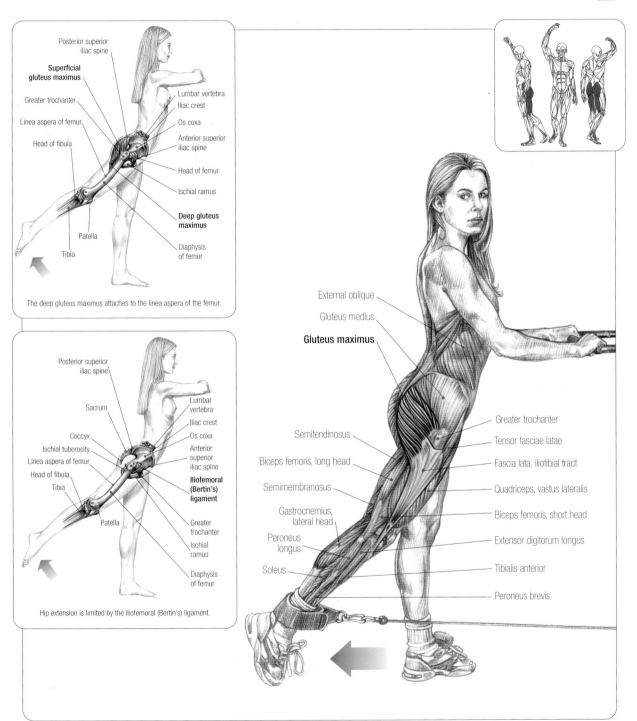

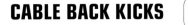

Posterior superior iliac spine

Superficial gluteus maximus

Greater trochanter

Linea aspera of femur

Head of fibula

Lumbar vertebra
Iliac crest

Os coxa

Anterior superior iliac spine

Head of femur

Ischial ramus

Deep gluteus maximus

Patella

Diaphysis of femur

Tibia

The deep gluteus maximus attaches to the linea aspera of the femur.

Posterior superior iliac spine

Sacrum

Coccyx

Ischial tuberosity

Linea aspera of femur

Head of fibula

Tibia

Patella

Lumbar vertebra

Iliac crest

Os coxa

Anterior superior iliac spine

Iliofemoral (Bertin's) ligament

Greater trochanter

Ischial ramus

Diaphysis of femur

Hip extension is limited by the iliofemoral (Bertin's) ligament.

External oblique

Gluteus medius

Gluteus maximus

Semitendinosus

Biceps femoris, long head

Semimembranosus

Gastrocnemius, lateral head

Peroneus longus

Soleus

Greater trochanter

Tensor fasciae latae

Fascia lata, iliotibial tract

Quadriceps, vastus lateralis

Biceps femoris, short head

Extensor digitorum longus

Tibialis anterior

Peroneus brevis

Stand on one leg facing the machine, the other leg attached to the ankle strap of the low pulley, and the pelvis tilted forward. Grasp the handle:

- Extend the hip and pull the leg back.
- Hip extension is limited by the tension of the iliofemoral (Bertin's) ligament.

This exercise mainly works the gluteus maximus and, to a lesser extent, the hamstrings (except the short head of the biceps femoris).

It helps develop the profile of the hips while firming the gluteal region.

4 MACHINE HIP EXTENSIONS

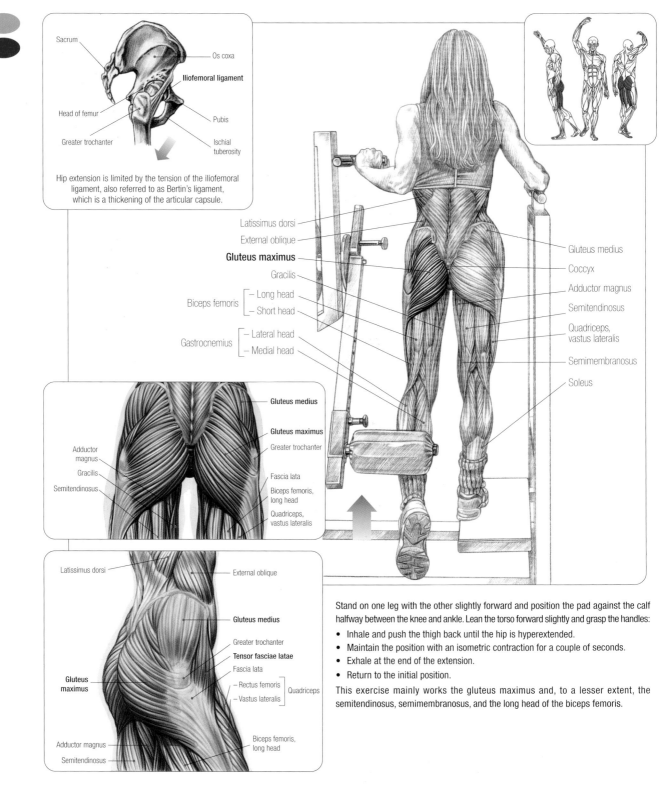

Sacrum

Os coxa

Iliofemoral ligament

Head of femur

Pubis

Greater trochanter

Ischial tuberosity

Hip extension is limited by the tension of the iliofemoral ligament, also referred to as Bertin's ligament, which is a thickening of the articular capsule.

Latissimus dorsi

External oblique

Gluteus maximus

Gracilis

Biceps femoris ⎧ – Long head
⎩ – Short head

Gastrocnemius ⎧ – Lateral head
⎩ – Medial head

Gluteus medius

Coccyx

Adductor magnus

Semitendinosus

Quadriceps, vastus lateralis

Semimembranosus

Soleus

Gluteus medius

Gluteus maximus

Greater trochanter

Fascia lata

Biceps femoris, long head

Quadriceps, vastus lateralis

Adductor magnus

Gracilis

Semitendinosus

Latissimus dorsi

External oblique

Gluteus medius

Greater trochanter

Tensor fasciae latae

Fascia lata

– Rectus femoris ⎫
⎬ Quadriceps
– Vastus lateralis ⎭

Gluteus maximus

Adductor magnus

Semitendinosus

Biceps femoris, long head

Stand on one leg with the other slightly forward and position the pad against the calf halfway between the knee and ankle. Lean the torso forward slightly and grasp the handles:

- Inhale and push the thigh back until the hip is hyperextended.
- Maintain the position with an isometric contraction for a couple of seconds.
- Exhale at the end of the extension.
- Return to the initial position.

This exercise mainly works the gluteus maximus and, to a lesser extent, the semitendinosus, semimembranosus, and the long head of the biceps femoris.

FLOOR HIP EXTENSIONS 5

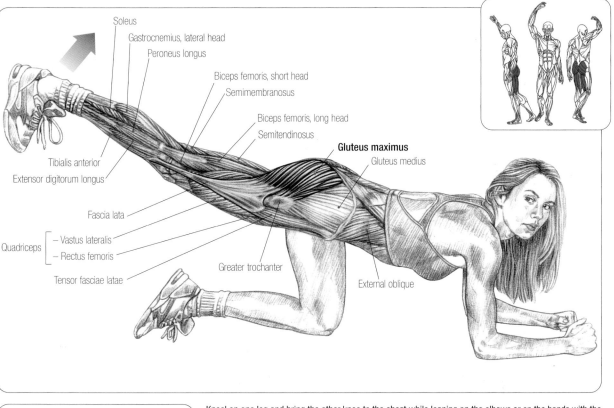

- Soleus
- Gastrocnemius, lateral head
- Peroneus longus
- Biceps femoris, short head
- Semimembranosus
- Biceps femoris, long head
- Semitendinosus
- **Gluteus maximus**
- Gluteus medius
- Tibialis anterior
- Extensor digitorum longus
- Fascia lata
- Quadriceps
  - − Vastus lateralis
  - − Rectus femoris
- Tensor fasciae latae
- Greater trochanter
- External oblique

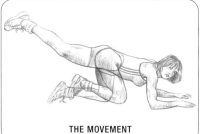

THE MOVEMENT

Kneel on one leg and bring the other knee to the chest while leaning on the elbows or on the hands with the arms extended:

- Extend the bent leg back with complete hip extension.

With the leg extended, this exercise uses the hamstrings and gluteus maximus. With the knee bent, only the gluteus maximus is used, and less intensely.

This exercise can be performed with higher or lower amplitude during the last part of the extension. You can maintain an isometric contraction for a couple of seconds at the end of the movement.

To increase the intensity, use ankle weights.

Its ease of execution and its effectiveness have made this exercise popular, and it is frequently used in group classes.

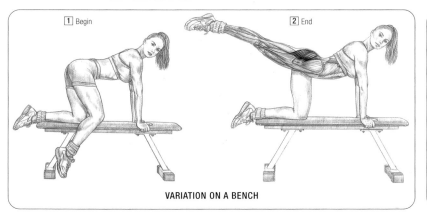

1 Begin   2 End

VARIATION ON A BENCH

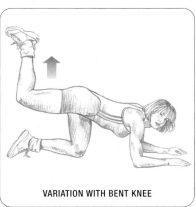

VARIATION WITH BENT KNEE

6 BRIDGING

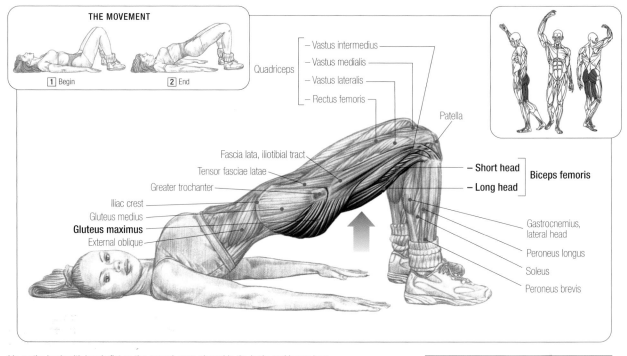

Lie on the back with hands flat on the ground, arms alongside the body, and knees bent:
- Inhale and lift the buttocks off the ground, pushing down through the feet.
- Maintain the position for a couple of seconds and lower the pelvis without touching the buttocks to the ground.
- Exhale and begin again.

This exercise mainly works the hamstrings and gluteus maximus.

Perform this exercise in long sets, making sure to contract the muscles at the top of the lift, when the pelvis is off the ground.

Comment: Because it is easy and effective, bridging has become part of most group exercise classes.

Variation 1

To perform bridging with the feet raised, lie on the back with hands flat at the sides, arms alongside the body, thighs vertical, and feet resting on a bench:
- Inhale and raise the pelvis off the ground; maintain the position for two seconds and lower without touching the buttocks to the ground.
- Exhale and begin again.

This exercise works the gluteus maximus and especially the hamstrings. The hamstrings are used more in this exercise than when bridging from the ground. Execute this exercise slowly, and focus on the muscle contraction.

Sets of 10 to 15 repetitions provide the best results.

Another variation is to perform bridging with the calves resting on the bench. This isolates the hamstrings even more intensely and also requires strong work from the gastrocnemius.

Variation 2

Limit the range of the movement by not lowering the pelvis as far to create a burn.

Comment: Bridging is actually extending the hips.

STRETCHING THE GLUTEUS MAXIMUS AND HAMSTRINGS

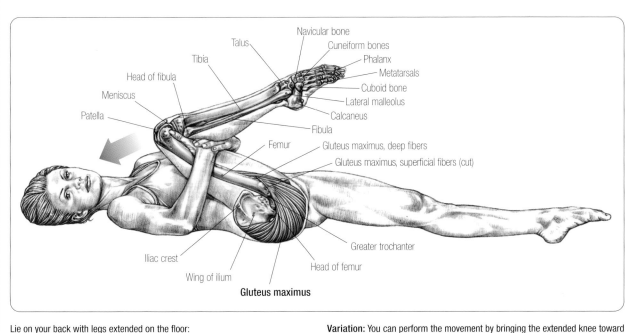

Talus
Navicular bone
Cuneiform bones
Tibia
Phalanx
Head of fibula
Metatarsals
Meniscus
Cuboid bone
Patella
Lateral malleolus
Calcaneus
Femur
Gluteus maximus, deep fibers
Gluteus maximus, superficial fibers (cut)
Fibula
Greater trochanter
Iliac crest
Head of femur
Wing of ilium
Gluteus maximus

Lie on your back with legs extended on the floor:

- Using your hands, gently bring one leg with the knee bent to your chest (to relax the hamstring muscles).
- Maintain the position, breathing slowly and trying to feel the stretching of the gluteus maximus muscle.
- Return to the initial position; change legs.

Variation: You can perform the movement by bringing the extended knee toward the chest. In this case, the stretch will be more intense on the hamstrings and less on the gluteus maximus. Note that tension on the hamstring muscles might strongly limit bending at the hip.

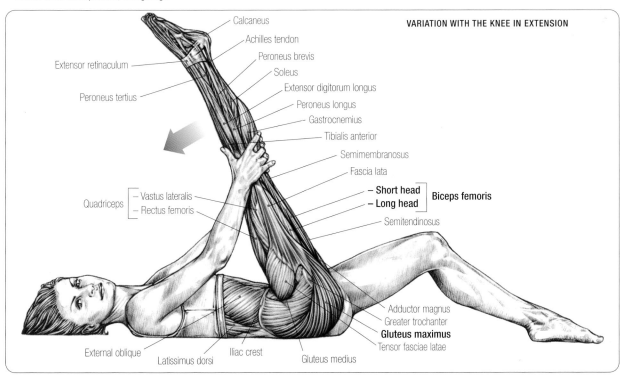

VARIATION WITH THE KNEE IN EXTENSION

Calcaneus
Achilles tendon
Peroneus brevis
Soleus
Extensor retinaculum
Extensor digitorum longus
Peroneus tertius
Peroneus longus
Gastrocnemius
Tibialis anterior
Semimembranosus
Fascia lata
Quadriceps
Vastus lateralis
Rectus femoris
– Short head
– Long head
Biceps femoris
Semitendinosus
Adductor magnus
Greater trochanter
Gluteus maximus
Tensor fasciae latae
External oblique
Latissimus dorsi
Iliac crest
Gluteus medius

7 CABLE HIP ABDUCTIONS

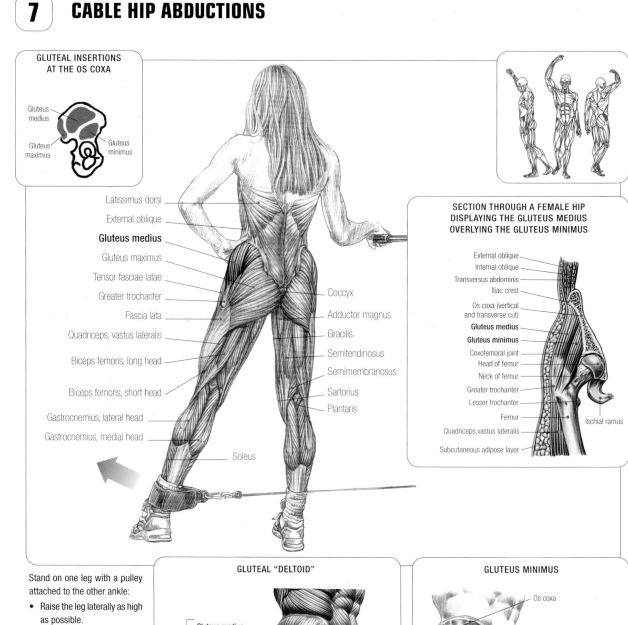

GLUTEAL INSERTIONS AT THE OS COXA

Gluteus medius
Gluteus maximus
Gluteus minimus

Latissimus dorsi
External oblique
Gluteus medius
Gluteus maximus
Tensor fasciae latae
Greater trochanter
Fascia lata
Quadriceps, vastus lateralis
Biceps femoris, long head
Biceps femoris, short head
Gastrocnemius, lateral head
Gastrocnemius, medial head
Soleus

Coccyx
Adductor magnus
Gracilis
Semitendinosus
Semimembranosus
Sartorius
Plantaris

SECTION THROUGH A FEMALE HIP DISPLAYING THE GLUTEUS MEDIUS OVERLYING THE GLUTEUS MINIMUS

External oblique
Internal oblique
Transversus abdominis
Iliac crest
Os coxa (vertical and transverse cut)
Gluteus medius
Gluteus minimus
Coxofemoral joint
Head of femur
Neck of femur
Greater trochanter
Lesser trochanter
Femur
Quadriceps, vastus lateralis
Subcutaneous adipose layer
Ischial ramus

Stand on one leg with a pulley attached to the other ankle:

- Raise the leg laterally as high as possible.

This exercise mainly works the gluteus medius and the deeper gluteus minimus.

Long sets until you feel a burn are most effective.

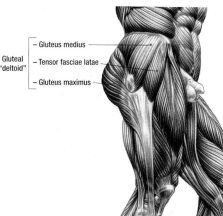

GLUTEAL "DELTOID"

Gluteal "deltoid"
– Gluteus medius
– Tensor fasciae latae
– Gluteus maximus

GLUTEUS MINIMUS

Os coxa
Gluteus minimus
Greater trochanter
Femur
Patella

Although located deep, the gluteus minimus contributes to the bulk of the upper buttock.

INDIVIDUAL VARIATIONS IN HIP MOBILITY

Regardless of individual muscle elasticity and ligamentous tension, it is mainly the shape of the bones of the coxofemoral joint that is responsible for hip mobility. The configuration of the bone is most important in hip abduction.

Examples

- When the neck of the femur is almost horizontal (coxa vara) and associated with a well-developed superior rim of the acetabulum covering the head of the femur, abduction movements are limited.
- When the neck of the femur is close to vertical (coxa valga) and associated with an undeveloped superior acetabular rim, abduction movements are facilitated.

Therefore, it is useless to try to raise the leg high laterally if your hip joint is not made for it.

Attention: If hip abduction is forced, the neck of the femur will butt up against the rim of the acetabulum, and the pelvis will tilt onto the head of the opposite femur to compensate for lateral extension of the leg. When some people perform sets of forced abductions, over time microtrauma may occur, which develops excessive growth of the superior rim of the acetabulum, limiting the mobility of the hip and risking painful inflammation.

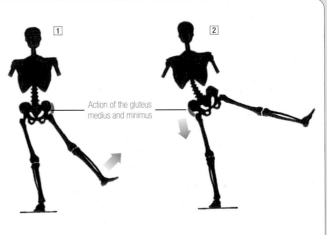

Action of the gluteus medius and minimus

1 Abduction of the hip (limited by the neck of the femur butting against the acetabulum)

2 Forced abduction of the hip (tilting the pelvis onto the head of the opposite femur)

VARIATIONS IN OSSEOUS HIP STRUCTURE

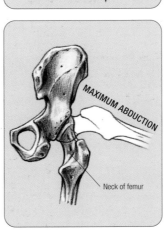

MAXIMUM ABDUCTION

Neck of femur

An almost horizontal neck of the femur is referred to as a coxa vara. It limits abduction movements because it butts up against the rim of the acetabulum sooner.

An almost vertical neck of the femur is referred to as **coxa valga**. It allows greater abduction movements.

Neck of femur

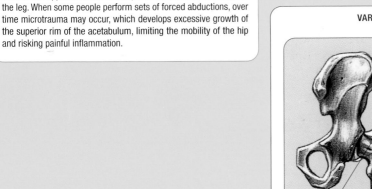

Os coxa

Greater trochanter

Head of femur

Lesser trochanter

Ischial spine

Ischion

Acetabulum

Neck of femur

ABDUCTION IS LIMITED BY THE NECK OF THE FEMUR BUTTING UP AGAINST THE RIM OF THE ACETABULUM.

8 STANDING MACHINE HIP ABDUCTIONS

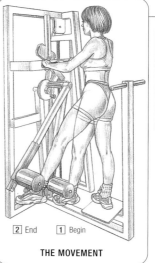

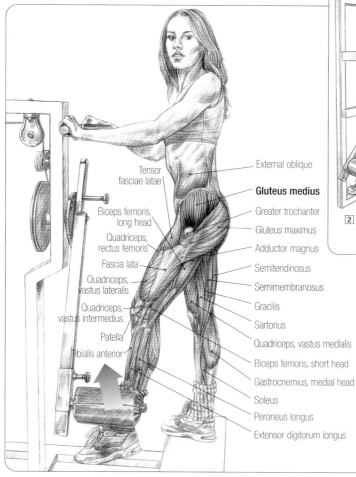

External oblique

Gluteus medius

Greater trochanter

Gluteus maximus

Adductor magnus

Semitendinosus

Semimembranosus

Gracilis

Sartorius

Quadriceps, vastus medialis

Biceps femoris, short head

Gastrocnemius, medial head

Soleus

Peroneus longus

Extensor digitorum longus

Tensor fasciae latae

Biceps femoris, long head

Quadriceps, rectus femoris

Fascia lata

Quadriceps, vastus lateralis

Quadriceps, vastus intermedius

Patella

Tibialis anterior

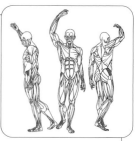

2 End   **1** Begin

THE MOVEMENT

Stand on one leg at the machine and place the other leg against the pad below the knee:

- Slowly raise the leg as high as possible.
- Return to the initial position.

Abduction is limited by how soon the neck of the femur butts up against the rim of the acetabulum.

This exercise develops the gluteus medius. It also develops the deeper gluteus minimus, whose function is the same as that of the anterior fibers of the gluteus medius. For best results, use long sets.

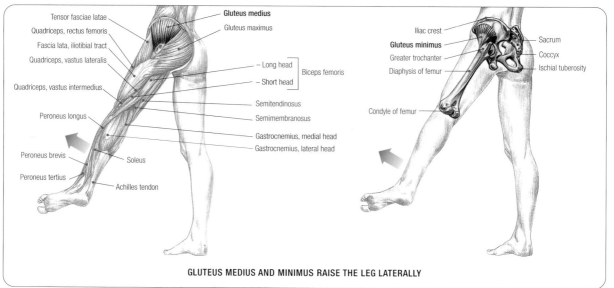

Tensor fasciae latae

Quadriceps, rectus femoris

Fascia lata, iliotibial tract

Quadriceps, vastus lateralis

Quadriceps, vastus intermedius

Peroneus longus

Peroneus brevis

Peroneus tertius

Soleus

Achilles tendon

Gluteus medius

Gluteus maximus

– Long head
– Short head } Biceps femoris

Semitendinosus

Semimembranosus

Gastrocnemius, medial head

Gastrocnemius, lateral head

Iliac crest

Gluteus minimus

Greater trochanter

Diaphysis of femur

Condyle of femur

Sacrum

Coccyx

Ischial tuberosity

GLUTEUS MEDIUS AND MINIMUS RAISE THE LEG LATERALLY

LYING HIP ABDUCTIONS 9

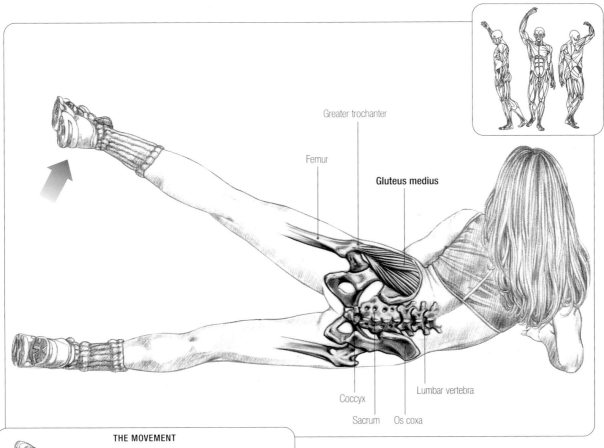

Greater trochanter

Femur

Gluteus medius

Coccyx

Lumbar vertebra

Sacrum   Os coxa

THE MOVEMENT

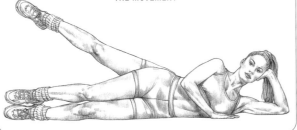

Lie on the side and support the head with the hand or rest the upper body on your elbow:

- Raise the leg laterally no more than 70 degrees, keeping the knee straight.

This exercise works the gluteus medius and minimus. You can vary how high you raise the leg. Hold the leg at the height of the movement for a few seconds with an isometric contraction.

You can raise the leg slightly to the front or the back or raise it vertically.

To increase the intensity, use ankle weights, an elastic band, or a low pulley.

THREE WAYS TO RAISE THE LEG

ISOLATED ZONES

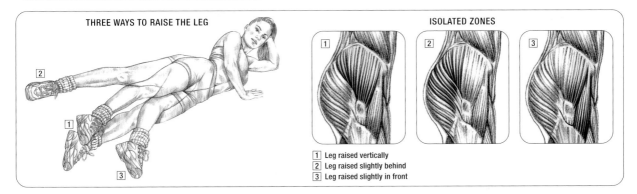

1 Leg raised vertically
2 Leg raised slightly behind
3 Leg raised slightly in front

10 SEATED MACHINE HIP ABDUCTIONS

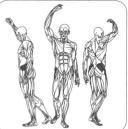

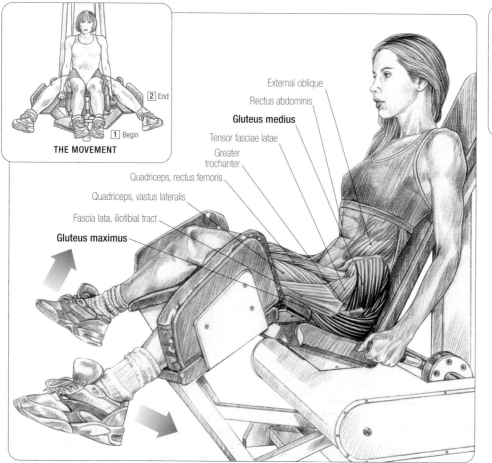

2 End

1 Begin

THE MOVEMENT

External oblique

Rectus abdominis

Gluteus medius

Tensor fasciae latae

Greater trochanter

Quadriceps, rectus femoris

Quadriceps, vastus lateralis

Fascia lata, iliotibial tract

Gluteus maximus

Sit at the machine:

• Spread the legs as wide as possible.

• Return to the initial position with a controlled movement.

The more angled the backrest, the more the gluteus medius is isolated. The more vertical the backrest, the more the gluteus maximus is worked. Ideally, lean forward or back to change the angle of the torso during a set.

Example: Perform 10 repetitions with the torso resting against the backrest and 10 repetitions with the torso leaning forward.

This exercise sculpts and firms the top of the hip, which makes the waistline look narrower.

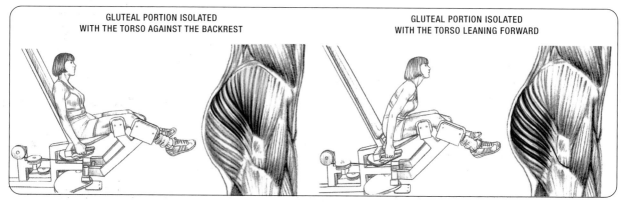

GLUTEAL PORTION ISOLATED
WITH THE TORSO AGAINST THE BACKREST

GLUTEAL PORTION ISOLATED
WITH THE TORSO LEANING FORWARD

STRETCHING THE GLUTEALS

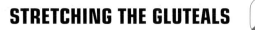

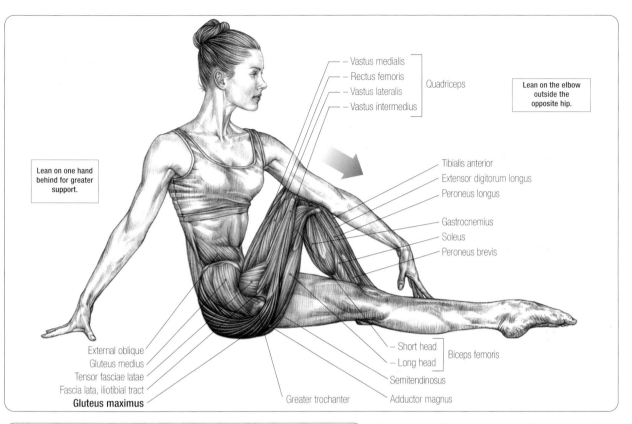

Vastus medialis
Rectus femoris
Vastus lateralis
Vastus intermedius

Quadriceps

Lean on the elbow outside the opposite hip.

Lean on one hand behind for greater support.

Tibialis anterior
Extensor digitorum longus
Peroneus longus

Gastrocnemius
Soleus
Peroneus brevis

External oblique
Gluteus medius
Tensor fasciae latae
Fascia lata, iliotibial tract
Gluteus maximus

Greater trochanter

— Short head
— Long head

Biceps femoris

Semitendinosus
Adductor magnus

VARIATION TO ACCENTUATE STRETCHING OF THE LUMBAR REGION

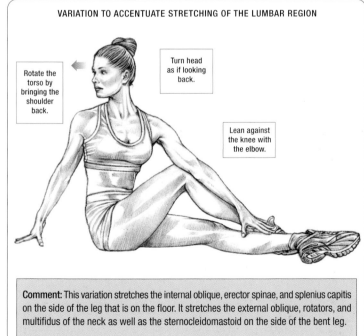

Rotate the torso by bringing the shoulder back.

Turn head as if looking back.

Lean against the knee with the elbow.

Comment: This variation stretches the internal oblique, erector spinae, and splenius capitis on the side of the leg that is on the floor. It stretches the external oblique, rotators, and multifidus of the neck as well as the sternocleidomastoid on the side of the bent leg.

Sit on the floor with one leg extended and the other bent with the foot on the floor outside the extended leg. Press to the inside against the external surface of the knee of the bent leg with the opposite elbow. This exercise mainly stretches the gluteus maximus muscle and deeper in the external hip rotator group (piriformis, gemelli, quadratus femoris, and obturator internus and externus).

Variation: Rather than use the elbow to put pressure against the knee, you can clasp it with both hands.

This exercise stretches the deep, small, external rotator muscles of the hip.

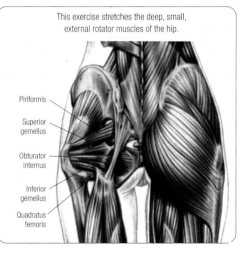

Piriformis
Superior gemellus
Obturator internus
Inferior gemellus
Quadratus femoris

7 ABDOMEN

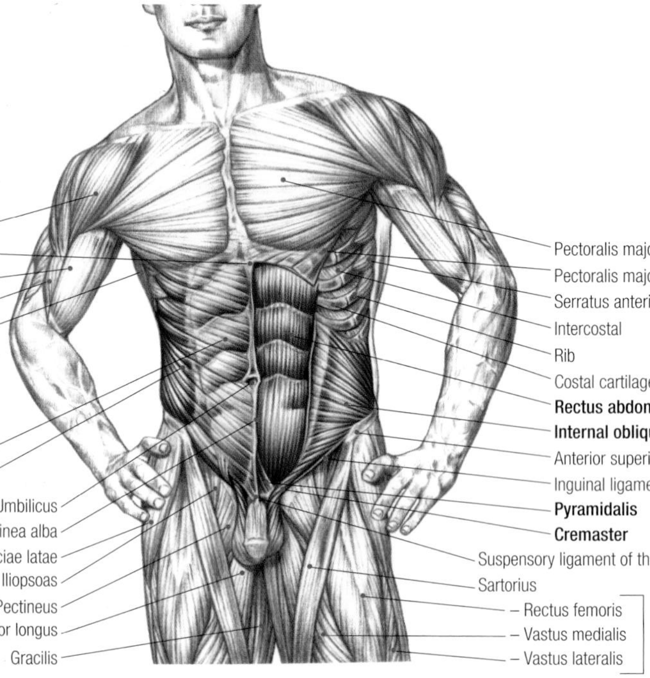

Deltoid
Xiphoid process
Biceps brachii
Brachialis
Latissimus dorsi

**Rectus abdominis,
under the aponeurosis**

External oblique

Umbilicus
Linea alba
Tensor fasciae latae
Iliopsoas
Pectineus
Adductor longus
Gracilis

Pectoralis major
Pectoralis major, abdominal part
Serratus anterior
Intercostal
Rib
Costal cartilage
Rectus abdominis
Internal oblique
Anterior superior iliac spine
Inguinal ligament
Pyramidalis
Cremaster
Suspensory ligament of the penis
Sartorius
– Rectus femoris
– Vastus medialis   Quadriceps
– Vastus lateralis

CORRECT POSITION FOR THE ABDOMINALS

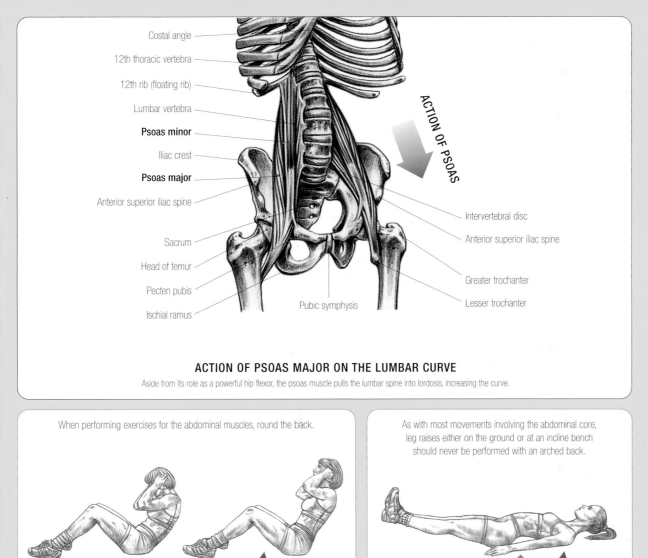

Costal angle	
12th thoracic vertebra	
12th rib (floating rib)	
Lumbar vertebra	
Psoas minor	
Iliac crest	
Psoas major	
Anterior superior iliac spine	Intervertebral disc
Sacrum	Anterior superior iliac spine
Head of femur	Greater trochanter
Pecten pubis	Lesser trochanter
Ischial ramus	Pubic symphysis

ACTION OF PSOAS

ACTION OF PSOAS MAJOR ON THE LUMBAR CURVE

Aside from its role as a powerful hip flexor, the psoas muscle pulls the lumbar spine into lordosis, increasing the curve.

When performing exercises for the abdominal muscles, round the back.

CORRECT POSITION, ROUNDED BACK   **INCORRECT POSITION, ARCHED BACK**

As with most movements involving the abdominal core, leg raises either on the ground or at an incline bench should never be performed with an arched back.

INCORRECT POSITION, ARCHED BACK

Unlike other weightlifting movements, exercises for the abdominal core and especially those for the rectus abdominis absolutely must be worked with a rounded back (rolling up the spine).

When performing exercises that roll the spine up off the floor, as in crunches, you hold the spine differently than when performing squats, deadlifts, or other standing movements.

If during exercises with additional weights, such as squats, deadlifts, or good mornings, the vertebral column is not arched at the lumbar spine, vertical pressure combined with rounding the back pushes the nucleus pulposus of the intervertebral disc posteriorly, which can compress the nerves and cause sciatica or a herniated disc.

On the other hand, when performing specific exercises for the abdomen, if the back is not rounded with intense contraction of the rectus abdominis and the internal and external obliques, the powerful psoas hip flexors will increase the lumbar curve, forcing the intervertebral discs forward.

This causes increased pressure at the posterior lumbar vertebral articulations, which can cause low back pain or, more seriously, articular compression or shearing.

1 CRUNCHES*

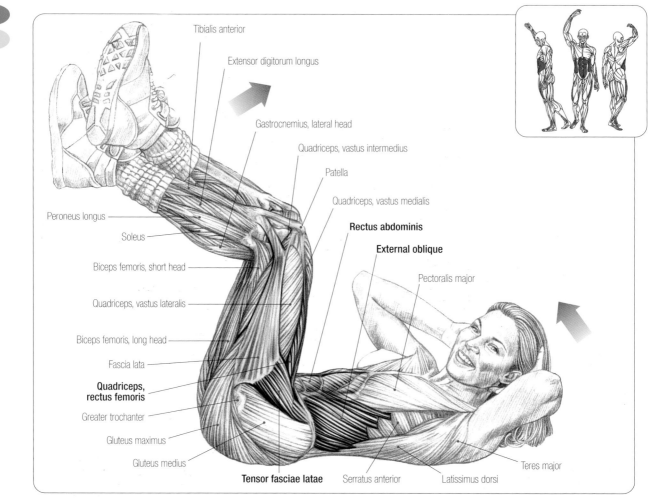

Lie on the back with hands behind the head, thighs vertical, and knees bent:

- Inhale and raise the shoulders off the ground, bringing the knees and head toward each other by crunching, which means rounding the back and rolling the spine up.
- Exhale at the end of the movement.

This exercise mainly uses the rectus abdominis.

To work the obliques more intensely, bring the right elbow to the left knee, then the left elbow to the right knee alternately with each crunch.

* Perform a crunch by rounding the back and rolling the spine up, bringing the pubis and sternum toward each through voluntary contraction.

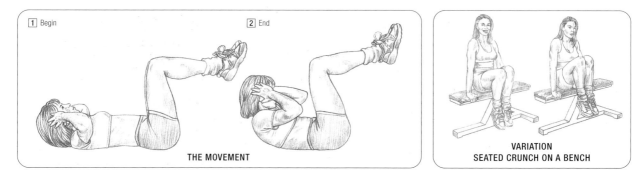

1 Begin   2 End

THE MOVEMENT

VARIATION
SEATED CRUNCH ON A BENCH

SIT-UPS 2

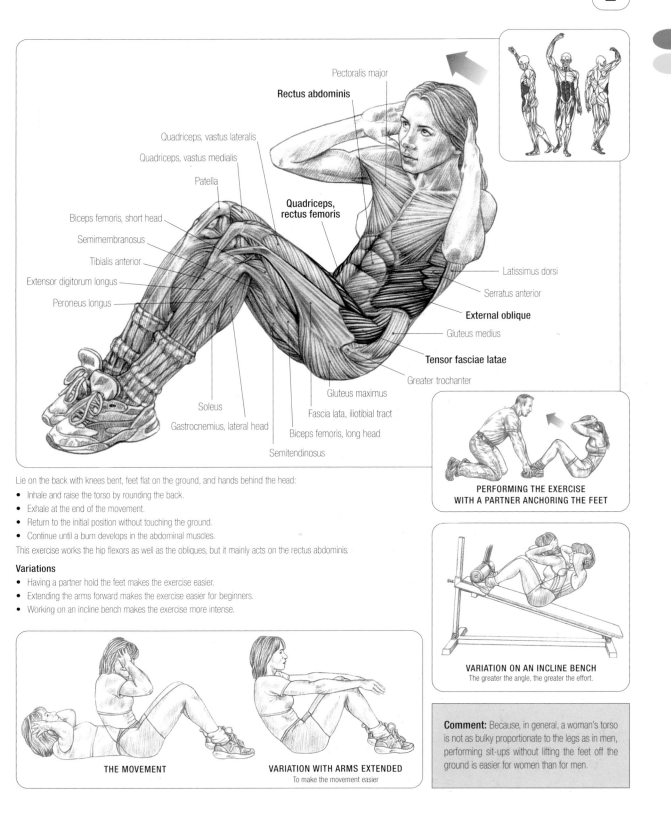

Pectoralis major

Rectus abdominis

Quadriceps, vastus lateralis

Quadriceps, vastus medialis

Patella

Quadriceps, rectus femoris

Biceps femoris, short head

Semimembranosus

Tibialis anterior

Extensor digitorum longus

Peroneus longus

Latissimus dorsi

Serratus anterior

External oblique

Gluteus medius

Tensor fasciae latae

Greater trochanter

Gluteus maximus

Fascia lata, iliotibial tract

Biceps femoris, long head

Semitendinosus

Soleus

Gastrocnemius, lateral head

PERFORMING THE EXERCISE WITH A PARTNER ANCHORING THE FEET

Lie on the back with knees bent, feet flat on the ground, and hands behind the head:

- Inhale and raise the torso by rounding the back.
- Exhale at the end of the movement.
- Return to the initial position without touching the ground.
- Continue until a burn develops in the abdominal muscles.

This exercise works the hip flexors as well as the obliques, but it mainly acts on the rectus abdominis.

Variations

- Having a partner hold the feet makes the exercise easier.
- Extending the arms forward makes the exercise easier for beginners.
- Working on an incline bench makes the exercise more intense.

VARIATION ON AN INCLINE BENCH
The greater the angle, the greater the effort.

THE MOVEMENT

VARIATION WITH ARMS EXTENDED
To make the movement easier

Comment: Because, in general, a woman's torso is not as bulky proportionate to the legs as in men, performing sit-ups without lifting the feet off the ground is easier for women than for men.

3 GYM LADDER SIT-UPS

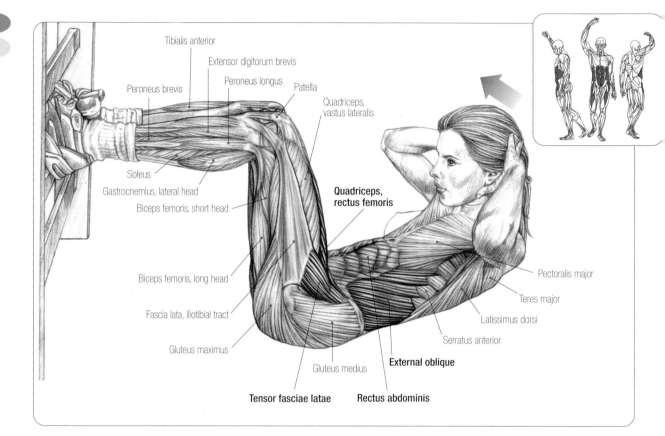

Tibialis anterior
Extensor digitorum brevis
Peroneus brevis
Peroneus longus
Patella
Quadriceps, vastus lateralis
Soleus
Gastrocnemius, lateral head
Biceps femoris, short head
Quadriceps, rectus femoris
Biceps femoris, long head
Pectoralis major
Teres major
Latissimus dorsi
Fascia lata, iliotibial tract
Serratus anterior
Gluteus maximus
External oblique
Gluteus medius
Tensor fasciae latae
Rectus abdominis

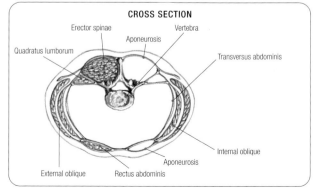

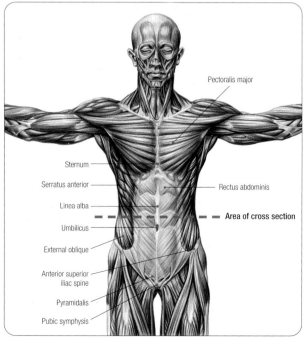

Pectoralis major
Sternum
Serratus anterior
Rectus abdominis
Linea alba
Area of cross section
Umbilicus
External oblique
Anterior superior iliac spine
Pyramidalis
Pubic symphysis

Lie faceup on the ground and position the feet between two bars in the ladder with the thighs vertical and hands behind the head:

- Inhale and raise the torso as high as possible, rounding the spine.
- Exhale at the end of the movement.

This exercise works the rectus abdominis and, to a lesser degree, the external oblique.

Position the feet lower on the ladder so that the pelvis can rock more and better contract the flexor muscles of the hip (iliopsoas, rectus femoris, and tensor fasciae latae) when lowering the torso.

CROSS SECTION

Erector spinae
Vertebra
Aponeurosis
Quadratus lumborum
Transversus abdominis
Internal oblique
Aponeurosis
External oblique
Rectus abdominis

CALVES OVER BENCH SIT-UPS 4

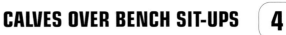

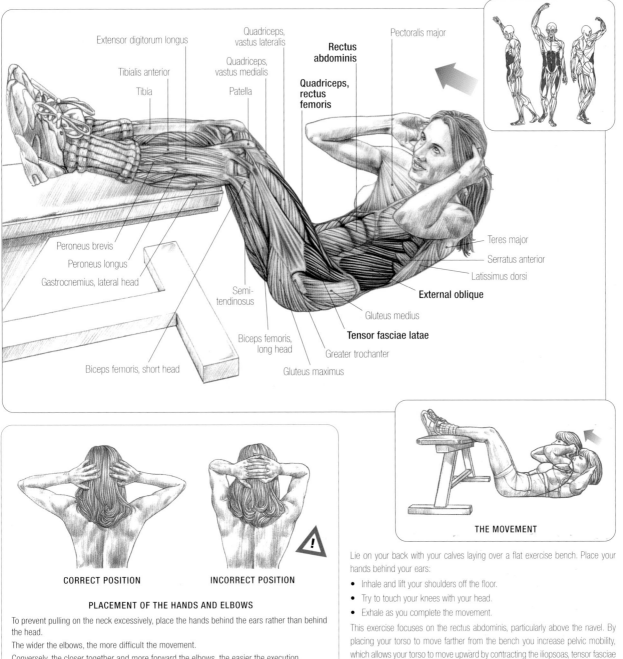

Extensor digitorum longus

Tibialis anterior

Tibia

Quadriceps, vastus lateralis

Quadriceps, vastus medialis

Patella

Rectus abdominis

Pectoralis major

Quadriceps, rectus femoris

Peroneus brevis

Peroneus longus

Gastrocnemius, lateral head

Semi-tendinosus

Biceps femoris, short head

Biceps femoris, long head

Gluteus maximus

Greater trochanter

Tensor fasciae latae

Gluteus medius

External oblique

Latissimus dorsi

Serratus anterior

Teres major

THE MOVEMENT

CORRECT POSITION

INCORRECT POSITION

PLACEMENT OF THE HANDS AND ELBOWS

To prevent pulling on the neck excessively, place the hands behind the ears rather than behind the head.

The wider the elbows, the more difficult the movement.

Conversely, the closer together and more forward the elbows, the easier the execution.

Lie on your back with your calves laying over a flat exercise bench. Place your hands behind your ears:

- Inhale and lift your shoulders off the floor.
- Try to touch your knees with your head.
- Exhale as you complete the movement.

This exercise focuses on the rectus abdominis, particularly above the navel. By placing your torso to move farther from the bench you increase pelvic mobility, which allows your torso to move upward by contracting the iliopsoas, tensor fasciae latae, and rectus femoris in order to flex the hips.

5 INCLINE BENCH SIT-UPS

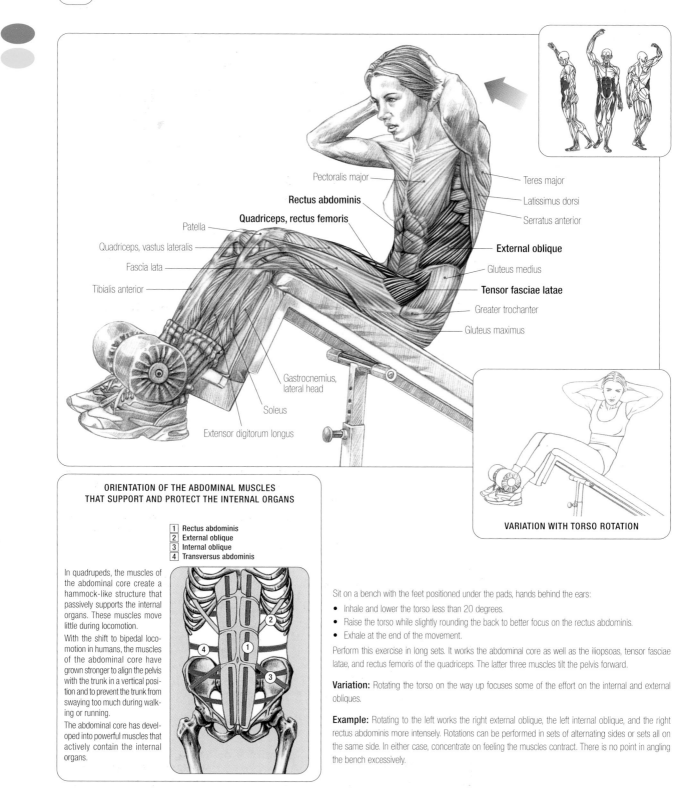

Pectoralis major

Rectus abdominis

Quadriceps, rectus femoris

Patella

Quadriceps, vastus lateralis

Fascia lata

Tibialis anterior

Teres major

Latissimus dorsi

Serratus anterior

External oblique

Gluteus medius

Tensor fasciae latae

Greater trochanter

Gluteus maximus

Gastrocnemius, lateral head

Soleus

Extensor digitorum longus

VARIATION WITH TORSO ROTATION

**ORIENTATION OF THE ABDOMINAL MUSCLES
THAT SUPPORT AND PROTECT THE INTERNAL ORGANS**

1 Rectus abdominis
2 External oblique
3 Internal oblique
4 Transversus abdominis

In quadrupeds, the muscles of the abdominal core create a hammock-like structure that passively supports the internal organs. These muscles move little during locomotion.

With the shift to bipedal locomotion in humans, the muscles of the abdominal core have grown stronger to align the pelvis with the trunk in a vertical position and to prevent the trunk from swaying too much during walking or running.

The abdominal core has developed into powerful muscles that actively contain the internal organs.

Sit on a bench with the feet positioned under the pads, hands behind the ears:

- Inhale and lower the torso less than 20 degrees.
- Raise the torso while slightly rounding the back to better focus on the rectus abdominis.
- Exhale at the end of the movement.

Perform this exercise in long sets. It works the abdominal core as well as the iliopsoas, tensor fasciae latae, and rectus femoris of the quadriceps. The latter three muscles tilt the pelvis forward.

Variation: Rotating the torso on the way up focuses some of the effort on the internal and external obliques.

Example: Rotating to the left works the right external oblique, the left internal oblique, and the right rectus abdominis more intensely. Rotations can be performed in sets of alternating sides or sets all on the same side. In either case, concentrate on feeling the muscles contract. There is no point in angling the bench excessively.

SUSPENDED BENCH SIT-UPS 6

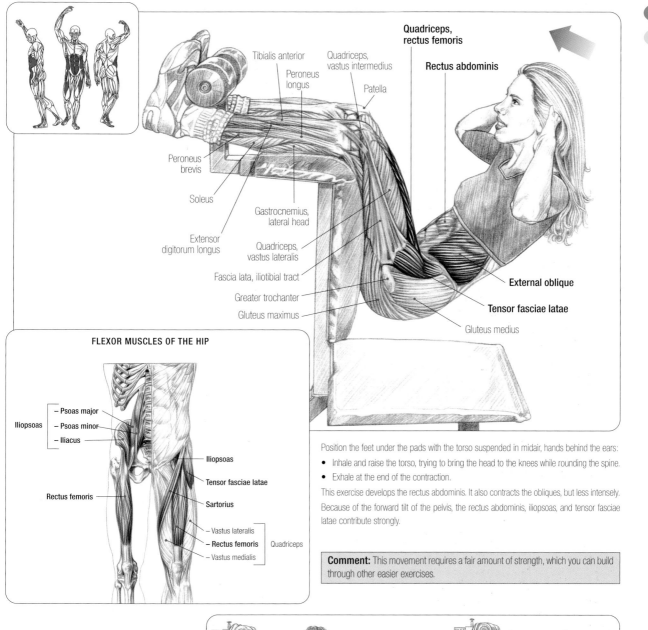

Quadriceps, rectus femoris

Rectus abdominis

Tibialis anterior

Quadriceps, vastus intermedius

Peroneus longus

Patella

Peroneus brevis

Soleus

Gastrocnemius, lateral head

Extensor digitorum longus

Quadriceps, vastus lateralis

Fascia lata, iliotibial tract

Greater trochanter

Gluteus maximus

External oblique

Tensor fasciae latae

Gluteus medius

FLEXOR MUSCLES OF THE HIP

Iliopsoas
– Psoas major
– Psoas minor
– Iliacus

Rectus femoris

Iliopsoas

Tensor fasciae latae

Sartorius

– Vastus lateralis
– Rectus femoris   Quadriceps
– Vastus medialis

Position the feet under the pads with the torso suspended in midair, hands behind the ears:

- Inhale and raise the torso, trying to bring the head to the knees while rounding the spine.
- Exhale at the end of the contraction.

This exercise develops the rectus abdominis. It also contracts the obliques, but less intensely.

Because of the forward tilt of the pelvis, the rectus abdominis, iliopsoas, and tensor fasciae latae contribute strongly.

Comment: This movement requires a fair amount of strength, which you can build through other easier exercises.

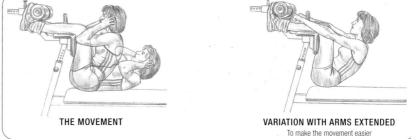

THE MOVEMENT

VARIATION WITH ARMS EXTENDED
To make the movement easier

7 HIGH-PULLEY CRUNCHES

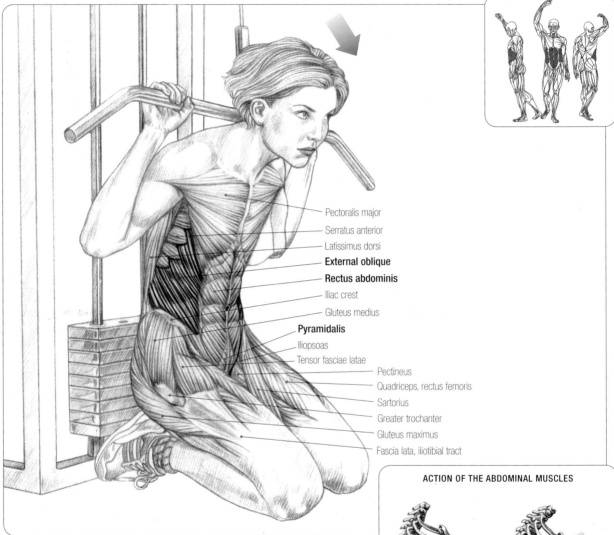

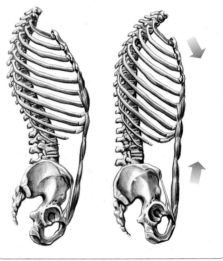

Pectoralis major
Serratus anterior
Latissimus dorsi
External oblique
Rectus abdominis
Iliac crest
Gluteus medius
Pyramidalis
Iliopsoas
Tensor fasciae latae
Pectineus
Quadriceps, rectus femoris
Sartorius
Greater trochanter
Gluteus maximus
Fascia lata, iliotibial tract

ACTION OF THE ABDOMINAL MUSCLES

Kneel in front of the machine and hold the handle behind the neck:

* Inhale.
* Exhale and roll the spine as you lower the sternum toward the pubis.

This movement is never performed with heavy weights. Concentrate on feeling the muscles contract, mainly the rectus abdominis, in order to focus the work on the abdominal core.

MACHINE CRUNCHES 8

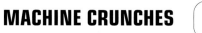

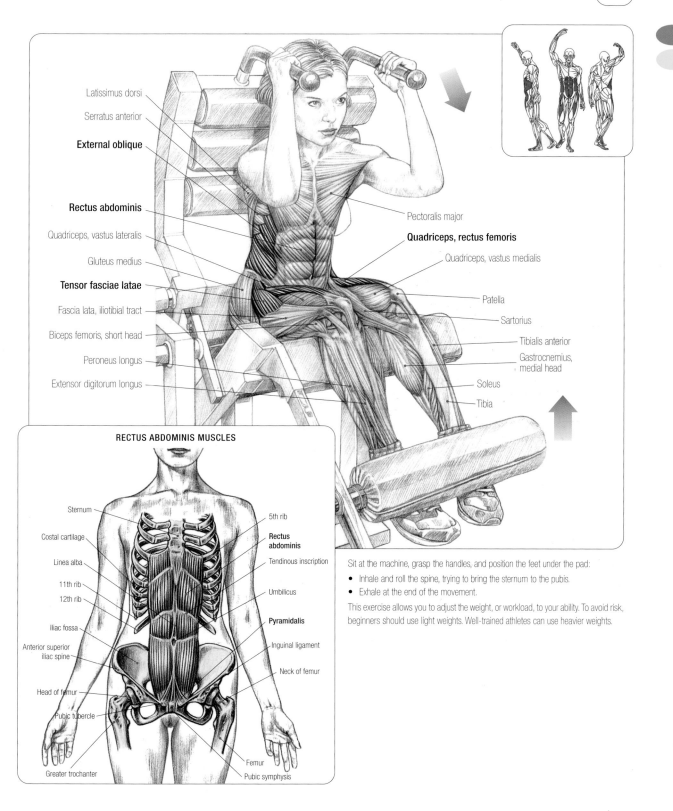

Latissimus dorsi

Serratus anterior

External oblique

Rectus abdominis

Quadriceps, vastus lateralis

Gluteus medius

Tensor fasciae latae

Fascia lata, iliotibial tract

Biceps femoris, short head

Peroneus longus

Extensor digitorum longus

Pectoralis major

Quadriceps, rectus femoris

Quadriceps, vastus medialis

Patella

Sartorius

Tibialis anterior

Gastrocnemius, medial head

Soleus

Tibia

RECTUS ABDOMINIS MUSCLES

Sternum

Costal cartilage

Linea alba

11th rib

12th rib

Iliac fossa

Anterior superior iliac spine

Head of femur

Pubic tubercle

Greater trochanter

5th rib

Rectus abdominis

Tendinous inscription

Umbilicus

Pyramidalis

Inguinal ligament

Neck of femur

Femur

Pubic symphysis

Sit at the machine, grasp the handles, and position the feet under the pad:

- Inhale and roll the spine, trying to bring the sternum to the pubis.
- Exhale at the end of the movement.

This exercise allows you to adjust the weight, or workload, to your ability. To avoid risk, beginners should use light weights. Well-trained athletes can use heavier weights.

9 INCLINE LEG RAISES

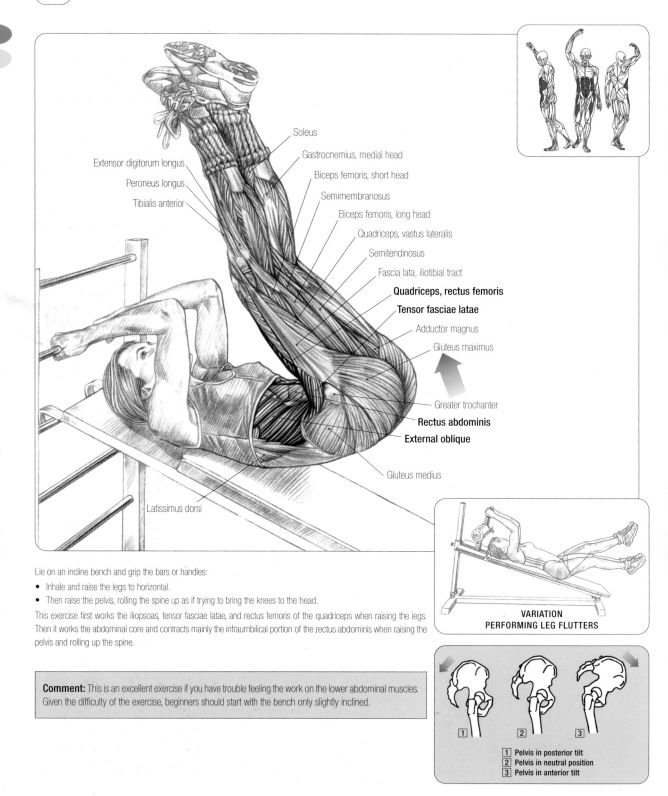

Soleus

Gastrocnemius, medial head

Biceps femoris, short head

Semimembranosus

Biceps femoris, long head

Quadriceps, vastus lateralis

Semitendinosus

Fascia lata, iliotibial tract

Quadriceps, rectus femoris

Tensor fasciae latae

Adductor magnus

Gluteus maximus

Greater trochanter

Rectus abdominis

External oblique

Gluteus medius

Extensor digitorum longus

Peroneus longus

Tibialis anterior

Latissimus dorsi

**VARIATION
PERFORMING LEG FLUTTERS**

① Pelvis in posterior tilt
② Pelvis in neutral position
③ Pelvis in anterior tilt

Lie on an incline bench and grip the bars or handles:

- Inhale and raise the legs to horizontal.
- Then raise the pelvis, rolling the spine up as if trying to bring the knees to the head.

This exercise first works the iliopsoas, tensor fasciae latae, and rectus femoris of the quadriceps when raising the legs. Then it works the abdominal core and contracts mainly the infraumbilical portion of the rectus abdominis when raising the pelvis and rolling up the spine.

Comment: This is an excellent exercise if you have trouble feeling the work on the lower abdominal muscles. Given the difficulty of the exercise, beginners should start with the bench only slightly inclined.

STRETCHING THE UPPER BODY

Stand with your legs wider apart than the pelvis and the back very straight:

- Extend the arms vertically, hands clasped together and palms facing the ceiling.
- Inhale and expand the chest, stretching the intercostal muscles and trying to push up. Keep the back and head very straight.
- Exhale slowly while relaxing, and repeat.

This is a general stretching exercise for the upper body and particularly for the intercostal muscles, rectus abdominis, latissimus dorsi, teres major, and the long portion of the triceps.

When bending to the side, the stretch becomes more intense on the external and internal obliques of the abdomen, quadratus lumborum, and the inferior and middle erector spinae muscles.

Comment: This stretch is excellent for relaxing and returning to a state of calm after an intense session of thigh presses, squats, or deadlifts when the rib cage and spine have been compressed.

It can on occasion replace or complement the stretch at a chin-up bar (see page 114) to equalize the pressures and tensions of the intervertebral articulations.

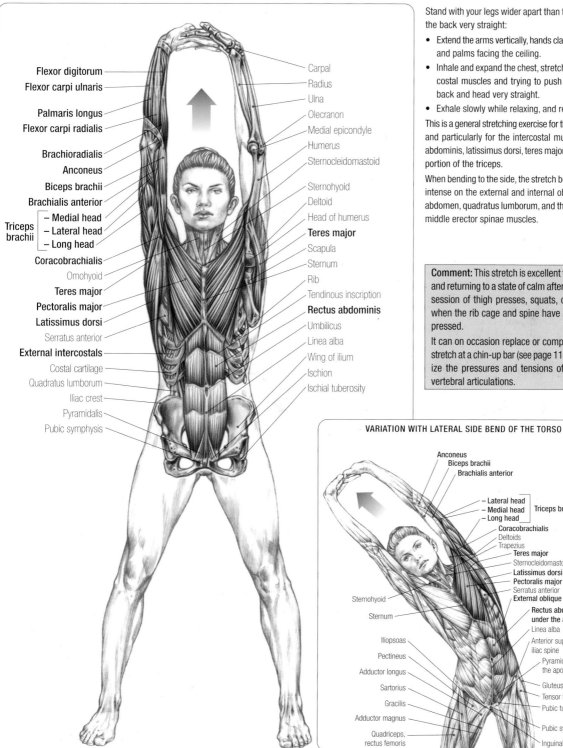

Flexor digitorum
Flexor carpi ulnaris
Palmaris longus
Flexor carpi radialis
Brachioradialis
Anconeus
Biceps brachii
Brachialis anterior
Triceps brachii
— Medial head
— Lateral head
— Long head
Coracobrachialis
Omohyoid
Teres major
Pectoralis major
Latissimus dorsi
Serratus anterior
External intercostals
Costal cartilage
Quadratus lumborum
Iliac crest
Pyramidalis
Pubic symphysis

Carpal
Radius
Ulna
Olecranon
Medial epicondyle
Humerus
Sternocleidomastoid
Sternohyoid
Deltoid
Head of humerus
Teres major
Scapula
Sternum
Rib
Tendinous inscription
Rectus abdominis
Umbilicus
Linea alba
Wing of ilium
Ischion
Ischial tuberosity

VARIATION WITH LATERAL SIDE BEND OF THE TORSO

Anconeus
Biceps brachii
Brachialis anterior
— Lateral head
— Medial head
— Long head
Triceps brachii
Coracobrachialis
Deltoids
Trapezius
Teres major
Sternocleidomastoid
Latissimus dorsi
Pectoralis major
Serratus anterior
External oblique
Rectus abdominis, under the aponeurosis
Linea alba
Anterior superior iliac spine
Pyramidalis, under the aponeurosis
Gluteus medius
Tensor fasciae latae
Pubic tubercle
Pubic symphysis
Inguinal ligament

Sternohyoid
Sternum
Iliopsoas
Pectineus
Adductor longus
Sartorius
Gracilis
Adductor magnus
Quadriceps, rectus femoris

10 LEG RAISES

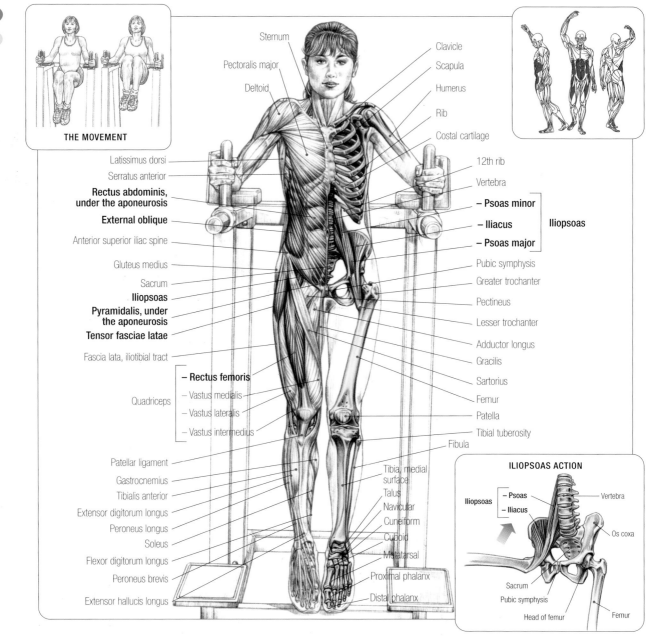

THE MOVEMENT

Sternum
Pectoralis major
Deltoid
Clavicle
Scapula
Humerus
Rib
Costal cartilage
Latissimus dorsi
Serratus anterior
Rectus abdominis, under the aponeurosis
External oblique
Anterior superior iliac spine
Gluteus medius
Sacrum
Iliopsoas
Pyramidalis, under the aponeurosis
Tensor fasciae latae
Fascia lata, iliotibial tract
– Rectus femoris
– Vastus medialis
Quadriceps
– Vastus lateralis
– Vastus intermedius
Patellar ligament
Gastrocnemius
Tibialis anterior
Extensor digitorum longus
Peroneus longus
Soleus
Flexor digitorum longus
Peroneus brevis
Extensor hallucis longus
12th rib
Vertebra
– Psoas minor
– Iliacus
– Psoas major
Iliopsoas
Pubic symphysis
Greater trochanter
Pectineus
Lesser trochanter
Adductor longus
Gracilis
Sartorius
Femur
Patella
Tibial tuberosity
Fibula
Tibial medial surface
Talus
Navicular
Cuneiform
Cuboid
Metatarsal
Proximal phalanx
Distal phalanx

ILIOPSOAS ACTION

Iliopsoas
– Psoas
– Iliacus
Vertebra
Os coxa
Sacrum
Pubic symphysis
Head of femur
Femur

Support the body by resting the elbows on the pads. Position the back against the back support:

- Inhale and raise the knees to the chest, rounding the back in order to contract the abdominal core.
- Exhale at the end of the movement.

This exercise works the hip flexors, mainly the iliopsoas, and the obliques. It intensely works the lower part of the rectus abdominis.

Variations

- To target the lower abdominal muscles, perform small flutters with the legs when rolling up the spine.
- To make the exercise more intense, extend the legs horizontally. However, this requires flexible hamstrings.
- Hold the knees to the chest for a few seconds with an isometric contraction.

HANGING LEG RAISES 〔11〕

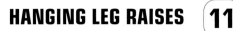

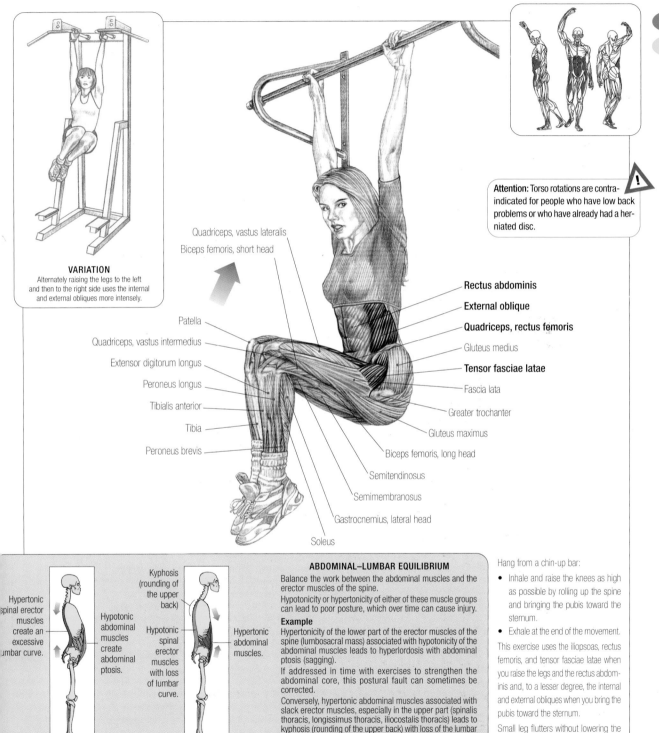

VARIATION
Alternately raising the legs to the left and then to the right side uses the internal and external obliques more intensely.

Attention: Torso rotations are contra-indicated for people who have low back problems or who have already had a herniated disc.

Quadriceps, vastus lateralis

Biceps femoris, short head

Patella

Quadriceps, vastus intermedius

Extensor digitorum longus

Peroneus longus

Tibialis anterior

Tibia

Peroneus brevis

Rectus abdominis

External oblique

Quadriceps, rectus femoris

Gluteus medius

Tensor fasciae latae

Fascia lata

Greater trochanter

Gluteus maximus

Biceps femoris, long head

Semitendinosus

Semimembranosus

Gastrocnemius, lateral head

Soleus

ABDOMINAL–LUMBAR EQUILIBRIUM

Balance the work between the abdominal muscles and the erector muscles of the spine.

Hypotonicity or hypertonicity of either of these muscle groups can lead to poor posture, which over time can cause injury.

Example

Hypertonicity of the lower part of the erector muscles of the spine (lumbosacral mass) associated with hypotonicity of the abdominal muscles leads to hyperlordosis with abdominal ptosis (sagging).

If addressed in time with exercises to strengthen the abdominal core, this postural fault can sometimes be corrected.

Conversely, hypertonic abdominal muscles associated with slack erector muscles, especially in the upper part (spinalis thoracis, longissimus thoracis, iliocostalis thoracis) leads to kyphosis (rounding of the upper back) with loss of the lumbar curve. This postural fault can be corrected with exercises to strengthen the erector muscles of the spine.

Hypertonic spinal erector muscles create an excessive lumbar curve.

Hypotonic abdominal muscles create abdominal ptosis.

Kyphosis (rounding of the upper back)

Hypotonic spinal erector muscles with loss of lumbar curve.

Hypertonic abdominal muscles.

Hang from a chin-up bar:

- Inhale and raise the knees as high as possible by rolling up the spine and bringing the pubis toward the sternum.
- Exhale at the end of the movement.

This exercise uses the iliopsoas, rectus femoris, and tensor fasciae latae when you raise the legs and the rectus abdominis and, to a lesser degree, the internal and external obliques when you bring the pubis toward the sternum.

Small leg flutters without lowering the knees below horizontal focus the effort on the abdominal core.

12 TRUNK ROTATIONS

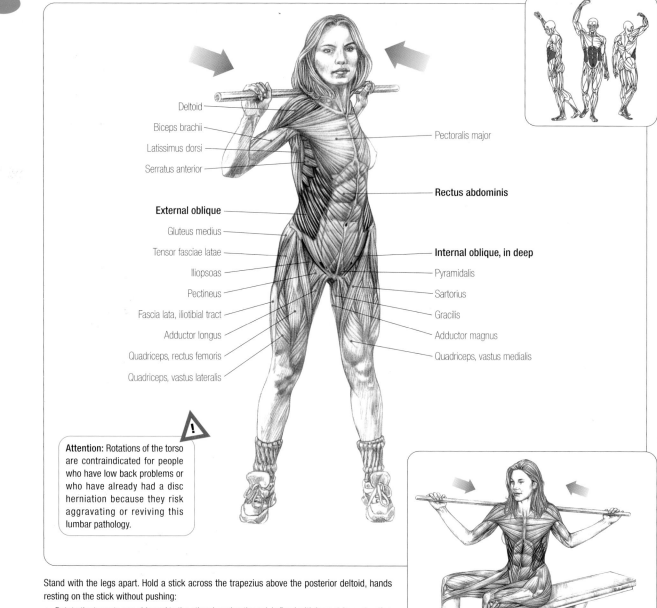

Deltoid

Biceps brachii

Latissimus dorsi

Serratus anterior

Pectoralis major

Rectus abdominis

External oblique

Gluteus medius

Tensor fasciae latae

Iliopsoas

Pectineus

Fascia lata, iliotibial tract

Adductor longus

Quadriceps, rectus femoris

Quadriceps, vastus lateralis

Internal oblique, in deep

Pyramidalis

Sartorius

Gracilis

Adductor magnus

Quadriceps, vastus medialis

! **Attention:** Rotations of the torso are contraindicated for people who have low back problems or who have already had a disc herniation because they risk aggravating or reviving this lumbar pathology.

Stand with the legs apart. Hold a stick across the trapezius above the posterior deltoid, hands resting on the stick without pushing:

• Rotate the torso to one side and to the other, keeping the pelvis fixed with isometric contraction of the gluteal muscles.

When the right shoulder is forward, this exercise works the right external oblique and, deep in, the left internal oblique and, to a lesser degree, the rectus abdominis, quadratus lumborum, and the extensor muscles of the spine on the left side.

To increase the intensity, round the back slightly.

You can also perform the movement while seated, which helps to fix the pelvis so that you can focus the effort on the abdominal core.

Best results are obtained with sets lasting several minutes.

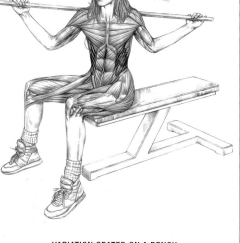

VARIATION SEATED ON A BENCH

DUMBBELL SIDE BENDS · 13

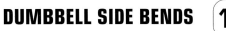

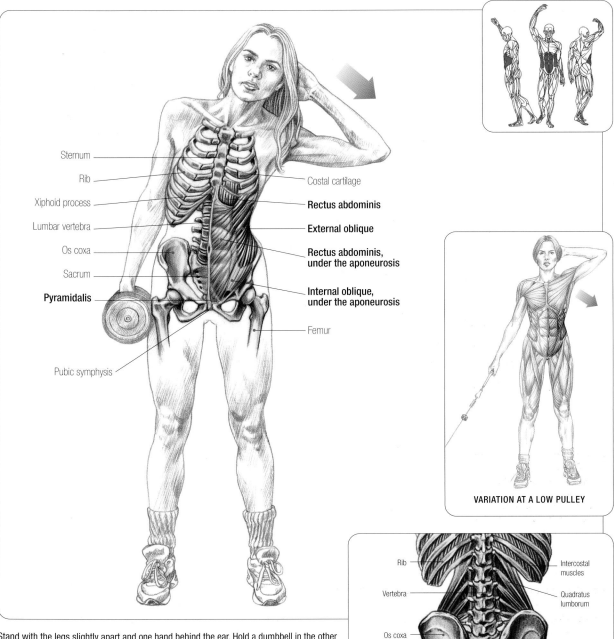

VARIATION AT A LOW PULLEY

QUADRATUS LUMBORUM MUSCLE

Stand with the legs slightly apart and one hand behind the ear. Hold a dumbbell in the other hand:

- Bend the torso to the side opposite to the dumbbell.
- Return to the initial position or beyond with passive flexion of the torso.
- Alternate sets, changing the side of the dumbbell without resting.

This exercise mainly works the obliques on the side the torso bends toward. It works the rectus abdominis, deep muscles of the back, and quadratus lumborum (back muscle that inserts on the 12th rib, the transverse processes of the lumbar vertebrae, and the iliac crest) less intensely.

14 ROMAN CHAIR SIDE BENDS

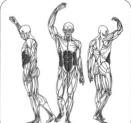

This exercise is performed on a bench originally designed for lumbar extensions.

Lie on your side with the hip on the bench, torso in the air, hands near the ears or on the chest, and feet positioned under the pads:

- Raise the side of the body toward the ceiling.

This exercise mainly works the obliques and rectus abdominis on the side that is bending, but the opposite obliques and rectus abdominis are also used in isometric contraction to prevent the torso from lowering below horizontal.

> **Comment:** The quadratus lumborum muscle is always used when bending the torso toward the side.

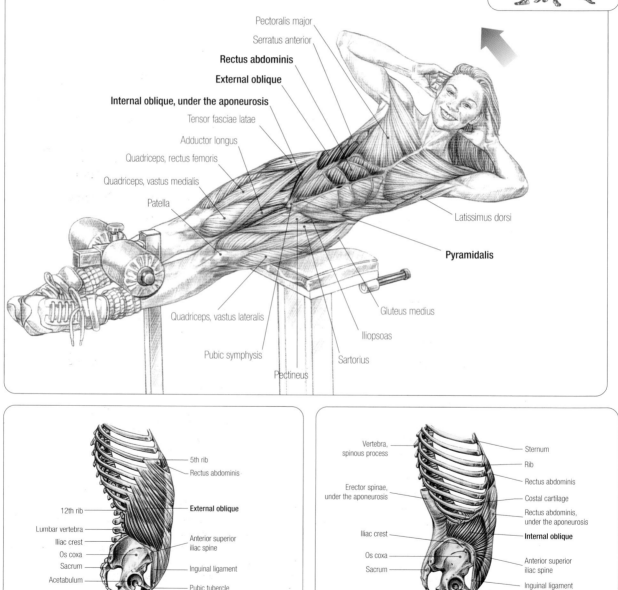

Pectoralis major

Serratus anterior

Rectus abdominis

External oblique

Internal oblique, under the aponeurosis

Tensor fasciae latae

Adductor longus

Quadriceps, rectus femoris

Quadriceps, vastus medialis

Patella

Quadriceps, vastus lateralis

Pubic symphysis

Pectineus

Sartorius

Iliopsoas

Gluteus medius

Pyramidalis

Latissimus dorsi

5th rib

Rectus abdominis

External oblique

12th rib

Lumbar vertebra

Iliac crest

Os coxa

Sacrum

Acetabulum

Anterior superior iliac spine

Inguinal ligament

Pubic tubercle

EXTERNAL OBLIQUE MUSCLE OF THE ABDOMEN

Vertebra, spinous process

Sternum

Rib

Rectus abdominis

Erector spinae, under the aponeurosis

Costal cartilage

Rectus abdominis, under the aponeurosis

Iliac crest

Internal oblique

Os coxa

Sacrum

Anterior superior iliac spine

Inguinal ligament

Pubic tubercle

Ischial tuberosity

INTERNAL OBLIQUE MUSCLE OF THE ABDOMEN

MACHINE TRUNK ROTATIONS 15

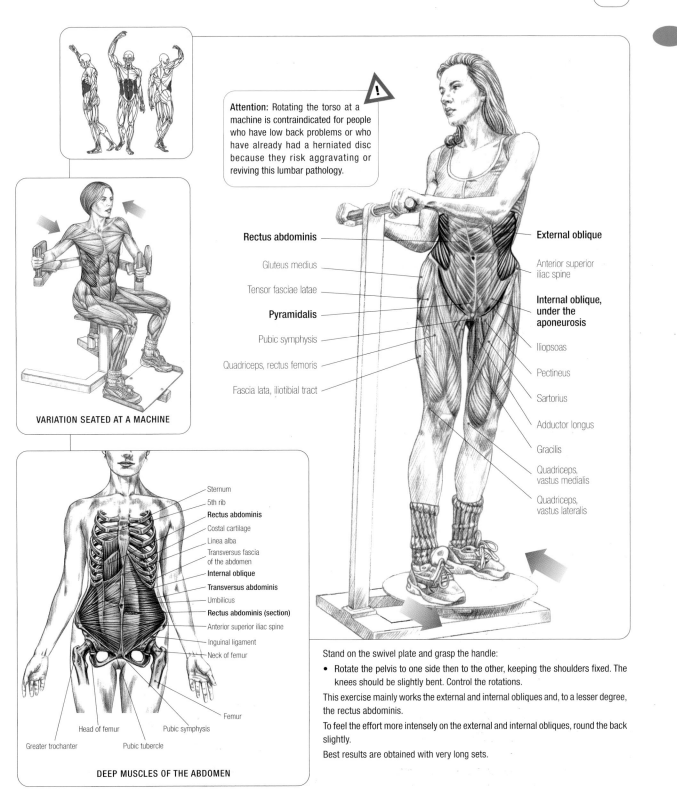

Attention: Rotating the torso at a machine is contraindicated for people who have low back problems or who have already had a herniated disc because they risk aggravating or reviving this lumbar pathology.

Rectus abdominis

Gluteus medius

Tensor fasciae latae

Pyramidalis

Pubic symphysis

Quadriceps, rectus femoris

Fascia lata, iliotibial tract

External oblique

Anterior superior iliac spine

Internal oblique, under the aponeurosis

Iliopsoas

Pectineus

Sartorius

Adductor longus

Gracilis

Quadriceps, vastus medialis

Quadriceps, vastus lateralis

VARIATION SEATED AT A MACHINE

Sternum

5th rib

Rectus abdominis

Costal cartilage

Linea alba

Transversus fascia of the abdomen

Internal oblique

Transversus abdominis

Umbilicus

Rectus abdominis (section)

Anterior superior iliac spine

Inguinal ligament

Neck of femur

Femur

Head of femur

Pubic symphysis

Greater trochanter

Pubic tubercle

DEEP MUSCLES OF THE ABDOMEN

Stand on the swivel plate and grasp the handle:

- Rotate the pelvis to one side then to the other, keeping the shoulders fixed. The knees should be slightly bent. Control the rotations.

This exercise mainly works the external and internal obliques and, to a lesser degree, the rectus abdominis.

To feel the effort more intensely on the external and internal obliques, round the back slightly.

Best results are obtained with very long sets.

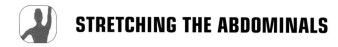

STRETCHING THE ABDOMINALS

Lie on your belly, resting on your hands with arms extended:

- Slowly raise the torso, tilting slightly back with your head.
- Maintain the position for a few moments, breathing slowly to really feel the stretch of the anterior part of the abdominal girdle.

Variations: You can stretch the abdominal muscles with your hands resting on a bench or your feet on the floor, or you can stretch backward on a Swiss ball.

Comment: Stretching the abdominal girdle is recommended in certain sports, such as throwing events in track and field, especially with the javelin, where good flexibility and good abdominal amplitude are essential for performing the movement perfectly.

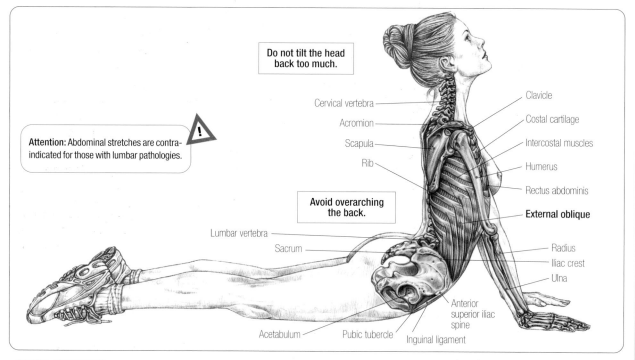

Do not tilt the head back too much.

Attention: Abdominal stretches are contra-indicated for those with lumbar pathologies.

Avoid overarching the back.

Cervical vertebra
Acromion
Scapula
Rib
Lumbar vertebra
Sacrum
Acetabulum
Pubic tubercle
Inguinal ligament
Anterior superior iliac spine

Clavicle
Costal cartilage
Intercostal muscles
Humerus
Rectus abdominis
External oblique
Radius
Iliac crest
Ulna

COMPARING THE PELVIC TILT IN WOMEN AND MEN

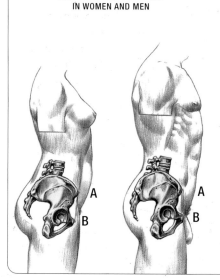

A
B
A
B

A: Anterior superior iliac spine

B: Pubic tubercle

TILT OF THE PELVIS

A woman's pelvis generally tilts more anteriorly than a man's. This anterior tilt pushes the gluteals back more and pulls the pubis in more between the thighs, which gives the impression that the lower belly is pushed out slightly. This small, typically feminine belly contrasts with the vertical abdominal wall that is more commonly seen in men, where the pelvis is tilted forward to a lesser degree.

The special position of the female pelvis prevents a fetus from excessively compressing the viscera during pregnancy as part of its weight presses against the abdominal wall.

SAGITTAL SECTION OF THE ABDOMEN OF A PREGNANT WOMAN

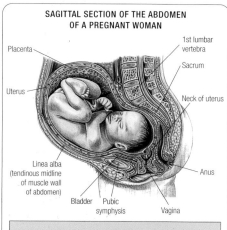

Placenta
Uterus
Linea alba (tendinous midline of muscle wall of abdomen)
Bladder
Pubic symphysis

1st lumbar vertebra
Sacrum
Neck of uterus
Anus
Vagina

Comment: The anterior tilt position (anteversion) of the pelvis in a woman allows part of the weight of the fetus to press against the abdominal wall. The muscles of the abdominal wall can be compared to a hammock.

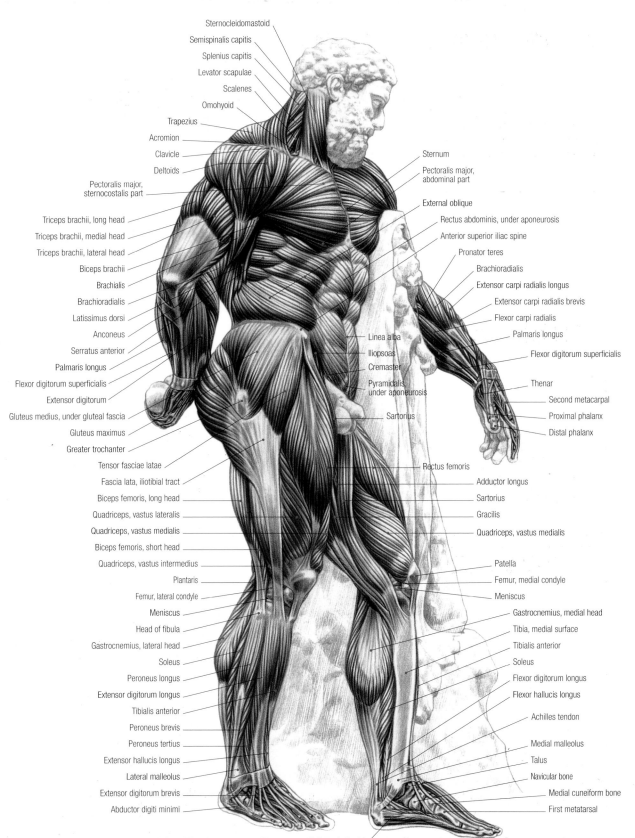

Sternocleidomastoid
Semispinalis capitis
Splenius capitis
Levator scapulae
Scalenes
Omohyoid
Trapezius
Acromion
Clavicle
Deltoids
Pectoralis major,
sternocostalis part
Triceps brachii, long head
Triceps brachii, medial head
Triceps brachii, lateral head
Biceps brachii
Brachialis
Brachioradialis
Latissimus dorsi
Anconeus
Serratus anterior
Palmaris longus
Flexor digitorum superficialis
Extensor digitorum
Gluteus medius, under gluteal fascia
Gluteus maximus
Greater trochanter
Tensor fasciae latae
Fascia lata, iliotibial tract
Biceps femoris, long head
Quadriceps, vastus lateralis
Quadriceps, vastus medialis
Biceps femoris, short head
Quadriceps, vastus intermedius
Plantaris
Femur, lateral condyle
Meniscus
Head of fibula
Gastrocnemius, lateral head
Soleus
Peroneus longus
Extensor digitorum longus
Tibialis anterior
Peroneus brevis
Peroneus tertius
Extensor hallucis longus
Lateral malleolus
Extensor digitorum brevis
Abductor digiti minimi

Sternum
Pectoralis major,
abdominal part
External oblique
Rectus abdominis, under aponeurosis
Anterior superior iliac spine
Pronator teres
Brachioradialis
Extensor carpi radialis longus
Extensor carpi radialis brevis
Flexor carpi radialis
Palmaris longus
Flexor digitorum superficialis
Thenar
Second metacarpal
Proximal phalanx
Distal phalanx

Linea alba
Iliopsoas
Cremaster
Pyramidalis,
under aponeurosis
Sartorius

Rectus femoris
Adductor longus
Sartorius
Gracilis
Quadriceps, vastus medialis
Patella
Femur, medial condyle
Meniscus
Gastrocnemius, medial head
Tibia, medial surface
Tibialis anterior
Soleus
Flexor digitorum longus
Flexor hallucis longus
Achilles tendon
Medial malleolus
Talus
Navicular bone
Medial cuneiform bone
First metatarsal

Abductor hallucis

189

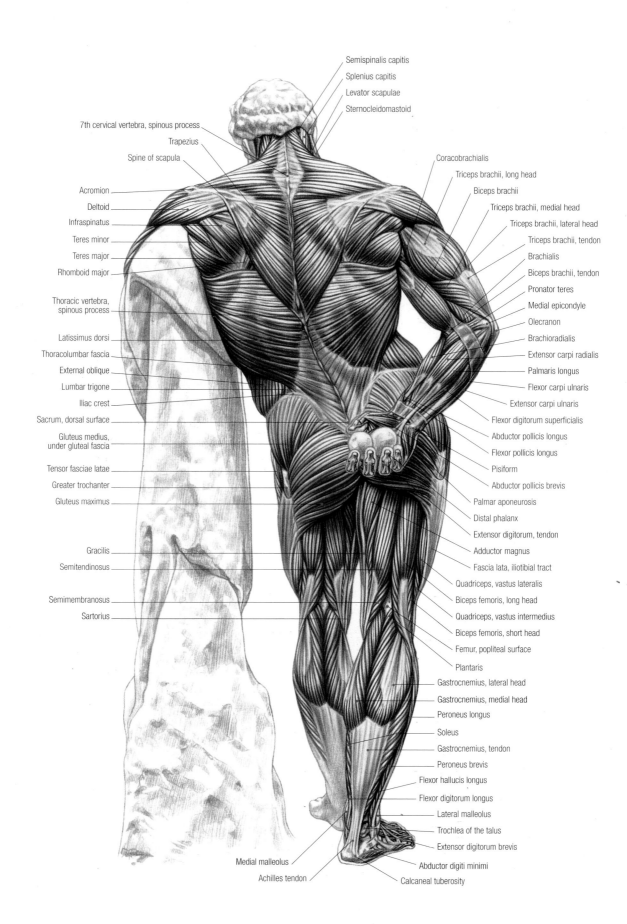

Semispinalis capitis

Splenius capitis

Levator scapulae

Sternocleidomastoid

7th cervical vertebra, spinous process

Trapezius

Spine of scapula

Coracobrachialis

Triceps brachii, long head

Biceps brachii

Acromion

Deltoid

Infraspinatus

Teres minor

Teres major

Rhomboid major

Triceps brachii, medial head

Triceps brachii, lateral head

Triceps brachii, tendon

Brachialis

Biceps brachii, tendon

Pronator teres

Medial epicondyle

Olecranon

Brachioradialis

Extensor carpi radialis

Palmaris longus

Flexor carpi ulnaris

Extensor carpi ulnaris

Flexor digitorum superficialis

Abductor pollicis longus

Flexor pollicis longus

Pisiform

Abductor pollicis brevis

Palmar aponeurosis

Distal phalanx

Extensor digitorum, tendon

Adductor magnus

Fascia lata, iliotibial tract

Quadriceps, vastus lateralis

Biceps femoris, long head

Quadriceps, vastus intermedius

Biceps femoris, short head

Femur, popliteal surface

Plantaris

Gastrocnemius, lateral head

Gastrocnemius, medial head

Peroneus longus

Soleus

Gastrocnemius, tendon

Peroneus brevis

Flexor hallucis longus

Flexor digitorum longus

Lateral malleolus

Trochlea of the talus

Extensor digitorum brevis

Abductor digiti minimi

Calcaneal tuberosity

Thoracic vertebra, spinous process

Latissimus dorsi

Thoracolumbar fascia

External oblique

Lumbar trigone

Iliac crest

Sacrum, dorsal surface

Gluteus medius, under gluteal fascia

Tensor fasciae latae

Greater trochanter

Gluteus maximus

Gracilis

Semitendinosus

Semimembranosus

Sartorius

Medial malleolus

Achilles tendon

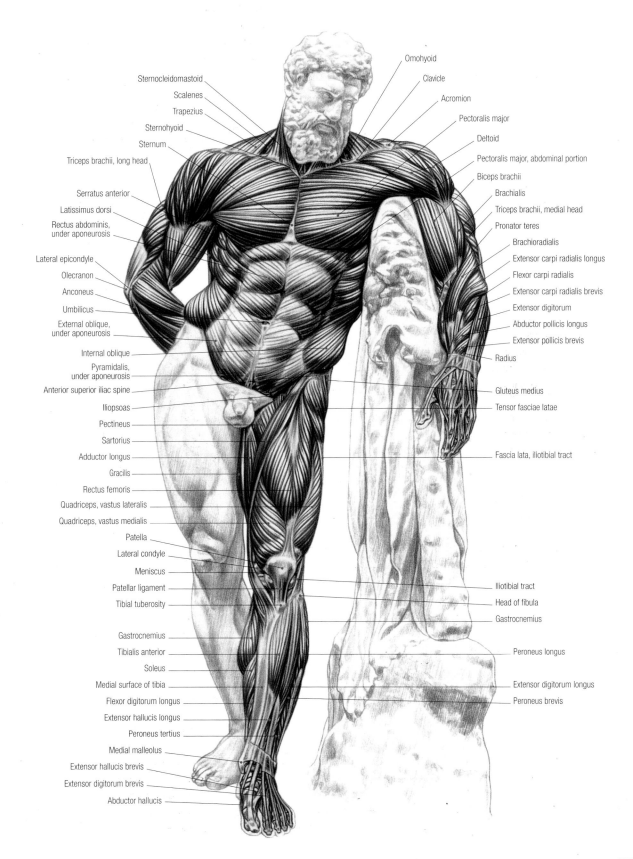

Sternocleidomastoid

Scalenes

Trapezius

Sternohyoid

Sternum

Triceps brachii, long head

Serratus anterior

Latissimus dorsi

Rectus abdominis,
under aponeurosis

Lateral epicondyle

Olecranon

Anconeus

Umbilicus

External oblique,
under aponeurosis

Internal oblique

Pyramidalis,
under aponeurosis

Anterior superior iliac spine

Iliopsoas

Pectineus

Sartorius

Adductor longus

Gracilis

Rectus femoris

Quadriceps, vastus lateralis

Quadriceps, vastus medialis

Patella

Lateral condyle

Meniscus

Patellar ligament

Tibial tuberosity

Gastrocnemius

Tibialis anterior

Soleus

Medial surface of tibia

Flexor digitorum longus

Extensor hallucis longus

Peroneus tertius

Medial malleolus

Extensor hallucis brevis

Extensor digitorum brevis

Abductor hallucis

Omohyoid

Clavicle

Acromion

Pectoralis major

Deltoid

Pectoralis major, abdominal portion

Biceps brachii

Brachialis

Triceps brachii, medial head

Pronator teres

Brachioradialis

Extensor carpi radialis longus

Flexor carpi radialis

Extensor carpi radialis brevis

Extensor digitorum

Abductor pollicis longus

Extensor pollicis brevis

Radius

Gluteus medius

Tensor fasciae latae

Fascia lata, iliotibial tract

Iliotibial tract

Head of fibula

Gastrocnemius

Peroneus longus

Extensor digitorum longus

Peroneus brevis

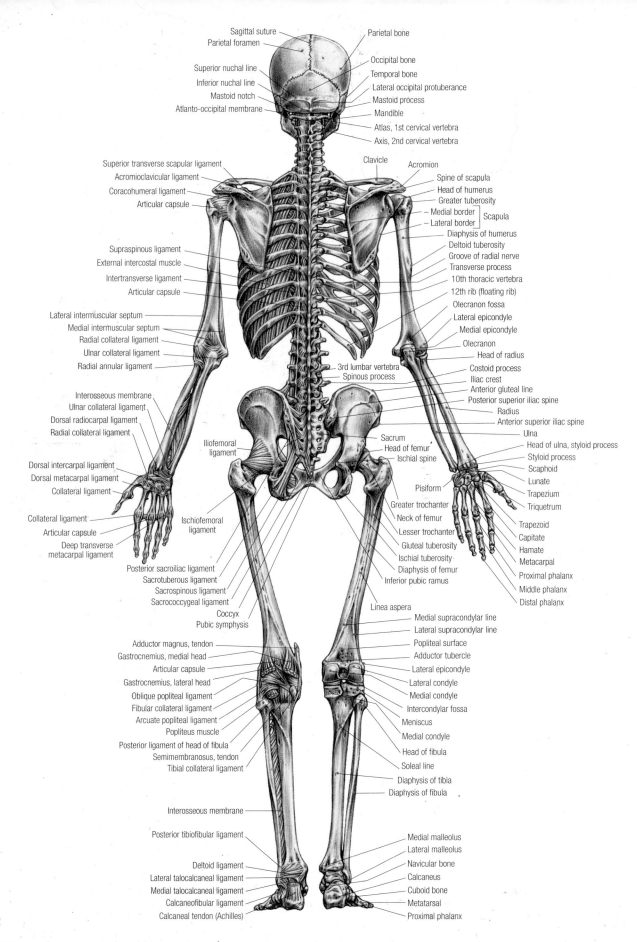

Sagittal suture
Parietal foramen
Superior nuchal line
Inferior nuchal line
Mastoid notch
Atlanto-occipital membrane

Parietal bone
Occipital bone
Temporal bone
Lateral occipital protuberance
Mastoid process
Mandible
Atlas, 1st cervical vertebra
Axis, 2nd cervical vertebra

Superior transverse scapular ligament
Acromioclavicular ligament
Coracohumeral ligament
Articular capsule

Clavicle
Acromion
Spine of scapula
Head of humerus
Greater tuberosity
Medial border
Lateral border
Scapula
Diaphysis of humerus
Deltoid tuberosity
Groove of radial nerve
Transverse process
10th thoracic vertebra
12th rib (floating rib)
Olecranon fossa
Lateral epicondyle
Medial epicondyle
Olecranon
Head of radius
Costoid process
Iliac crest
Anterior gluteal line
Posterior superior iliac spine
Radius
Anterior superior iliac spine
Ulna
Head of ulna, styloid process
Styloid process
Scaphoid
Lunate
Trapezium
Triquetrum
Trapezoid
Capitate
Hamate
Metacarpal
Proximal phalanx
Middle phalanx
Distal phalanx

Supraspinous ligament
External intercostal muscle
Intertransverse ligament
Articular capsule

Lateral intermuscular septum
Medial intermuscular septum
Radial collateral ligament
Ulnar collateral ligament
Radial annular ligament

Interosseous membrane
Ulnar collateral ligament
Dorsal radiocarpal ligament
Radial collateral ligament

Iliofemoral
ligament

Dorsal intercarpal ligament
Dorsal metacarpal ligament
Collateral ligament

Collateral ligament
Articular capsule
Deep transverse
metacarpal ligament

Ischiofemoral
ligament

3rd lumbar vertebra
Spinous process

Sacrum
Head of femur
Ischial spine

Pisiform

Greater trochanter
Neck of femur
Lesser trochanter
Gluteal tuberosity
Ischial tuberosity
Diaphysis of femur
Inferior pubic ramus

Posterior sacroiliac ligament
Sacrotuberous ligament
Sacrospinous ligament
Sacrococcygeal ligament
Coccyx
Pubic symphysis

Linea aspera

Adductor magnus, tendon
Gastrocnemius, medial head
Articular capsule
Gastrocnemius, lateral head
Oblique popliteal ligament
Fibular collateral ligament
Arcuate popliteal ligament
Popliteus muscle
Posterior ligament of head of fibula
Semimembranosus, tendon
Tibial collateral ligament

Medial supracondylar line
Lateral supracondylar line
Popliteal surface
Adductor tubercle
Lateral epicondyle
Lateral condyle
Medial condyle
Intercondylar fossa
Meniscus
Medial condyle
Head of fibula
Soleal line
Diaphysis of tibia
Diaphysis of fibula

Interosseous membrane

Posterior tibiofibular ligament

Deltoid ligament
Lateral talocalcaneal ligament
Medial talocalcaneal ligament
Calcaneofibular ligament
Calcaneal tendon (Achilles)

Medial malleolus
Lateral malleolus
Navicular bone
Calcaneus
Cuboid bone
Metatarsal
Proximal phalanx